# Growth Disorders in Infants, Children, and Adolescents

# Growth Disorders in Infants, Children, and Adolescents

**MARVIN L. RALLISON, M.D.**
**Associate Professor of Pediatrics**
**University of Utah School of Medicine**
**Salt Lake City, Utah**

**A Wiley Medical Publication**
**JOHN WILEY & SONS**
**New York • Chichester • Brisbane • Toronto • Singapore**

**Library of Congress Cataloging in Publication Data**

Rallison, Marvin L.
  Growth disorders in infants, children, and
adolescents.

  (A Wiley medical publication)
  Includes index.
  1. Infants—Growth.  2. Children—Growth.
3. Youth—Growth.  4. Growth disorders.  I. Title.
II. Series.  [DNLM: 1. Child Nutrition.  2. Growth.
3. Growth Disorders—in adolescence.  4. Growth
Disorders—in infancy & childhood.  5. Nutrition—'
in adolescence.  WK 550 R163g]

RJ131.R28  1986    618.92    85-6487
ISBN 0-471-08567-7

Printed in the United States of America

10  9  8  7  6  5  4  3  2  1

# Preface

It is evident to every physician providing care for children that the changes in body size, shape, and configuration (which we call growth), are the most characteristic and fascinating events of childhood. We spend a great deal of our time examining and measuring each child to ascertain whether growth is normal or aberrant and we find that growth is affected, sometimes temporarily, by most disease states of children. Although growth patterns of individual children tend to be consistent and predictable, there is a great deal of variability inherent in the growth process. It is vital that we understand the normal processes of growth so that we are able to recognize normal variations in growth. We must be aware of disorders that may cause deviation from normal growth processes and be able to recognize and correct aberrations.

This book reviews the normal growth of children from the fetal growth period through adolescence and draws attention to disease states that influence normal growth and may bring about growth aberrations. Growth deviations are examined by age groups in this book. Those most likely to occur in infancy include skeletal dysplasias, dysmorphic syndromes, intra-uterine growth retardation, and congenital endocrine disorders. Those characteristic of childhood include constitutional delayed and accelerated growth, Turner's syndrome and other chromosomal imbalance syndromes, endocrine deficiencies such as hypothyroidism and hypopituitarism, and systemic disorders including asthma, celiac disease, and renal disease. Growth deviations peculiar to adolescence are those that accompany delayed or precocious puberty. The division of growth problems into age-related groups will help physicians by showing the finite number of disease states (or variants of normal) most likely to occur at a given age. In organizing our knowledge of growth problems in this manner, I have tried to keep in mind the needs of medical students, pediatric housestaff officers, and primary care physicians providing care mainly to children.

For the material dealing with normal growth in children I am indebted to Tanner, Prader, Lowrey, and others who have enriched our knowledge of the normal growth patterns of children through their thoughtful study, tabulations, and interpretations of growth. The clinical sections of the book reflect my experiences in clinics and consultations in endocrinology over the past 20 years, supplemented by observations of many other students of growth problems, including Smith, Prader, Sizonenko, Rimoin, Root, and Frasier. Dave Smith, whose recent death leaves us all a little poorer, has left us a legacy of outstanding clinical examples of growth problems.

The material for this book was reviewed in part by many of my colleagues, but particularly by Dr. Frank Tyler, Professor of Medicine, University of Utah, who served as my mentor in helping me reduce the vast amount of material available on growth problems to a reasonable and accurate representation. Kathy Fagan, Terry Smith, and Lisa Mitchell aided me in preparing the manuscript by checking references, typing and revising the text (a monumental task even with a word processor), and obtaining permissions for use of tables and illustrations. Illustrations were prepared by Julian Maack (illustrator) and Steven Leitch (photographer). I acknowledge a special debt for the patience, understanding, and support of my wife, Beth, and my children, Scott, Mark, Todd, and Lisa, who lived with an often distracted, sometimes short-tempered, and frequently absent father during the several years required for completion of this work. I hope it will be found useful by all students of children's growth.

MARVIN L. RALLISON

*Salt Lake City, Utah*
*June 1985*

# Contents

Growth Disorders
in Infants,
Children,
and Adolescents

# 1

# The Nature
# of Growth

*Growth* is a term used to describe the process of growing—the increase in size and development of a living organism from a simple to a more complex form or from its earliest stage of being to maturity (1). *Development* implies increase in skill and complexity of function, that is, a series of changes by which an individual embryo becomes an organism. Development, therefore, includes *differentiation* of various parts of the body to perform different functions and alterations of the body as a whole, as well as the formation of individual organs and systems (2). Growth can be accomplished by an increase in the number of cells (*hyperplasia*), by increase in the size of cells (*hypertrophy*), or by an increase in the amount of intercellular material (*accretion*). Growth is not simply a uniform process of becoming taller and larger, however. It involves changes in shape and body composition and may involve replacement of tissues (the ductus arteriosus), tissue substitution (cartilage/bone), and alteration or modification of specific tissues (puberty).

## CELLULAR GROWTH AND DIFFERENTIATION

The human body consists of cells and intercellular matrix. The rate of growth of an organ or of an individual is fundamentally determined by the rate of cellular division. After the formation of a cell, there occurs a resting phase in which no growth occurs (but, of course, there is metabolic activity by which the cell serves the purpose for which it was formed). In response to some intrinsic or chemical stimulus there is growth of cytoplasm and duplication of DNA. When the cell achieves optimal size, cell division (mitosis) occurs, followed again by a resting phase. Each phase is modifiable and the process is sensitive to disruptive or stimulatory influences.

Beginning with the fertilized ovum, the growth process is initially one of cell division to form two daughter cells, each containing about half the

1

material of the parent cell. In these initial generations there is reduplication of chromatin material derived from cellular cytoplasm and a reduction in the amount of cytoplasm per daughter cell. After a few generations cells do not divide until optimal amounts of nuclear and cytoplasmic material have been generated. The stimulus that initiates cell division is unknown, but cell size is not the only determinant. Cells can be stimulated to divide at less than maximum size, though there is a level below which no division can occur. The stimulus appears to originate within the cytoplasm, for in multinucleated cells all nuclei enter mitosis synchronously (2).

The amount of nuclear material available is obviously crucial in determining the time of cell division. A cell cannot divide until there is adequate chromatin material for two daughter cells. Because each cell contains a constant amount of nuclear material, the number of cells being synthesized may be determined by measuring the amount of DNA being produced. An increase in DNA content of a tissue or an organ thus indicates cellular hyperplasia.

There are periods in the growth of tissues or organs in which cellular hyperplasia or hypertrophy predominate. Initial growth of most tissues is characterized by rapid increase in cell numbers with formation of less cytoplasm per cell and an increase in the cellular DNA/protein ratio. As the adult organ size is approached, growth consists almost entirely of hypertrophy of cells with little change in cell number. This may be identified by a decrease of DNA/protein ratio of the tissue because of further increases in cytoplasmic protein without changes in DNA content of the tissue. At maturity, a state of equilibrium is achieved in which there are nearly constant amounts of both DNA and cytoplasmic protein (3, 4) (Figure 1-1).

The stage of cellular hyperplasia, in which the number of cells increases rapidly, represents a "critical growth period," that is, a period in which the organ is most susceptible to permanent damage, malformation or aberrant growth (5). The timing of this period of rapid cell division varies from one tissue to another and hence the period of vulnerability also varies (6). The majority of brain cells are already present by 6 months of age so the period of vulnerability of the brain to factors affecting growth occurs during fetal life and early infancy. Skeletal cells, by contrast, continue to be formed until 15–20 years of age. The skeletal system displays vulnerability to factors adversely affecting growth, not only during early formative periods, but throughout childhood and adolescence.

In some tissues the space between cells becomes filled with a viscous substance, such as hyaluronic acid or chondroitin sulfate (e.g., cartilage), giving it a jelly-like consistency enabling it to hold large amounts of fluid and to assume a firm shape. In most tissues, as connective tissue cells appear, collagen and elastic fibers are laid down. They provide structure and elasticity to the tissues. Formation of matrix and fibers continues

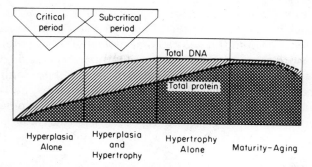

**Figure 1-1.** Stages of growth and differentiation of an organ tissue depicting periods of predominantly cellular hyperplasia versus cellular hypertrophy. DNA content is an index of cell number and protein content is an index of cell number and size. In the early stages of growth, characterized by cellular hyperplasia, organs or tissues tend to be more vulnerable to damaging influences that causes permanent growth deficiencies. (Reproduced by permission from Smith DW: *Growth and its Disorders*, Philadelphia, WB Saunders Co, 1977, adapted from Winick M: Fetal malnutrition and growth processes. *Hosp Pract* **5**(May):33, 1970.)

throughout the period of growth and is vital for repair of injuries and regeneration of tissues throughout the organism's life.

Initial growth produces daughter cells that are totipotential, but as growth proceeds the cells begin to *differentiate* into cells of more specific function. They lose their totipotential capacity and begin to assume specialized functions that give rise to specific tissues, such as bone, muscle, or blood-forming tissues. A differentiated cell usually acquires new functions but at the same time loses old ones. The more specialized the cell becomes, the less likely it is to retain capacity to multiply. A cell may be spoken of as fully differentiated when it is reduced to a specific form and retains only certain functions. The red blood cell is derived from a stem cell which retains potential for self-propagation. The fully developed red blood cell acquires a peculiar shape fitting it to its function, which is restricted to the transport of oxygen and carbon dioxide in the blood. It has no further capacity to grow, divide, or change function, but has reached its ultimate form and function.

Another form of differentiation may be seen in specific responses to growth-promoting substances. At puberty sex hormones affect genitalia, sexual hair follicles, bone, muscle, and fat in a specific manner, suggesting that such tissues have been programmed to react to specific stimuli during their differentiation into specific cell types.

## THE DYNAMIC NATURE OF GROWTH

Growth is a dynamic process. Not all tissues of the body grow at the same rate nor stop growing simultaneously. Some tissues continue to grow throughout our lifetime, while others reach full development early and remain relatively static thereafter. There is a constant interchange of building materials within the body so that most molecules entering as food stay only a short time. Different substances turn over at different rates. The average nitrogen atom (muscle) remains in the body only a week or two, a molecule of calcium (bone) a matter of months, and cholesterol (nerve sheaths) may remain a lifetime. This constant turnover of tissue constituents requires energy which represents part of our basal energy requirement, that is, energy we use when totally at rest (4).

## Tissue Turnover

Though there is a constant turnover of living material, the manner and rate of formation and turnover of different tissues varies widely. Tissues may be roughly classified into: (a) those in which there is very active turnover of cell populations, (b) those with a moderate turnover, and (c) those with essentially none.

To the first group belong those tissues in which cells are constantly being lost or removed but which maintain a constant mass. This group might include epidermis, lining of the gut, endometrium, transitional epithelium, blood-forming tissues, and male sex cell precursors. In such tissues a "bank" of relatively undifferentiated stem cells is preserved by multiplication, which constantly or on demand produces the highly functional differentiated line of cells (2).

In the second group belong such organs as the liver, kidney, and the endocrine glands. In these there is not an obligatory loss of tissue during functional activity. Growth occurs by division of functional cells and turnover is relatively slow, but growth by hypertrophy and/or hyperplasia can occur under appropriate stimuli, particularly in repair of injuries. Endocrine organs may undergo severalfold increases in size under the influence of endogenous or exogenous stimuli.

In the third group belong muscle and nerve tissue which achieve most of their cellular hyperplasia in the early period of their growth. After the period of hyperplasia, further growth is achieved by enlargement of existing cells, which remain theoretically unchanged in number throughout the life of the organism. Such tissues, however, retain the capacity to regenerate injured or atrophic parts. The axon of a nerve will regenerate if the nerve sheath is restored or remains intact—a destroyed nerve cell, however, will not be replaced. Similarly, injured or atrophic muscle fibers may regenerate within the sarcolemmal sheath—there may be increase in syncytium and in nuclei, but no new fibers will be formed (4).

## Growth of Bone

Bone represents a unique tissue, both because of its growth characteristics, and because of its profound effect on the size of the organism. A limb bone is formed first in cartilage. At the center of the cartilaginous bone

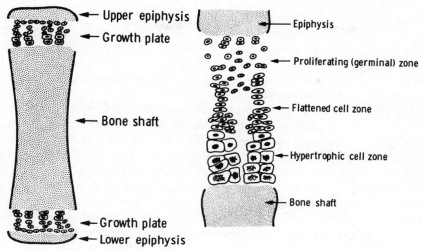

**Figure 1-2.**  (*Left*) Diagram of limb bone with upper and lower epiphyses. (*Right*) Magnified view of the growth plate to show zones of cells within the growth plate. New cells are formed in the proliferating or germinal zone and are replaced by bone in the hypertrophic cell zone next to the bone shaft. (Reproduced by permission from Tanner JM: *Fetus into Man.* Cambridge, MA, Harvard University Press, 1978.)

the cartilage cells undergo degeneration to be replaced by the primary ossification center. In most bones this process begins to take place in early fetal life. Shortly before birth, secondary centers of ossification appear at the ends of long bones called *epiphyses*. The area between the epiphysis and the shaft of the bone is termed the *growth plate* (Figure 1-2). Immediately under the epiphysis is the zone of proliferating cartilage cells. Cells in this area divide and are arranged into flattened longitudinal columns. As they approach the end of the main shaft of the bone, they become larger and are surrounded by intercellular substance forming a sleeve or tube. The cells gradually lose their flat stacked arrangement, eventually die, and are replaced by bone (4, 7).

As growth at the epiphyseal plates slows, the plate gets thinner until finally the area is replaced by bone completely and the epiphysis is said to be closed or fused to the main shaft. When the growth plate is gone, no more growth in length of the long bone is possible and the bone is said to be mature. The long bones generally have growth plates (epiphyses) at both ends. Growth occurs at some epiphyses more readily than at others. The femur grows mainly through the epiphyses at the knee and very little at the hip. The humerous grows chiefly at the shoulder end, forearm bones mainly at the wrist, and the tibia and fibula about equally at the knee and ankle (4).

The growth in width of limb bones takes place by deposition of new layers of bone on the outside of existing bone (appositional growth). The inner layer of the periosteum (the fibrous covering of the bone), called the "cambium", consists of cells which lay down new bone. Growth of bones of the skull and of the face, which are membranous bones, also take place by appositional growth.

A growing bone has to be continually remodeled. Large areas of bone are broken down and absorbed or reformed. The final shape of a bone depends not only on growth in length and in width, but also on muscle pulls and positioning of adjacent structures. The formation of the jaw for the proper bite, for example, requires considerable remodeling and the final shape of the femur and pelvis depends on normal muscular attachments and weight bearing. Even after full adult size and shape have been achieved, continuous remodeling and daily interchange of minerals which form the solid portions of the bones continue.

## FACTORS AFFECTING GROWTH

The "harmony" of growth lies in the intricate orchestration of growth processes so that each tissue is found in the right amount at the right time and that differentiation of each tissue is accomplished as needed so that each function of the growing organism can be served (8).

### Local Growth Stimulation and Inhibition

The precise mechanisms by which cell division and differentation are regulated are largely unknown. Specific humoral substances which limit mitotic activity in particular tissues have been described (9). A specific humoral protein within liver cells seems to be responsible for regulating mitosis occurring during repair of liver tissue. When the optimal number of liver cells is present, a substance termed a *chalone* accumulates to inhibit further mitotic growth, in effect, representing a cellular growth negative feed-back system. These tissue-specific substances act to keep the liver at its optimal size for the organism. Similar negative feed-back systems to regulate growth of spleen and kidney have been suggested (10).

Some tissue-specific factors have also been described which enhance growth. Somatomedins, produced in the liver and other tissues primarily under stimulation of human growth hormone, accelerate cartilaginous growth. Other factors promote growth of the nerve cells (nerve growth factor), epiphyseal cells (epiphyseal growth factor), and fibroblasts. The fibroblast growth factor is a peptide secreted locally in the area in which it is needed (a paracrine effect). Many of these locally active growth factors seem to be interrelated in terms of size, shape, type of activity, and immunologic characteristics, though each exerts a specific action on a specific tissue (3, 11).

In addition to endocrine and paracrine growth regulators, tissue growth requires provision of adequate substrate (especially protein), a vascular supply to provide oxygen and substrate to the tissues, innervation (tissues deprived of innervation undergo atrophy), and use of tissues (most particularly muscle or bone) (3).

## Genetic Factors Affecting Growth

The growth of a child is the result of complex interactions of genetic and environmental factors. Certain peoples are taller than others, largely the consequence of multiple genetic differences, though nutrition may play some role as well. The pigmies of the Congo, one of the world's smallest races, appear to have a genetically determined inability to respond to somatomedin. Black children tend to be larger and more advanced in skeletal maturation than white children. Asiatic children tend to be smaller than black or white children (12).

Twin studies have shown that body size, body shape, and patterns of growth are strongly influenced by genetic factors (2). The average difference in height of monozygotic twins is 2.8 cm versus a 12 cm difference for dizygotic twins of the same sex (3). The stature to which a child attains as an adult correlates best to mid-parent height but appears to have a polygenic mode of inheritance. Offspring of one tall and one short parent are, on the average, about the same size as those born to two average size parents, but there is more variation in the size of offspring born to parents of disparate height than those born to parents both of whom are of medium height (3).

The rate of development reflected by bone age, dental development, time of sexual maturation, and neurological milestones is also heavily influenced by genetic control (2). Tempo of growth or maturation rate is often reflected in a family pattern. The age at which adolescent development begins is quite variable and the age at which final height and maturity is reached may vary by as much as a third between the fast and slow maturing youth. The level of maturation of bones represents a biological or physiological age which can be used as a marker to help determine the tempo of growth of an individual and may be of some use in interpreting the growth and ultimate potential of the child (3).

Some observations suggest that the sex genes themselves may affect growth. There is a sex difference in tempo of growth and time of adolescent growth spurt. The noticeable and consistent advancement of girls over boys in respect to skeletal maturation has been attributed to a retarding action of genes located on the Y chromosome of the male (3). Males with Klinefelter syndrome (XXY) still follow a male time pattern of growth and development. Size correlation among girls is closer than among boys with less variability in the sequence of osseous maturation between sisters than between brothers (13).

## Neural Control of Growth

It has been suggested that there may be a growth center in the brain, possibly in the hypothalamus, that is responsible for keeping the child in his or her genetically determined growth curve. If a child deviates from a growth pattern for a period of time because of malnutrition or illness, a period of accelerated or "catch-up" growth brings him back to the "predetermined" curve (4). This phenomenon implies some sort of central control mechanism. Although such a neural control center for growth has not yet been demonstrated, the hypothalamus would be the most logical location because of its proximity to and connection with the pituitary gland with its basic hormonal control of growth. Peripheral nerves may also play some part in control of growth. Many structures, including muscles, nails, and taste buds undergo atrophy when denervated. It is suggested that peripheral nerve fibers exert a trophic effect on structures they supply. A chemical may be liberated at endings of nerve fibers which in some way modifies growth and stimulates repair of structures so innervated.

## Hormonal Influence on Growth

Most of the endocrine glands influence growth in some way but some have a greater influence than others. *Human growth hormone* produced by the anterior pituitary gland is necessary for normal growth throughout infancy and childhood. Growth hormone promotes synthesis of protein, inhibits synthesis of fat and carbohydrate, and is necessary for the proliferation of cartilage leading to bone growth. As such, it is a major determinent of height achievement. Growth hormone must be present for androgens to exert their full effect during the adolescent growth spurt. The growth promoting effects of growth hormone are mediated through *somatomedins* which enhance the rate of mitosis of cartilage cells at the epiphyseal plate (14). *Insulin* appears to be a major growth regulating hormone and together with somatomedins, some of which have insulin-like activity, influences the complex growth of the fetus (15). Insulin probably contributes primarily to growth by regulating the supply of substrate to cells for metabolism. *Thyroid hormone* is essential to normal growth and development of the skeleton and of the central nervous system and is essential for complete expression of human growth hormone's effect on cartilage and bone formation. *Testosterone* and other *androgenic hormones* mediate the growth spurt of puberty. There occurs an increase in muscle mass, acceleration of bone growth and maturation, growth and maturation of male sexual organs, and appearance of male secondary sexual characteristics. The marked effect of androgens on osseous maturation produces rapid fusion of epiphyses and cessation of linear growth. *Estrogens* produce a widening of the hips and stimulate growth of female sexual organs and secondary sexual characteristics. Estrogens accelerate osseous maturation without stimulating linear growth as much as testosterone.

## Nutrition in Growth

Adequate food to provide substrate for energy and synthesis of protein is essential for normal growth. Observations of growth in humans during famine have shown a lack of normal growth, but most of our knowledge of the relationship of nutrition to growth derives from animal work. Rats and mice cease to grow when fed a diet deficient in calories. Growth is restored when calories are once again offered. Maximal size of experimental animals is achieved by feeding a diet a little less than that chosen by appetite from free-feeding (2). In the first year of life the baby requires about twice as many calories per kilogram as a male adult and a growing adolescent may require as many calories as a heavy manual worker. In the diet suitable for normal growth there must be an adequate supply of protein and appropriate amounts of specific amino acids. Absence of any of the essential amino acids will result in disordered or stunted growth. Undernutrition at any given stage of development seems to unmask the normal differential of growth, that is, the most vital growth is affected first and most profoundly. In dietary deprivation the growth of bones is affected more than that of teeth, and bones grow better than muscle or fat. In the brain, myelinization is affected less than brain cell hyperplasia. During puberty, undernutrition affects sexual organs less than other tissues (2).

Specific nutritional deficiencies may also interfere with growth. A lack of zinc, a constituent of many enzymes involved in protein metabolism, has been associated with growth failure. Formation of bone requires an adequate supply of calcium, phosphorus and trace amounts of magnesium and manganese. Iron is required for hemoglobin and copper for normal growth of the blood-forming organs. Iodine is required for thyroxine formation and fluoride for proper formation of tooth enamel and bone (2). Vitamin A deficiency results in shortened, thickened bones and pressure on nerves which pass through bony canals. Vitamin C deficiency results in deficient formation of intercellular substance of bone and fragility (scurvy). Too little Vitamin D results in inadequate calcification of the bones resulting in softening and bending of the bones with shortness of stature (rickets).

## Miscellaneous Factors Affecting Growth

*Oxygen* is understandably required for optimal growth. Children born with cyanotic congenital heart disease may experience interference with growth until the lesion is corrected. Children in top socioeconomic groups are taller than children of unskilled laborers—the lower the social class or *social/economic status* of the mother, the smaller the baby and child. Children in large families tend to be smaller and lighter than children in smaller

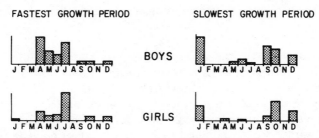

**Figure 1-3.**  Fastest and slowest growth periods for boys and girls. Distribution of months in which individual boys or girls completed their fastest and slowest periods of growth measured at 3-month intervals. (Adapted with permission from Marshall WA: Evaluation of growth rate in height over periods of less than one year. *Arch Dis Child* **46:**414, 1971.)

families. Later children may not receive the same nutrtion, especially in those with large families. Parents in low socio-economic groups tend to be small, reflecting their own limitations and deprivations (2). Growth in height of children is faster in the spring than in the autumn; whereas, growth in weight is faster in autumn (16) (Figure 1-3). The reason for this *seasonal difference* is unknown. Such seasonal variations make it essential to measure a child suspected of growth failure over at least a full year to distinguish seasonal changes from true growth failure (2). Whether *climate* has an effect on growth is doubtful. Effects initially attributed to climate may be a reflection of racial, dietary, or disease factors, for though tall whites originate in cold northern areas, tall aborigines are found in tropical Australia (3). *Generalized disease*, such as tuberculosis or kidney disease, may affect growth in about the same manner as malnutrition. Just how disease alters the growth pattern is not completely known, though there is some evidence that somatomedin production or activity is reduced or that somatomedin antagonists may be formed during certain disease states. During generalized illness there is a decrease in the mitotic index of cartilage cells at the epiphyseal plates; the plates become thinner and the number of cartilage cells reduced (2).

## CANALIZATION AND CRITICAL PERIODS OF GROWTH

The growth of a child or any other organism is, under normal circumstances, a very regular process. This regularity of growth is a result of a dynamic and complex system of control. Prader has likened the child's growth curve to the course of a ship or of a guided missile (17). Just as a ship is steered along a course or channel, so a child's growth is said to be *canalized*, a term suggested by Waddington (18), which means that the growth of any growing organism has a tendency to return to its original path or channel even though illness or malnutrition might temporarily push it off course. Waddington used the term *homeorrhesis* (meaning to flow back together) for the tendency of animals to return to their paths of growth after deviating from them (18). According to Tanner, growth is self-stabilizing and seeks a target supposedly determined by genetic traits (4). The power to stabilize or return to a predetermined growth curve after being pushed off track persists throughout the period of growth, though return to the normal target is limited by severity, length, and timing of the insult to growth (4).

## Catch-Up or Lag-Down Growth

Children demonstrate the tendency to "canalization" of their growth quite dramatically. During periods of illness, hormone deficiency, or starvation, growth is slowed. Removal of the cause of the illness, starvation, or hormonal dysequilibrium, however, results in a period of accelerated growth, so that the child returns to his original growth curve (Figure 1-4). Prader has called this phenomenon "Aufholwachstum" or "catch-up growth" (17). If the period of catch-up growth is plotted on a growth velocity curve, it assumes a characteristic pattern of a rapid early phase followed by gradual deceleration and resumption of normal velocity when the original growth channel is reached (Figure 1-5).

The reverse of catch-up occurs when a child recovers from a period of accelerated growth such as might occur with congenital adrenal hyperplasia. This reverse growth phenomenon has been called a "lagging-down growth" (19) (Figure 1-5). Both of these phenomena can be seen in normal infants during the first 18 months to 2 years of life. Smith has shown that small infants frequently demonstrate an accelerated pattern of growth and large infants a decelerated pattern crossing channels of growth until they achieve their target (channel) which is believed to represent their genetically determined growth channel (20).

## Critical Periods of Growth

In animal experimentation, the amount of growth recovery or catch-up growth depends on the cause, duration, and severity of the injury to growth, as well as the age of the animal. In general, catch-up growth is less complete if growth retardation is severe and of long duration or if the animal is very immature or very old. This latter observation suggests that there may be "critical" periods in the growth of animals and that injury during a critical period of growth may lead to a permanent growth deficit (19). Mosier has shown that damage to or malformation of the central nervous system is characteristically associated with growth impairment that is permanent and lacking a catch-up phase. He suggests that the central nervous system houses a growth control center within the hypothalamus–limbic system, damage to which precludes achievement of the genetic growth potential. This growth impairment is uninfluenced by levels of human growth hormone, somatomedins, or good nutrition (21).

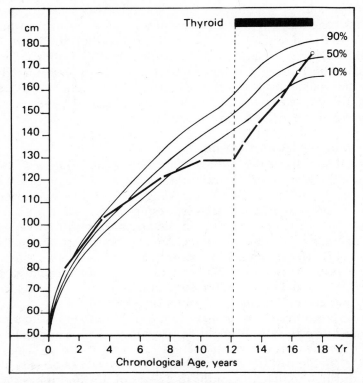

**Figure 1-4.** *Catch-up growth* in an individual with hypothyroidism. Height may be seen to be falling away after age 4 to a position well below the 10th percentile by age 12. Catch-up growth with return to the 75th percentile by age 17 with thyroid therapy. (Reproduced by permission from Prader A, Tanner JM, Harnack GA: Catch-up growth following illness or starvation: An example of developmental canalization in man. *J Pediatr* **62:**646, 1963.)

The child's catch-up capacity seems also to be limited as either he or she approaches maturity as in older animals. Complete catch-up does not occur if damage to the growth process occurs at or after puberty.

## Regulators of Catch-Up Growth

The factors which are responsible for the phenomena of *catch-up* or *lag-down* growth are not completely known. Growth hormone, insulin, and androgens are the best known growth-promoting factors, but there is no evidence yet linking them with the catch-up growth phenomenon. We are just beginning to discover and understand the serum growth factors, such as the somatomedins and related specific tissue growth factors, which appear to have a more direct effect on the growth of specific tissues than the classical growth hormones. We do not know much yet concerning

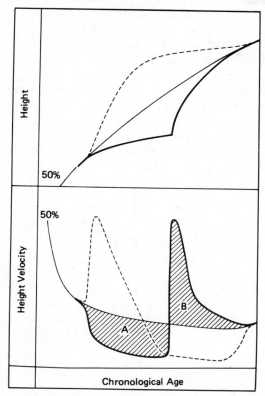

**Figure 1-5.** Schematic illustrations of "catch-up" and "lag-down" growth phenomena on distance and velocity growth curves for height. "Catch-up" growth is illustrated by the heavy lines. The section marked "A" represents the slowing of growth and the section marked "B" the period of catch-up growth. "Lag-down" growth is illustrated by the broken lines with early rapid growth and a subsequent lagging down of growth to resume the appropriate channel of growth. (Reproduced by permission from Prader A: Catch-up growth. *Postgrad Med J* **54**:141, 1978.)

cellular responses and receptors. It is possible that during catch-up growth the sensitivity of tissues to growth factors is enhanced or, as suggested by Prader, that cells are simply programmed for a certain amount of growth and that they will follow that program as soon as inhibitory factors are removed, providing the necessary hormones and growth factors are present (19).

Perhaps equally as mysterious is the question of how the body knows when catch-up growth is complete and normal growth velocity can be resumed. A child's catch-up velocity is high at the beginning and decreases progressively as the target growth curve is approached. Tanner suggests that growth velocity may be regulated by a signal of discrepancy between

the target curve and the actual achieved growth. The genetically programmed curve is visualized as being stored within the brain, possibly in
the hypothalamus, which perceives by some as yet to be explained process,
when the programmed growth curve has been achieved and regulates the
progressive deceleration of growth toward normal (4). It is now known
that in states of hormone excess there is down-regulation of numbers of
receptors specific to the action of the hormone and that in states of
hormone deficiency, an up-regulation of receptor number occurs. Both
catch-up and lag-down growth regulation may be mediated by means of
up- and down-regulation of receptors for somatomedin, human growth
hormone, or tissue growth factors.

## SECULAR TRENDS IN GROWTH PATTERNS

During the past two hundred years there has been a noticeable change in
the tempo of growth and maturation and to a lesser extent the ultimate

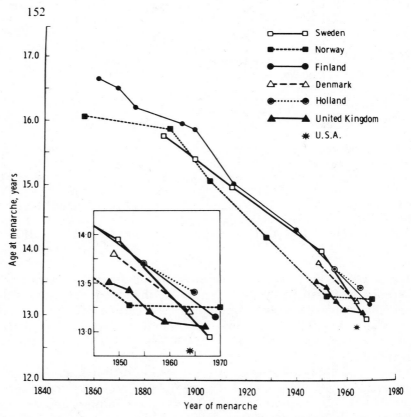

**Figure 1-6.**   Secular trend in age at menarche from 1860 to 1970. (Reproduced
by permission from Tanner JM: *Fetus into Man.* Cambridge, MA, Harvard University Press, 1978.)

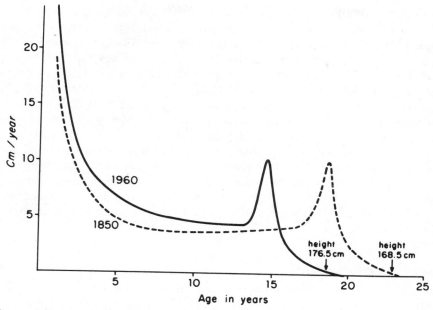

**Figure 1-7.** Accelerated maturation in Netherlands' males between 1850 and 1960. Note that in 1960, peak height velocity is achieved at an earlier age, and there is a greater height achievement in the adult. (Reproduced by permission from Smith DW: *Growth and its Disorders.* Philadelphia, WB Saunders Co, 1978.)

size of individuals. Faster maturation has led to noticeable differences in size for children of all ages. Between 1880 and 1950 the average height of children between ages 5 and 7 years has increased by 10 cm in North American and Western European countries (22). The average height of 16-year-old English boys has increased by more than 1.3 cm per decade between 1873 and 1943 (4).

The increased tempo of maturation has led to earlier advent of adolescence and of final height achievement. A century ago the average male did not achieve final height until the age of 23 years. He now achieves it by 17 years of age. The change in the age of menarche provides one of the most striking features of a secular trend in maturation (Figure 1-6). The figures for Western Europe show a decline of menarche from about 17 to 13 years over the past century (4). A similar trend has been noticed in the United States over the past century but this trend now seems to be leveling off (3).

Some of the reports of changes in population height are influenced by the increased tempo of maturation and give an inaccurate picture of the changes in ultimate height achievement. The average 14-year-old boy today may be at about the same maturational level as an 18-year-old of 100 years ago. Oppers compared the stature of 19 and 25-year-old Dutch recruits from the 1850s with those of the 1960s showing an increase of 16 cm in the 19-year-olds but only a 6 cm difference between 25-year-olds (23) (Figure 1-7). Shifts in adult height between 1854 and 1935 are also reported by Lenz and Kellner from Munich. They reported a mean height of 165 cm for males in their mid-20s in Munich in 1935, compared to a mean height of 158 cm in 1854 (24).

The cause or causes of this interesting trend in growth and maturation are not known. The most popular hypothesis is that it is a combination of genetic outbreeding with greater hybrid vigor combined with better nutrition and freedom from illness during childhood allowing people over several generations to achieve their full genetic potential. An observation perhaps supporting this hypothesis is that the average age of menarche in Lap women, whose culture and living conditions have changed little over the past century, was 16.5 years in 1930, the same as it had been in 1870 (3).

## PERIODS OF GROWTH

Growth is a continuous process, but in studying growth it is often informative to distinguish phases or periods of growth. When we speak of phases or periods, however, we acknowledge that all phases blend almost imperceptibly into each other and that growth continues smoothly even though we view it in terms of more or less distinct periods (25).

*Intrauterine growth* includes growth and development of the embryo and of the fetus. The early embryo is the period in which most rapid growth occurs and the period in which growth is most dependent on the mother and her health. During the embryonic period, rapid differentiation takes place and organ systems are established. During fetal growth the functional activities of the organ systems are developed and there is rapid increase in body mass.

*Infancy* is a period of rapidly changing growth rate. At birth, dependence upon mother and placenta is abruptly discontinued, requiring major changes in function of respiratory, circulatory, digestive, and excretory systems. Rapid growth and maturation, especially of the central nervous system, continue during infancy, but at a decelerating rate. After birth, the infant shifts from a growth rate predominately determined by maternal factors to one related to genetic background and extrauterine environment.

*Childhood* is a period of stabilized growth. Early shifts in growth patterns have generally been accomplished by two years of age and growth proceeds at a constant rate. Major brain growth is complete, lymphoid tissue growth is at a maximum, and general growth is slow but steady. There is increasing coordination of function and development of skills and intellectual processes.

*Adolescence* heralds the onset of the final growth spurt mediated through the sex hormones. Adolescence is a period of accelerated growth in height and weight with maturation of the reproductive system and appearance of sexual characteristics culminating in ability to reproduce. Growth proceeds through a deceleration phase and is finally terminated by union of the epiphyses of the bones.

*Adulthood and Old Age* represent phases of growth characterized by functional activity of fully differentiated tissues. Size change is accomplished primarily by hypertrophy or atrophy of preexisting cells and growth is restricted to repair or replacement of cells and tissues. In old age cells are lost without replacement and eventually degeneration leads to death of the organism.

## REFERENCES

1. *American Heritage Dictionary of the English Language*, William Morris (ed). Boston, Houghton Mifflin Company, 1979.
2. Sinclair D: *Human Growth after Birth*. London, Oxford University Press, 1978, pp 1–15, 140–159.
3. Smith DW: Basics and nature of growth, in *Growth and Its Disorders*. Philadelphia, WB Saunders Co., 1977, pp 1–17.
4. Tanner JM: *Fetus into Man: Physical Growth from Conception to Maturity*. Cambridge, Harvard University Press, 1978, pp 24–36, 117–154, 155–165.
5. Winick M: Fetal malnutrition and growth processes. *Hosp Pract* 5(May):33, 1970.
6. Smith DW, Berman EL: *Biologic Ages of Man*. Philadelphia, WB Saunders Co., 1973.
7. Rimoin DL, Horton WA: Short stature, Part I. *J. Pediatr* **92**:523–528, 1978.
8. Widdowson EM: Harmony of growth. *Lancet* **1**:901–905, 1970.
9. Weiss P, Kavanaugh JL: A model of growth and growth control in mathematical terms. *J Gen Physiol* **41**:1, 1957.
10. Bullough WS: Chalone control mechanisms. *Life Sci* **16**:323, 1975.
11. Nevo Z, Laron Z: Growth factors. *Am J Dis Child* **133**:419, 1979.
12. Barr GD, Allen CM, Shinefield HR: Height and weight of 7500 children of three skin colors, Pediatric Multiphasic Program, Report #3. *Am J Dis Child* **124**:866, 1972.
13. Garn SM, Rohmann CG: X-linked inheritance of developmental timing in man. *Nature* **196**:695, 1962.
14. Zapf J, Schmid Ch, Froesch ER: Biological and immunological properties of insulin-like growth factors (IGF) I and II. *Clin Endocr Metab* **13**:3, 1984.
15. Underwood LE, D'Ercole AJ: Insulin and insulin-like growth factors/somatomedins in fetal and neonatal development. *Clin Endocr Metab* **13**:69, 1984.
16. Marshall WA: Evaluation of growth rate in height over periods of less than one year. *Arch Dis Child* **46**:414, 1971.
17. Prader A, Tanner JM, Harnack GA: Catch-up growth following illness or starvation: An example of developmental canalization in man. *J Pediatr* **62**:646, 1963.
18. Waddington CH: *The Strategy of the Genes*. London, George Allen and Unwin Ltd., 1957.
19. Prader A: Catch-up growth. *Postgrad Med J* **2**(54):133, 1978.
20. Smith DW, Truog W, Rogers JE, et al: Shifting linear growth during infancy: Illustration of genetic factors in growth from fetal life through infancy. *J Pediatr* **89**:225, 1976.
21. Mosier HD: Catch-up and proportionate growth. *Med Clin North Am* **62**:337, 1978.
22. Graham GG: Environmental factors affecting the growth of children. *Am J Clin Nutr* **25**:1184, 1972.

23. Oppers VM: Analyse van de acceleratte van de manselije lengtegroei door bepaling van het tijdstip van de groeifasen, Amsterdam. *Academisch Proefschrift*, 1963.

24. Lenz W, Kellner H: Die Körperliche Akzeleration. *Deutsches Jugend Institut*, Munich, 1965, p 35.

25. Lowrey GH: *Growth and Development of Children*, ed 7. Chicago, Yearbook Medical Publishers Inc., 1978, pp 11–17.

# 2
# Fetal Growth and Development

Intrauterine growth begins after fertilization of the ovum by the sperm and implantation of the fertilized ovum within the uterus. Fertilization of the ovum occurs within 48 hours after ovulation; in a woman with regular periods every 28 days this occurs 2 weeks after the last normal menstrual period. The time of the onset of the last normal menstrual period is often used for calculation of the duration of gestation, known as (post) menstrual age, but because many women have irregular timing of periods and menstrual flow after conception is fairly common, precision in timing is often uncertain (1). In the discussion of fetal growth in this chapter estimated true gestational age will be used to denote the age of the developing organism unless menstrual age is specified.

## STAGES OF INTRAUTERINE GROWTH

Prenatal growth from ovum to infant can be divided into three stages. The initial period describes growth of the *ovum* from fertilization to formation of the embryonic plate. In this period of two weeks there is rapid cellular division and formation of the anlage for placenta and embryo. The *embryonic period*, beginning 12–14 days after fertilization, lasts approximately 6 weeks. It is a period of rapid growth and differentiation to form the tissues, organs, and organ systems of the developing organism. The remainder of the pregnancy, 28–30 weeks, is termed the *fetal period*. During this period, rapid growth in mass occurs. Functional development of the tissues, organs, and systems occurs mainly during this period.

## INTRAUTERINE GROWTH

Intrauterine growth is phenomenally rapid. From conception to birth there occurs a 6 billion fold increase in size, whereas from birth to maturity only a 20 fold increase in size occurs (2).

## Growth of the Ovum

Fertilization of the ovum takes place within the fallopian tube, which receives the egg from the ovary. At the moment that a single sperm enters the ovum additional sperm are prevented from entering the egg. When the nucleus of the sperm unites with the nucleus of the egg fertilization takes place. This union provides the combination of chromosomes and genes which will determine the heritable characteristics of the developing organism, including the sex of the child. Many ova are fertilized but fail to develop into a fetus. Some 10% fail to implant, and of those which implant, about 50% are aborted spontaneously. Often those ova that are lost spontaneously are abnormal in their development. About 5–10% of fertilized ova have a chromosomal abnormality, but chromosomal abnormalities are present in only 0.5% of live born infants. The remaining ova with chromosomal abnormalities are lost early in their development, often before the mother is even aware she is pregnant (1).

After fertilization of the ovum, there is a rapid cellular division. The resulting cluster of cells moves slowly down the fallopian tube to the uterus. During the journey of four or five days down the fallopian tube, the cells have been dividing to form a *blastocyst* consisting of about 150 cells by the time of implantation. Up to this time there is very little change in total mass, so an increase in the number of cells results in a progressive decrease in the size of individual cells.

After implantation within the uterus, two layers of cells are formed within the blastocyst. From the outer layer, the trophoblast, the placenta is formed. The embryo develops from the embryonic plate formed from the inner layer (Figure 2-1). By the end of this period the inner cell mass forms a flattened, dish-shaped mass of cells (blastodisc) that subdivides into specialized groups of cells (germ layers) which will eventually form specific tissues within the embryo (3).

## Development of the Placenta

The placenta is an extraordinary organ in that it simultaneously performs the functions of intestinal mucosa, liver, lung, kidney, and several endocrine organs. It provides nourishment for the embryo and fetus, clears away waste products, provides protection against toxins and infectious agents, and elaborates hormones that regulate growth and metabolism of the developing organism. The placenta stores glycogen for energy requirements of rapid growth, transports lipids from maternal stores or forms lipids from glucose, provides for passage of amino acids for protein synthesis by the fetus, and synthesizes gonadotrophins, progesterone and estrogen to maintain the pregnancy. It provides an immunologic barrier between mother and fetus allowing passage of protective immunoglobulins to the fetus but protecting the fetus from destruction by the mother's immune system. Human chorionic somatomamammotrophin (hCS) or placental lactogen, a growth hormone-like substance formed by the

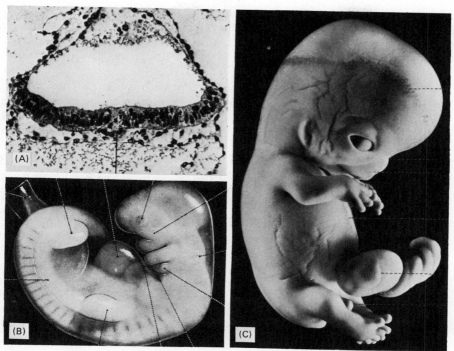

**Figure 2-1.** Stages of embryonic development. (A) In a photomicrograph of an early stage of embryonic development (Horizon VI of Streeter) is depicted the *embryonic disc* from which the embryo develops. Below the disc is seen the developing yolk sac and above, the amniotic cavity and attachment of the embryo to the developing placenta. (Reproduced by permission from Blechschmidt E: *The Stages of Human Development Before Birth.* Philadelphia, WB Saunders Co, 1961.) (B) Embryo of approximately 30 days gestation (Horizon XIII). The head is forming, limb buds just appearing, and the yolk sac and "tail" are still prominent. (Reproduced by permission of Macmillan, London and Basingstoke from Hamilton WJ, et al: *Human Embryology.* Baltimore, Williams and Wilkins Company, 1952.) (C) The embryo in a final stage of development (Horizon XXII) shows rudimentary development of major organs and systems. The brain is well developed and the face is forming. The limbs are formed and fingers and toes are distinct. Part of the bowel still lies within the umbilical cord. (Reproduced by permission from Blechschmidt E: *The Stages of Human Development Before Birth.* Philadelphia, WB Saunders Co, 1961.)

placenta, mobilizes maternal fat stores, maintains a positive nitrogen balance in the mother, and increases serum glucose levels within the mother to assure adequate supplies of food to the placenta and fetus. This placental hormone performs most of the functions of pituitary growth hormone in the fetus (4).

Placental growth generally preceeds fetal growth. Peak placental growth usually occurs within the first trimester and very little change in size occurs in the third trimester when fetal growth reaches its peak velocity. Whether defects in placental growth are the cause of much fetal growth retardation is not certain, but low birth weight may be correlated with low functional placental mass. The same factors which reduce the fetal growth may also affect placental growth, particularly if the noxious factors are active early in the uterine growth period.

## Growth and Differentiation of the Embryo

While the placenta is growing in size and complexity, the embryo is also growing very rapidly. During the embryonic period the embryo loses its flat shape and takes on a rounded body configuration (3). Regions such as head, trunk, and extremities appear and there is differentiation into organs and specialized tissues, such as muscle and nerve. This is a critical period of prenatal development "because the embryo is extremely vulnerable . . . to factors that are capable of disrupting the developmental process . . ." (3). Stages of development of the embryo can be expressed as "horizons" as described by Streeter (5). Horizon VI, reached at 12–14 days after fertilization, represents the beginning of the embryonic period of growth. Horizon XXIII represents completion of the embryonic development and beginning of the fetal period (Figure 2-1).

The 30-day-old embryo (Horizon XIII) has begun to form a head and body with the beginning of a brain. The embryo has four buds where arms and legs will grow (Figure 2-1). There is a tube-shaped heart which is beating and circulating blood. Blood is being formed in the yolk sac, which is about as large as the embryo. The embryo itself is already 10,000 times larger than the fertilized egg (6).

By 56 days (Horizon XXIII) the general shape of the organism is present with arms, legs, feet, eyes, ears, nose, and lips recognizable (Figure 2-1). Trunk and limb musculature are present with some intrinsic tone and capability of limited movement. Flexion of the trunk and extension of the head are possible. The skeleton has begun to develop with formation of cartilage as models of the bones to come. The heart has been beating for about 4 weeks and is beginning to change shape in anticipation of chamber formation. From this point on, the growing organism is termed a fetus (6).

## Growth of the Fetus

Reliable growth curves of the fetus are difficult to construct. From the study of products of conception removed from the uterus by therapeutic abortion it is possible to obtain reliable measurements of size from about 8 to 16 weeks of gestational age, and studies of infants born prematurely, from 26 to 28 weeks onward, provide information about growth in the last trimester of intrauterine life. There is a paucity of information concerning the growth of the fetus in the period from 16 to 28 weeks (1, 7).

Growth curves showing average length and weight velocity in the prenatal and immediate postnatal period are drawn by Tanner (Figure 2-2). Figure 2-2A shows a striking increase in length velocity during the first trimester, reaching a peak velocity of nearly 10 cm per 4 week period at about 18 weeks postmenstrual age (16 weeks gestational age), with an equally dramatic deceleration of length velocity during the last part of the final trimester (Figure 2-2A). The velocity of length increments levels off somewhat after birth, though it continues to fall rapidly throughout infancy (1). A similar curve of velocity of weight gain, expressed in kilograms per year, shows a peak weight gain at about 34 weeks postmenstrual age followed by a steep fall in velocity of weight gain until after birth. This fall is most likely occasioned by uterine restraint on growth, that is, limitation of growth because of limitation in the size which the uterus can accommodate (Figure 2-2B). Immediately after birth there is a brief acceleration of weight velocity, lasting about 8 weeks, and followed by a more gradual deceleration of weight gain velocity throughout early infancy (1).

When the fetus is 60 days of age, differentiation is almost completed; it now has the appearance of a human infant with brain, heart, lungs, stomach, intestines, nerves, and bladder all in place. Eyes, ears, nose, mouth, and a bulging forehead are recognizable as a human face. The muscles work and the fetus can "swim" in the fluid of the amniotic sac. In the *third month* (60–90 days) amniotic fluid is swallowed to be secreted again into the fluid sac by the now functional kidneys. The heart has assumed a definite shape by as early as 45 days and will become four-chambered by 120 days gestation. Blood formation begins in the bone marrow by the end of the third month (90 days gestation) but oxygen is obtained, as needed, from the placenta. The fetus practices breathing and the lungs, which have assumed a definite shape, are filled with liquid. Islands of pancreatic tissue appear during this month and bile is secreted by the liver. By the end of the first trimester (90 days) discrete reflexes appear and the fetus makes brief jerky movements of legs and head without stimulation (4, 6).

The *fourth month* (90–120 days) is a month of rapid growth. The fetus adds about 300 gms of weight and 13 cm of length. Sweat and sebaceous glands of the skin form, the duodenum and colon assume their proper position, and accessory nasal sinuses are developing. By 120 days, sucking reflexes are present and regular respiratory movement can be detected (4, 6). By the *fifth month* (120–150 days) internal genitalia are formed and

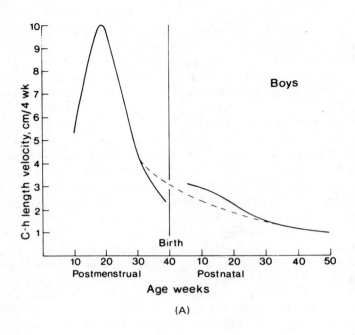

(A)

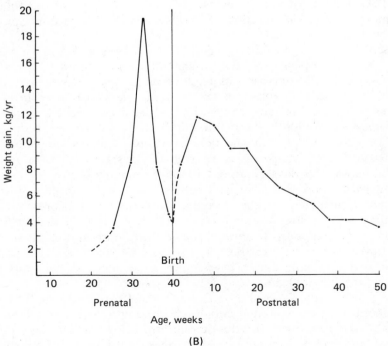

(B)

**Figure 2-2.** (A) Diagramatic prenatal and early postnatal velocity curve in cm/4 wk for growth in body length. Solid lines represent actual crown–heel length

24

external genitalia are beginning to differentiate. Commissures of the brain are complete and myelinization of the cord begins. It is thought that very few new nerve cells are formed after 150 days. By the *sixth month* (150–180 days) typical cortical layering of the central nervous system is completed and primordia of permanent teeth have begun to form. Hair begins to grow on the arms, legs, and back. The skin is thin and wrinkled but contains three layers as at birth. The fetus floats in the amnionic sac and by the sixth month somersaults, kicks and swings arms and legs, often distinctly perceived by the mother (4).

By the *seventh month* (180–210 days) the baby has developed enough function to live, even though born prematurely (age of *viability*). All body functions are present, though still immature and some are untried. Blood is being circulated, muscles are developed, the digestive system is ready for the first meal, the testes descend into the scrotum, permanent teeth primordia are completed, and the spleen assumes its final internal structure. The eyelids are open. Neurologic development is progressing rapidly and systematically and seems after 180 days to progress at the same rate whether within or outside of the uterus. Because of this, the status of neurologic development may be helpful in determining maturational age (4). During the last 3 months of prenatal growth the fetus gains most of its weight. At 180 days the fetus weighs about 1000 g and measures 36 cm—by birth the average infant weighs about 3400 g and measures 50 cm. The final month is one of slowing of growth because the limits of the uterus are being approached and uterine restraint prevents continued rapid growth. Functional progress of the fetus during the final trimester of intrauterine existence is reflected in behavior observed in the premature infant (Table 2-1.)

## Growth and Development of the Fetal Brain

Growth and development of the brain occurs, to a large extent, during the intrauterine period. Growth of the brain is reflected indirectly in growth of the skull, which can be measured in utero by use of ultrasound. Peak velocity of head breadth is reached as early as 11–12 weeks of gestational age and continues at a high velocity until about 28 weeks. Head circumference reaches its peak velocity a little later, at about 13–15 weeks of gestational age, perhaps because the earliest growth is of the cerebrum

---

velocity; the interrupted line, the theoretical curve if no uterine restraint took place. (Reproduced by permission from Tanner JM: *Fetus into Man*. Cambridge, MA, Harvard University Press, 1978.) (B) Weight gain curve for growth in body weight in kg/yr in prenatal and early postnatal periods. Note the effect of uterine restraint on weight gain during the third trimester and the brief acceleration of weight velocity for a few weeks after birth. (Reproduced by permission from Tanner JM: The regulation of human growth. *Child Development* **34**:817, 1963, copyright The Society for Research in Child Development, Inc.)

**Table 2-1. Behavior in the Premature Infant (Fetus), Gestational Ages
28–40 Weeks**

*Infant (Fetus) at 28–32 Weeks*[a]
Movements meager, fleeting, poorly sustained.
Lack of muscular tone.
Mild avoidance responses to bright light and sound.
In prone position turns head to side.
Palmar stimulation elicits barely perceptible grasp.
Breathing shallow and irregular.
Sucking and swallowing present but lack endurance.
No definite waking and sleeping pattern.
Cry may be absent or very weak.
Inconstant tonic neck reflex.

*Infant (Fetus) at 32–36 Weeks*[a]
Movements sustained and positive.
Muscle tone fair under stimulation.
Moro reflex present.
Strong but inadequate response to light and sound.
In prone position turns head, elevates rump.
Definite periods of being awake.
Palmar stimulation causes good grasp.
Good hunger cry.
Fairly well established tonic neck reflex.

*Infant (Fetus) at 36–40 Weeks*[a]
Movements active and sustained.
Muscle tone good.
Brief erratic following of objects with eyes.
Moro reflex strong.
In prone position attempts to lift head.
Active resistance to head rotation.
Definite periods of alertness.
Cries well when hungry and disturbed.
Appears pleased when caressed.
Hands held as fists much of time, good grasp.
Tonic neck reflex more pronounced to one side (usually right) than to the other.
Good, strong sucking reflex.

Reproduced with permission from Lowrey GH: *Growth and Development of Children*, ed 7.
Copyright © 1978 by Year Book Medical Publishers, Inc., Chicago.

[a] Note: The time periods of the table correspond to the 7th to 9th months of gestation [180–266 days] as described in text.

and midbrain structures which affect head breadth most prominently; this is followed by cerebellar growth which would provide the later increase in circumference. Head circumference continues its rapid growth velocity until 30–32 weeks gestational age, after which it experiences a rapid deceleration in growth. This slowing down of head growth continues after birth, though for the first 6 months of postnatal life there is still considerable head and brain growth. The velocity curve for the weight of the brain reaches its peak at around 30 weeks gestational age (8).

The early development of the brain means that the head appears large in a fetus or infant compared to the rest of the body. At birth the brain has already achieved 25% of its adult weight. By contrast, the total body is 5% of its adult weight at birth (8). Different parts of the brain grow at different rates and there are maturity gradients in brain development, much like those seen in the bones and skeleton. The spinal cord, midbrain, and hindbrain mature first, followed by the cerebrum and finally the cerebellum. Most of the neurons in the cerebrum are formed by 16 weeks of gestational age. Growth of axons and dendrites comes later, sometimes much later. Glial cells, the support cells of the central nervous system, begin formation in the cerebrum at about 13 weeks gestational age and continue until about 2 years postnatally. Growth continues in the cerebellum until about 15 months (1). Functional maturity of the brain is accomplished in infancy and early childhood and will be discussed in ensuing chapters.

Although most formation of nerve cells ceases shortly after birth of the infant, a dynamic state of turnover of nerve cell constituents is preserved throughout life. The turnover of amino acids in the brain is as high as it is in the liver and higher than in most other tissues of the body. Since the brain does not itself transform amino acids into fuel for energy, but depends almost exclusively on glucose for energy, the rapid amino acid turnover must be related to a very active synthesis and degradation of neural transmittors, peptides, and proteins within the nerve cells. Despite this rapid *replacement activity*, new cells are not formed when a nerve cell has been destroyed.

### *Prenatal Sex Differentiation*

During the earliest stages of development, only examination of the chromosomes tells us whether the embryo is male or female. Chromosomal sex is determined by the sex chromosome of the sperm which unites with the ovum at the time of fertilization. An ovum or a sperm contains only one member of each chromosome pair (haploid number) from the parent. When they join at fertilization, the fertilized egg will contain 23 pairs of chromosomes, one of each pair from the sperm and one of each pair within the nucleus of the egg. These include 22 pairs of homologous or similar chromosomes and one pair of sex chromosomes. The ovum always contains an X chromosome. The sperm may carry either an X or a Y

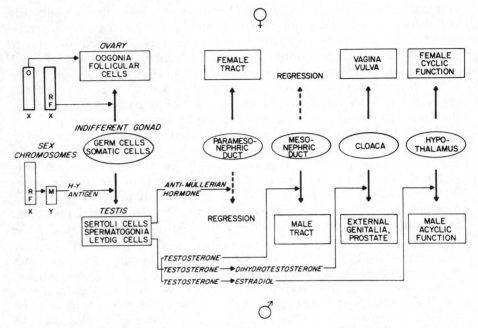

**Figure 2-3.** Regulatory mechanisms in prenatal sexual differentiation. The indifferent stages are shown in the middle oval blocks. Female structures differentiate upwards and male structures downwards. Regulatory factors and their source and target are indicated by thin arrows. Regression is indicated by dashed arrows. F = gene for ovarian differentiation, M = structural gene for testicular differentiation, O = the gene for further ovarian development, R = regulatory gene for testicular differentiation. (Reproduced by permission from Pelliniemi LJ, Dym M: The fetal gonad and sexual differentiation in Tulchinsky D, Ryan KJ, (eds), *Maternal–Fetal Endocrinology*. Philadelphia, WB Saunders Co, 1980.)

chromosome. If the sperm carrying a Y chromosome unites with the egg, the child will be male; if the sperm has an X chromosome, it will be a female.

The reproductive system and sex-related organs develop from a common indifferent primordium. The medullary portion of the primordial gonad has the potential for development into a testes and the cortical portion into an ovary. The female phenotype appears to be the basic pattern in human (mammalian) sexual differentiation (9). A male phenotype (male somatic sex) will develop only if the primordia are acted upon by male organizing factors. A person's sexual characteristics are the result of a series of successive developmental events that occur mainly in the prenatal period. Genetic coding appears to be responsible for gonadal differentiation, but only the testes regulate development of the genital

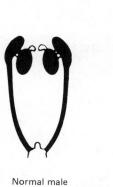 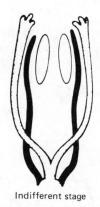 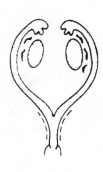

Normal male                    Indifferent stage                    Normal female

**Figure 2-4.**  Differentiation of gonadal ducts. In the indifferent stage both the mesonephric duct (in black) and the paramesonephric duct (stippled) are shown. Differentiation of the male genital tract from the mesonephric duct and the differentiation of the female internal structures from the paramesonephric duct are shown with regression of the nondominant ductal system. (Reproduced by permission from Pelliniemi LJ, Dym M: The fetal gonad and sexual differentiation in Tulchinsky D, Ryan KJ, (eds), *Maternal–Fetal Endocrinology*. Philadelphia, WB Saunders Co, 1980.)

ducts and external genitalia. In the absence of testicular hormones in the fetal period female structures will be formed (10).

Sex-determining genetic material is located on the sex chromosomes. A *testes-organizing gene*, located on the Y chromosome, seems to be responsible for differentiation of the medullary portion of the primordial gonad into a *testis* (11). The gene for the H-Y (histocompatibility-Y) antigen, located on the Y chromosome, may be the testes organizer gene (12). In addition to these two genes, full testicular development seems to require genes for establishment of specific H-Y antigen receptors on gonadal cells and another gene which regulates final testicular size (10) (Figure 2-3). Between 7 and 8 weeks after fertilization the male gonad becomes recognizable as a testis. Any failure of the testicular differentiation genes to act at the proper time or place will result in differentiation of the primordial gonad in the female direction. Ovarian differentiation from the primordial gonadal tissue occurs about 2 weeks later under the genetic influence of the *sex-determining genes of the X chromosomes* (13) (Figure 2-3). It appears that the "ovary gene" can act only if the "testes gene" is not active. For the primary differentiation of the *ovary* only one gene and one X chromosome appear to be necessary, but the ovary of the 45 X individual degenerates before birth, suggesting that a second gene and X chromosome are necessary for maintenance of or further development of ovarian tissue (10).

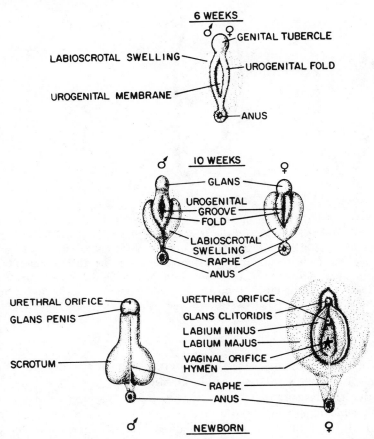

**Figure 2-5.** Differentiation of external genital structures. The primordial indifferent genito–urinary structure is shown at 6 weeks gestation, with separate male and female development at 10 weeks gestation and at birth. (Reproduced by permission from Pelliniemi LJ, Dym M: The fetal gonad and sexual differentiation in Tulchinsky D, Ryan KJ, (eds), *Maternal-Fetal Endocrinology*. Philadelphia, WB Saunders Co, 1980.)

About 7 weeks after fertilization, Leydig cells appear in the testes of the male fetus and begin to secrete testosterone. Testosterone from the fetal testis induces development of *male internal genital structures* (epididymis, ductus deferens, and seminal vesicles) from the mesonephric (or Wolffian) duct (Figure 2-4). Without adequate fetal testicular testosterone the mesonephric duct degenerates by the end of the fourth month (10). The *female (Müllerian) ducts* differentiate autonomously without any known external regulating factors. The paramesonephric duct gives rise to the oviduct (fallopian tube), uterus, and proximal vagina (Figure 2-4). In the male, regression of the Müllerian duct is induced by a testicular factor called Müllerian inhibitory factor (MIF) shortly before 8 weeks. Differentiation of the ductal systems is complete by about 13 weeks after fertilization.

The *external genital structures* arise from the same primordia as do the urinary organs. Female differentiation will occur, whatever the genetic or gonadal sex, at about 12 weeks after fertilization if testosterone is not present. Under the influence of testosterone the prostate gland is formed as a derivative of the vesicourethral canal and the urogenital folds fuse to form a urethra extending up the phallus (penis), which is formed by growth of the genital tubercle (Figure 2-5). The scrotum is formed from the labio-scrotal swelling. Testes descend into the inguinal canal at about 6 months and enter the scrotal swelling shortly before birth. Gonadotropin stimulation seems to regulate testicular descent (14). In the female infant the genital tubercle becomes the clitoris; the urogenital groove remains open to allow opening of the urethra and vagina. Labia minora and the distal portion of the vagina are formed from the urogenital folds. The labio-scrotal swelling becomes the labia majora (Figure 2-5). Barring accidents of development, the internal and external genitalia are consistently male or female in pattern.

In animals, and to some extent in man, differentiation of the gonads into testes and ovaries is accompanied by differentiation of the hypothalamus into a male or female oriented system capable of providing appropriate signals for later development of distinct male versus female sex hormone patterns. In this sense, endocrine maleness resides in the hypothalamus and not in the testes or pituitary. Tanner points out an irony in this differentiation. Testosterone has to be transformed to estradiol in the cells of the hypothalamus in order to exert its action in imprinting *male* patterns in the brain (1). Rat brain differentiation provides an excellent example of "critical periods" of sensitivity. Testosterone must be secreted by the infant rat testicles during the first few days after birth to provide the male imprint. Thereafter, it is too late, and earlier it is ineffective. The transformation of the gonad into a testes and the development of internal–external genitalia of a male fetus seem also to require rather precise timing to effect the changes necessary to produce a fully developed male infant.

## FACTORS THAT INFLUENCE FETAL GROWTH

Growth of the fetus results from a complex interplay of placental, maternal, and fetal factors which include provision of an adequate supply of nutrients from the mother both in quantity and in quality, ability of the placenta to effect transfer of the required nutrients to the fetus, and the genetic and endocrine control of growth within the fetus.

## Genetic Factors That Influence Fetal Growth

The growth of the fetus may be influenced by the genetic endowment from the parents of the fetus, or by the occurrence of genetic or chromosomal abnormalities which affect part, or all, of the growth process.

There is little doubt that the *parental genotype* has some influence on fetal growth. There is an obvious truth to the oft-quoted statement that "Great Danes cannot be expected from the union of Scotty dogs." Animal studies are commonly invoked to demonstrate that intrauterine growth is more closely related to the size of the mother and hence, by inference, to mother's genotype. In the mating of a Shire horse with a Shetland pony, Walton and Hammond reported that the foal of the Shetland mother and the Shire father was considerably smaller at birth than the foal of the Shire mare and the Shetland sire (15). Though there was some differential growth after birth, tending toward equalization in size, maternal size was still paramount in determining fetal growth. In studies of human populations, the relationship between maternal size and intrauterine growth is more difficult to demonstrate. Baird (16) and Jones (17) found a strong correlation between maternal height and birth weight of an infant, whereas Weiss and Jackson (18) and Tiisala and Kantero (19) failed to find any such correlation. Thomson found that individual mothers tend to produce babies of similar birth weights unrelated to maternal size (20). Although maternal genotype may have an influence on fetal growth, it is generally recognized that size of an infant at birth is not strongly correlated with eventual height or weight in childhood.

Studies of *racial differences* in intrauterine growth are often complicated by differences in maternal environment as well, so that clear cut genetic racial differences are not always evident. However, the black baby tends to be smaller at birth and matures more rapidly than the white baby. Roberts reported smaller infants in India than in Europe, which he felt represented a racial difference, even taking into consideration differences in maternal size and nutrition (21).

The *fetal genome* may also influence fetal growth. The most consistent chromosomal influence on fetal growth is seen in the difference in overall growth in boys and girls. The male fetus grows faster than the female fetus after 32 weeks gestation. Although not proven, this difference may be related to testosterone produced by the male infant's gonads (17). Infants with XO gonadal dysgenesis are, on the average, smaller than their XX female counterparts, but multiple X chromosomes also seem to limit intrauterine growth. It has been suggested that extra X chromosomes decrease cellular division and result in a fetus with fewer cells (22). Trisomy-21 is regularly associated with low birth weight (17) and infants with Trisomy-13 and Trisomy-18 have even more profound intrauterine growth retardation. Extra chromosomes may inhibit general cell growth or may reduce the number of brain cells and interfere with the influence which brain development may have over growth of other fetal tissues (22).

Many dysmorphic syndromes associated with fetal growth retardation do not have identifiable chromosomal aberrations, nor known genetically determined disturbances, but because of established inheritance patterns, can be said to be the result of gene abnormality. Specific gene disorders tend to influence fetal size less than do chromosomal aberrations. However, a gene mutation leading to a deficient synthesis of a hormone (somatomedin) can result in impairment of fetal growth (Laron dwarfism). Growth retardation may occur because of lack of substrate provision (glycogen storage diseases), or by production of toxic by-products (galactosemia) which may interfere with cellular division.

## Nutritional Needs of the Fetus

Though it is clear that the growth of the fetus depends on a continuing supply of nutrients required to make tissues and provide energy, it is less clear how much the fetus suffers when the mother's nutritional intake is suboptimal. It was commonly assumed by early physiologists that the infant might be deprived from any limitation in maternal diet, but it is now recognized that the fetus is a remarkably efficient parasite and is protected against the effects of maternal deprivation unless it becomes extremely severe (20). A striking example of such protection is shown in the Dutch famine of 1944–1945 in which Stein et al. reported a birth weight reduction of only 9%, although the famine was severe enough to produce a dramatic decrease in conception rate and to prevent mothers from gaining weight during pregnancy (23). However, poor nutrition during pregnancy and low weight gain during pregnancy are correlated with fetal growth retardation (24). Beneficial effects on fetal size have been demonstrated from improving the diets of pregnant women in deprived rural communities in Guatemala. Women given food supplements during pregnancy had larger babies than women who did not receive supplements (25).

## Placental Function and its Effect on the Fetus

Since the placenta plays a pivotal role in transferring necessary nutrients from the mother to the fetus and must act both as selector and filter to assure the fetus of optimal substrate of all kinds, it seems natural to assume that anything that interferes with the placental function would profoundly affect growth and development of the fetus. However, it is difficult to ascribe poor fetal growth to "placental insufficiency"; unless obvious pathology distorts the placental structure compromising large functional areas of the placenta. A massive placental infarction might be expected to reduce placental perfusion and substrate transfer sufficiently to impair fetal growth.

Animal studies have shown that interference with blood supply to the placenta by any of a variety of experimental procedures has produced growth retardation in fetuses (26), but extensive compromise of blood supply to the placenta is not a common phenomenon in man. The difficulty, as expressed by Thompson, is that we have no reliable way to measure "placental insufficiency". The weight of the placenta is not necessarily a measure of its efficiency. Though infants born light-for-dates often have placentas that are small and light, the placental weight of light-for-dates infants is not lower on the average than that of a prematurely born baby of similar weight (20). It is possible that small placentas may be the result, rather than the cause, of fetal growth retardation, or that whatever limits fetal growth may also limit placenta size.

## Maternal Influences on Fetal Growth

In addition to the influences of maternal size and maternal nutritional state on the developing fetus, maternal disease may have a profound effect on fetal growth. Maternal hypertension tends to retard fetal growth, whereas diabetes in the mother results in a very large infant. Women whose first pregnancies end in stillbirth tend to have smaller babies in subsequent pregnancies (20). Cigarette smoking or alcohol ingestion in the mother are associated with diminution of birth weight. (See Chapter 8.)

## Hormonal Regulation of Fetal Growth

Hormones normally produced by the mother, the placenta, and the fetus can all potentially influence the growth and maturation of the fetus. Selective movement of hormones to and from the fetus across the placental barrier limits effects of maternal hormones on fetal growth. Insensitivity of fetal tissues to hormones may further limit the hormone's effect on growth of fetal tissues. With the exception of insulin, there is little evidence that "traditional" hormones secreted by fetal endocrine glands have significant effect on fetal growth. Human growth hormone appears to be of minimal importance in regulating fetal growth, but chorionic somato-mammotrophin (hCS), also called placental lactogen, a hormone structurally homologous to pituitary growth hormone, may promote fetal growth, mediated by the somatomedins (27).

### Human Growth Hormone

Maternal growth hormone does not cross the placenta in early pregnancy and appears to have relatively little influence on the growth of the fetus. Infants born to hypophysectomized mothers or to mothers having isolated growth hormone deficiency or acromegaly appear to be unaffected by mothers' human growth hormone levels (28).

Although growth hormone is formed in the fetal pituitary gland after about five weeks of gestation (29), a definitive need for growth hormone in the fetus has not yet been demonstrated. Levels of fetal growth hormone remain above maternal levels throughout fetal life. In term infants there is a brief postnatal rise and thereafter a fall to childhood levels; in premature infants a prolonged postnatal rise may occur (30). There is, however, evidence to suggest a lack of dependence of the human fetus and very young infant on growth hormone. In a 1960 review by Seckel, apituitary and acephalic fetuses were of normal or near normal size if corrected for lack of brain tissue (31). Others have also reported normal sized infants with agenesis of the pituitary (32, 33), but some authors have disagreed with Seckel's observations, claiming that birth weight of anencephalic or acephalic fetuses was significantly less than that of control infants (34, 35).

When Ducharme and Grumbach (36) administered human growth hormone in higher than usual dosages to premature infants, they found elevation of the blood sugar and serum phosphate, but effects of human growth hormone on growth were lacking. They suggested that tissues of the fetus and newborn are relatively insensitive to human growth hormone and that growth hormone has little effect on fetal growth. This insensitivity changes gradually after birth so that by later infancy growth hormone assumes an increasingly important role in growth (30, 36).

### Somatomedins

There are several lines of evidence to suggest that somatomedins, peptides with growth-stimulating properties, may be involved in growth regulation in utero: somatomedin stimulates proliferation of fetal cells in vitro; multiple fetal tissues possess somatomedin receptors and can synthesize somatomedin; and somatomedin in cord blood correlates with birth size (27).

In fetal tissues, somatomedins stimulate mitosis of human embryonic fibroblasts (37), growth of fetal rat cartilage (38), and growth of mesenchymal cells from fetal mouse limb buds (39). Receptors for somatomedin C (insulin-like growth factor, IGF 1) are found on membranes of many fetal and placental tissues (40). There is no transplacental passage of somatomedin C (Sm C), but the peptide can be synthesized in fetal limb bud mesenchyme, heart, kidney, liver, intestine, and lung tissue (27). This suggests the possibility that the primary action of somatomedins might be exerted locally at the site of their origin (27).

Compared to maternal sera, somatomedin concentration in fetal and cord sera are low, but despite this, somatomedin concentrations in cord blood correlate closely with birth size (41). Very low levels are seen in infants small-for-gestational-age (SGA) (42). In the rat, MSA (multiplication stimulating activity), equivalent to IGF II in the human, is very high, suggesting that the major fetal somatomedin might be IGF II (27), but IGF II levels have not been shown to be elevated in the human fetus (43). Fetal tissues may be unusually sensitive to low circulating levels of somatomedin, or the actions of somatomedin may not be reflected too precisely by measurements of circulating somatomedins (27). While growth hormone appears to be the primary hormonal regulator of somatomedin in postnatal life, other growth-hormone-like peptides, such as chorionic somatomammotrophin (hCS) or prolactin, appear more likely to be regulators of fetal somatomedin activity (44). Administration of ovine placental lactogen (analogous to hCS) causes an increase in Sm C in hypophysectomized rats (45). Levels of Sm C rise during pregnancy in concert with levels of hCS, suggesting a pre-eminent role for hCS in regulation of somatomedin in mother and fetus (27).

A number of other peptide growth factors appear to be essential for specific fetal tissue growth and differentiation. Those identified so far include epidermal growth factor (46), fibroblast growth factor, and nerve growth factor, which is critical for growth and development of human nerve cells (47) and may be stimulated by thyroxine (48).

### Insulin

Insulin, one of the organism's most important anabolic hormones, appears in the fetal pancreas as early as the 10th week of gestation (49), and receptors for insulin are detectable on a variety of tissues from early in gestation (50). During the last half of gestation, insulin may assume a pivotal role in fetal metabolism and growth (51). Fetal glucose is derived almost entirely from the mother, but fetal insulin is needed for formation and storage of glycogen, uptake and utilization of amino acids for protein synthesis, and for lipogenesis and storage of fat (52). Syndromes associated with high insulin levels are characterized by fetal macrosomia while infants with diabetes or pancreatic agenesis and low or absent insulin levels are characteristically small and light for gestational age (53). It was been suggested that insulin may stimulate somatomedin activity (54), but it is more likely that insulin exerts only a permissive effect on fetal growth by stimulating uptake and utilization of substrates necessary for growth.

### Thyroid Hormones

Thyroid tissue is formed in the human fetus by about six weeks. Uptake of iodine and thyroxine production are usually established by about 15 weeks (55). The placenta appears to be relatively impermeable to thyroxine, the hormone product of the thyroid gland, but not impermeable to thyroid stimulating hormone (TSH) or thyroid stimulating immunoglobulins. Except under pathologic circumstances, most of the thyroxine available to the fetus derives from the fetus's own thyroid gland which is released under stimulation of TSH from the fetus's own pituitary gland. TSH release is dependent on thyrotrophin releasing hormone (TRH), a tripeptide found in various parts of the fetal brain (24).

Serum concentrations of thyroxine ($T_4$) and free $T_4$ ($FT_4$) are high in the fetus, partly due to increase in thyroid-binding globulin (TBG) and to increased affinity of TBG for $T_4$. Triiodothyronine ($T_3$), by contrast, is usually undetectable until shortly before term, though capacity for peripheral conversion of $T_4$ to $T_3$ has been demonstrated (56). Reverse $T_3$

(RT$_3$), an inactive thyroxine metabolite, has been detected at high levels in the serum of the fetus; though its function in fetal life is not known, it has been suggested that RT$_3$ is formed to protect the fetus from high levels of T$_3$. At the time of birth, T$_3$ levels rise rapidly while RT$_3$ levels fall. At term, the concentraiton of FT$_4$ in cord blood is slightly higher than levels observed in the mother (55).

Thyroxine deficiency in the human fetus does not appear to retard linear growth or weight gain (27). The hypothyroid infant tends to be slightly heavier at birth than control infants. Both dental and osseous maturity are delayed at birth and may be recognized in utero by as early as 28 weeks gestation. Thyroxine does appear to be essential for normal development of nerve and brain cells (47). The critical role played by thyroid hormone in the development of the fetal and neonatal brain may be mediated through thyroxine stimulation of nerve growth factor (27). The most serious consequence of intrauterine hypothyroidism is the risk of mental retardation, which reaches significant proportions in as many as 40%. The severity of the intellectual handicap depends to some extent on the time after birth at which treatment with thyroid replacement medication is started (57). Since clinical features of hypothyroidism are not always obvious in early postnatal life, T$_4$ should be measured in all infants soon after birth, a procedure being followed now in many areas of the world.

### Adrenal Gland

The fetal adrenal gland is unique both morphologically and functionally. A very large inner "fetal" zone develops in the adrenal cortex comprising 80% of the total volume near term. The major secretory product of the fetal adrenal is the weak androgen, dehydroepiandrosterone sulfate (DHEAS), which serves primarily as a precursor for placental estrogen synthesis. The fetus derives cortisol from the mother, some of which is converted to cortisone by the placenta (58), but the outer, "definitive" zone of the fetal adrenal cortex also actively secrets cortisol. During the latter half of pregnancy the secretions from the adrenal are increasingly regulated by endogenous ACTH. Absence of the adrenal gland in utero produces no evident defects in fetal development or growth, possibly because of transplacental supply of adrenal glucocorticoids and androgens. Soon after birth there is rapid involution of the "fetal" zone of the adrenal cortex (59).

### The Kidney in Fetal Growth

The *fetal kidney* affects growth of the fetus through its regulation of fetal electrolyte and water metabolism. Homeostasis between fetal fluid compartments and the amniotic fluid is achieved by the fetal kidney. Infants with bilateral renal agenesis (Potter's syndrome) manifest general growth retardation and pulmonary hypoplasia. One reason for this restraint on growth with agenesis of the kidneys may be the role which the fetal kidney plays in formation of somatomedin. It is thought, at least in animals, that the kidney represents one of the major sources of somatomedin. Bilateral nephrectomy in a fetal animals is followed by reduction in fetal somatomedin levels and fetal growth failure (60). Oligohydramnios, resulting from renal agenesis, leads to restraints on fetal growth also, with shortening and contracture of limbs and typical facies.

## HOW FETAL GROWTH IS MEASURED

Measurements of fetal growth must be regarded only as approximations, no matter how accurate the physical measurements themselves, because of potential error in calculation of gestational age. Variations in length of menstrual cycle, time of ovulation within the cycle, and time of conception with relation to ovulation can produce errors of at least 5 days in gestational age estimates based on menstrual history. Errors may also occur due to inaccuracy of mother's memory in recalling the date of her last normal menstrual period or to the common event of vaginal bleeding during early pregnancy.

Initially, fetal growth was approximated simply by measurements of infants at birth (61, 62). In 1966 Lubchenko et al. published standards for birth weight, length and head circumference by gestational age and popularized the concept of use of special standards for postnatal growth of prematurely born infants, immatures, or offspring of multiple pregnancies (62). From the use of such information arose the concepts of appropriate (AGA), small (SGA) or large-for-gestational age (LGA) based on curves for intrauterine weight or length by week of gestation (Figure 2-6).

In 1969 Usher and MacLean published standards obtained from measurements of newborn Caucasian infants from the Montreal region ranging from 24 to 44 weeks gestation. They included mean values for measurements of weight, length, foot length, head, chest, abdomen, and thigh circumference, and double skin thickness (63) (Table 2-2). The authors emphasized the need to standardize techniques for measurement of live born fetuses and provided specific instructions for measurements.

The measurements of Lubchenko et al. and Usher et al. are generally applicable to live fetuses in the later months of gestation, but acceptable measurements of fetal growth in earlier phases of gestation must be obtained from aborted fetuses. Measurements of crown–rump length in aborted fetuses can be made with a millimeter rule without undue manipulation of the fetus. In Figure 2-7, data collected by Shepherd (7) are superimposed upon the mean of values earlier reported by Streeter (5) for fetuses ages 20–120 days. Though there is some variation in gestational ages, the data generally complement each other. Foot length and fetal weight can still be used with considerable accuracy in the very

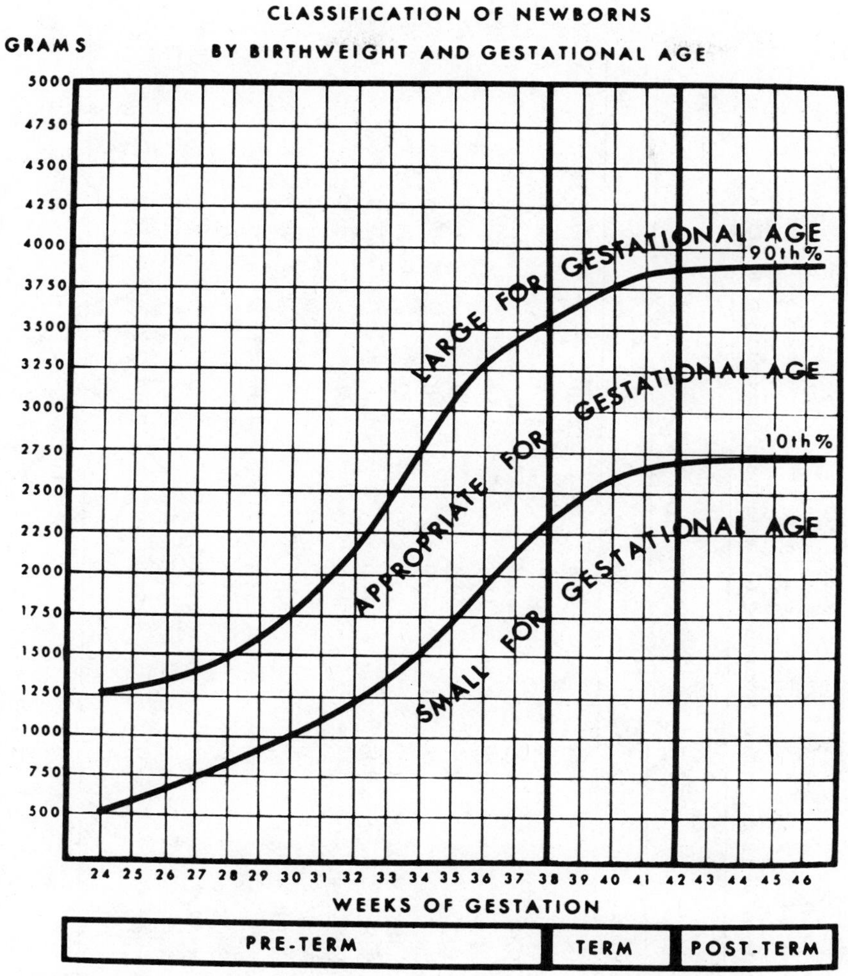

**CLASSIFICATION OF NEWBORNS BY BIRTHWEIGHT AND GESTATIONAL AGE**

**Figure 2-6.** Percentiles of intrauterine weight showing measurements considered to be appropriate (AGA), small (SGA), or large (LGA) for gestational age. (Reproduced by permission from Lubchenco LO, Hansman C, Boyd E: Intrauterine growth in weight, length, and head circumference as estimated from live births at gestational ages from 26 to 42 weeks. *Pediatrics* **37**:403, 1966, copyright American Academy of Pediatrics 1966.)

**Table 2-2. Measurements in Newborn Infants According to Gestational Age (Menstrual Age)**

| Gestation (weeks) | No. infants | Weight (g) | | Length (cm) | | Foot Length (mm) | |
|---|---|---|---|---|---|---|---|
| | | Mean | SD | Mean | SD | Mean | SD |
| 24–26 | 13 | 853 | 188 | 34.6 | 2.46 | 50.1 | 3.33 |
| 27–28 | 20 | 1115 | 151 | 37.3 | 1.84 | 55.4 | 3.08 |
| 29–30 | 12 | 1261 | 113 | 38.8 | 1.21 | 57.7 | 2.12 |
| 31–32 | 11 | 1632 | 218 | 41.8 | 1.48 | 62.6 | 3.32 |
| 33 | 11 | 1943 | 227 | 44.3 | 1.59 | 67.4 | 4.78 |
| 34 | 18 | 2095 | 238 | 45.0 | 1.86 | 69.6 | 3.76 |
| 35 | 13 | 2382 | 429 | 46.2 | 1.32 | 71.4 | 3.76 |
| 36 | 20 | 2482 | 305 | 46.6 | 1.56 | 72.8 | 4.12 |
| 37 | 20 | 2961 | 516 | 49.2 | 2.21 | 78.0 | 3.91 |
| 38 | 20 | 3231 | 391 | 50.2 | 2.13 | 78.2 | 4.11 |
| 39 | 25 | 3310 | 432 | 50.2 | 2.12 | 77.3 | 3.56 |
| 40 | 47 | 3477 | 461 | 51.4 | 1.97 | 78.4 | 3.45 |
| 41 | 27 | 3548 | 513 | 51.8 | 1.77 | 79.8 | 3.49 |
| 42 | 20 | 3348 | 470 | 51.0 | 2.89 | 78.9 | 4.60 |
| 43 | 11 | 3420 | 455 | 51.3 | 2.06 | 80.0 | 2.80 |
| 44+ | 12 | 3396 | 510 | 51.0 | 1.68 | 78.0 | 3.83 |

| Gestation (weeks) | Head circumference (cm) | | Chest circumference (cm) | | Abdominal circumference (cm) | | Double skin thickness (mm) | |
|---|---|---|---|---|---|---|---|---|
| | Mean | SD | Mean | SD | Mean | SD | Mean | SD |
| 24–26 | 23.2 | 1.86 | 19.8 | 1.79 | 16.2 | 1.58 | 2.34 | 0.43 |
| 27–28 | 25.8 | 1.23 | 21.5 | 1.24 | 18.0 | 1.16 | 2.72 | 0.38 |
| 29–30 | 26.7 | 0.81 | 22.3 | 0.90 | 19.0 | 0.97 | 2.67 | 0.36 |
| 31–32 | 29.2 | 1.55 | 24.6 | 1.61 | 20.8 | 1.63 | 3.35 | 0.85 |
| 33 | 31.3 | 1.40 | 26.8 | 1.57 | 22.5 | 1.30 | 3.75 | 0.80 |
| 34 | 30.8 | 1.36 | 27.7 | 1.79 | 23.0 | 1.57 | 3.89 | 0.68 |
| 35 | 32.3 | 1.37 | 29.2 | 1.73 | 24.3 | 1.85 | 4.51 | 1.20 |
| 36 | 32.8 | 1.11 | 29.2 | 1.24 | 24.4 | 1.22 | 3.86 | 0.72 |
| 37 | 33.6 | 1.29 | 30.9 | 2.07 | 26.0 | 2.16 | 4.58 | 0.87 |
| 38 | 34.7 | 1.37 | 32.2 | 1.66 | 27.6 | 1.79 | 4.85 | 0.81 |
| 39 | 34.7 | 0.98 | 32.5 | 1.66 | 28.1 | 1.93 | 5.19 | 0.98 |
| 40 | 34.7 | 1.14 | 33.4 | 1.47 | 28.8 | 1.91 | 5.41 | 1.12 |
| 41 | 35.2 | 0.89 | 33.6 | 1.58 | 29.1 | 2.08 | 5.24 | 1.14 |
| 42 | 35.0 | 1.11 | 32.8 | 1.77 | 27.8 | 1.85 | 4.70 | 0.94 |
| 43 | 35.0 | 0.91 | 32.8 | 1.64 | 28.2 | 1.80 | 4.84 | 0.85 |
| 44 + | 34.6 | 0.89 | 33.0 | 1.94 | 28.3 | 2.26 | 4.73 | 1.20 |

Reproduced with permission from Usher R, McLean F: Intrauterine growth of live-born Caucasian infants at sea level: Standards obtained from measurement in 7 dimensions of infants born between 25 and 44 weeks of gestation. J Pediatr **74**:901, 1969.

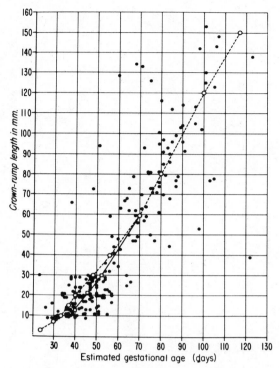

**Figure 2-7.** Estimated gestational age plotted against crown–rump length of specimens obtained from therapeutic abortion. The dotted line is from mean crown–rump length, reported by Streeter in 1951. The solid line is the best fit from the plotted measurements by Shepherd. (Reproduced by permission from Shepherd TH: Growth and development of the human embryo and fetus in Gardner L (ed), *Endocrine and Genetic Diseases of Childhood and Adolescence*. Philadelphia, WB Saunders Co, 1975.)

young fetus and head width and circumference can be calculated from ultrasound measurements in utero.

Brenner et al. have recently reconstructed fetal growth curves for weight at sea level in the United States (64). Their data are derived from measurements of 430 fetuses aborted with prostaglandins at 8–20 weeks gestation, defined as weeks since last menstrual period, and from 30,772 live born infants, 21–44 weeks gestation. A figure demonstrating fetal weight percentiles from 28 to 44 weeks (menstrual age) was constructed from these data (Figure 2-8) with inserts showing the available growth curve data from 8 to 28 weeks and corrections in the mean fetal weight during the fetal period of 36–42 weeks affected by parity, race, or sex of the infant.

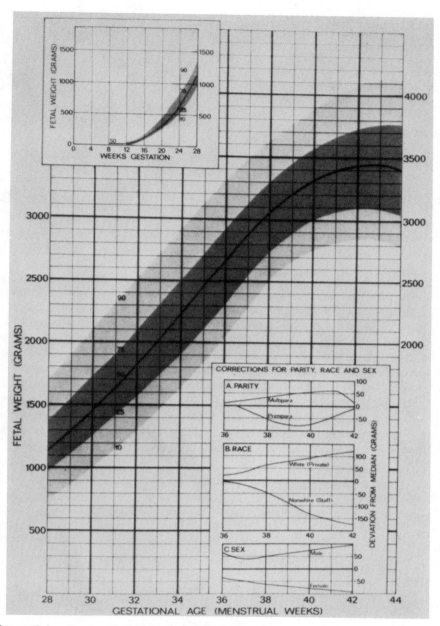

**Figure 2-8.** Fetal weight in grams plotted against gestational (menstrual) age showing smooth curve centiles for fetal weight from 28 to 44 weeks. The inset at the top of the figure shows smooth curve percentiles from available growth data for earlier fetal growth from 12 to 28 weeks gestation (menstrual) age. In the lower inset are shown corrections for birth weight for parity, race, and sex for menstrual ages of 36–42 weeks. (Reproduced by permission from Brenner WE, Edleman DA, Hendricks CH: A standard of fetal growth for the United States of American. *Am J Obstet Gynecol* **126**:555, 1976.)

Miller and Merritt call attention to the fact that most reports of fetal measurement include many infants whose growth has been compromised by factors known to affect fetal growth. They present data on live born, white infants excluding all infants with known fetal or maternal growth-retarding conditions as well as gestational diabetes or diabetes mellitus (24). In their data, gestational age was calculated in completed weeks from the first day of the mother's last menstrual period. Gestational age was also estimated by obstetrical examinations in the first trimester and was further refined by measurements of biparietal head diameter by ultrasound between 20 and 28 weeks of pregnancy. After birth, use was made of the criteria prepared by Dubowitz et al. to define gestational age neurologically (65). The data of Miller and Merritt on 1200 infants are listed in Tables A-1 and A-2 in the Appendix.

## BIRTH—THE END OF INTRAUTERINE EXISTENCE

By the end of nine months the baby is ready to live outside the uterus. He has grown from one to over 200 billion cells and has developed from a unicellular organism to a masterpiece of efficiency. Birth brings to a close the growth within the uterus with its simple extraction of all necessities for growth from the placenta. The infant must now change from a parasitic existence, in which all his needs were met by the placenta of his mother, to self-sufficient cardiorespiratory and digestive excretory systems capable of immediate oxygen—carbon dioxide exchange and of receiving and handling appropriate nutrients for further growth. The sojourn within the uterus affects directly the subsequent growth and development of the infant, which will be taken up in succeeding chapters.

## REFERENCES

1. Tanner JM: *Fetus into Man: Physical Growth from Conception to Maturity.* Cambridge, Harvard University Press, 1978, pp 37–51, 52–59, 103–116.

2. Malina RM: *Growth and Development, the First Twenty Years in Man.* Minneapolis, Burgess Publishing Co., 1976, p 6.

3. Crowley LV: Survey of Embryonic and Fetal Development, in *An Introduction to Clinical Embryology.* Chicago, Year Book Medical Publications, 1974, pp 63–72.

4. Lowrey GH: The Placenta and Fetal Development, in *Growth and Development of Children,* ed 7. Chicago, Year Book Medical Publishers Inc., 1978, pp 47–68.

5. Streeter GL, Heuser CH, Corner GW: Developmental horizons in human embryos, description of age groups XIX–XXIII, *Contrib Embryology.* pp 197, 199, 211, 230, Reprint Volume 2, 1951.

6. How a Baby Develops, *Life Cycle Library for Young People.* Chicago, Parent and Child Institute, 1969, pp 141–157.

7. Shepard TH: Growth and development of the human embryo and fetus, in Gardner L (ed), *Endocrine and Genetic Diseases of Childhood,* ed 2. Philadelphia, WB Saunders Co., 1975.

8. Cheek DB: in *Fetal and Postnatal Cellular Growth*. New York, John Wiley & Sons, 1975.

9. Jost A, Vigier B, Prepin J, et al: Studies on sex differentiation in mammals. *Recent Prog Horm Res* **29**:1, 1973.

10. Pelliniemi LJ, Dym M: The fetal gonad and sexual differentiation, in Tulschinsky D, Ryan KJ (eds), *Maternal–Fetal Endocrinology*. Philadelphia, WB Saunders Co., 1980, pp 252–280.

11. Welschone WJ, Russell LV: The Y-chromosome as the bearer of male determining factors in the mouse. *Proc Natl Acad Sci USA* **45**:560, 1959.

12. Wachtel SS, Ohno S, Koo GC, et al: Possible role for H-Y antigen in the primary determination of sex. *Nature* **257**:235, 1975.

13. Boczkowski K: Sex determination and gonadal differentiation in man: A unifying concept of normal and abnormal sex development. *Clin Genet* **2**:379, 1971.

14. Hadziselimovic F, Girard J: Pathogenesis of cryptorchidism. *Horm Res* **8**:76, 1977.

15. Walton A, Hammond J: The maternal effects on growth and conformation in shire horse-shetland pony crosses. *Proc R Soc* [Biol] **125**:311, 1938. Cited by Jones OW: Genetic factors in the determination of fetal size. *J Reprod Med* **21**:305, 1978.

16. Baird D: in Reed DM, Stanley FJ (eds), *The Epidemiology of Prematurity*. Baltimore, Erbin and Schwarzenburg, 1977.

17. Jones OW: Genetic factors in the determination of fetal size. *J Reprod Med* **21**:305, 1978.

18. Weiss W, Jackson EC: Maternal factors affecting birth weight, in *Perinatal Factors Affecting Human Development*. Washington, DC, Pan American Health Organization, 1969, p 54.

19. Tiisala R, Kantero RL: Some parent–child correlations for height, weight and skeltal age up to ten years. *Acta Paediatr Scand* [Suppl] **220**:42, 1971.

20. Thomson AM: Clinical and environmental determinants of fetal growth. *Postgrad Med J* **54**(Suppl 2):43, 1978.

21. Roberts DF: Environment and the fetus, in Roberts DF, Thompson AM (eds), *The Biology of Human Fetal Growth*. London, Taylor and Francis Ltd., 1976, pp 267–283.

22. Naeye RL: Prenatal organ and cellular growth with various chromosomal disorders. *Biol Neonate* **11**:248, 1967.

23. Stein Z, Susser M, Saenger G, et al: in *Famine and Human Development: The Dutch Hunger Winter of 1944/45*. New York, Oxford University Press, 1975.

24. Miller HC, Merritt TA: *Fetal Growth in Humans*. Chicago, Year Book Medical Publishers, 1979, pp 9–24, 31–56.

25. Lechtig A, Yarbrough C, Delgado H, et al: Influence of maternal nutrition on birth weight. *Am J Clin Nutr* **28**:1223, 1975.

26. Dawes GS: The physiological determinants of fetal growth. *J Reprod Fertil* **47**:183, 1976.

27. Underwood LE, D'Ercole AJ: Insulin and insulin-like growth factors/somatomedins in fetal and neo-natal development. *Clin Endocrinol Metab* **13**:69, 1984.

28. Little B, Smith OW, Jesseman AG, et al: Hypophysectomy during pregnancy with cancer of the breast: Case report with hormone studies. *J Clin Endocrinol Metab* **18**:425, 1958.

29. Siler-Khodr TM, Morgenstern LL, Greenwood FC: Hormone synthesis and release from human fetal adenohypophyses in vitro. *J Clin Endocrinol Metab* **39**:891, 1974.

30. Gluckman PD, Grumbach MM, Kaplan SL: The human fetal hypothalamus and pituitary gland, in Tulchinsky D, Ryan KJ (eds), *Maternal–Fetal Endocrinology*. Philadelphia, WB Saunders Co., 1980, pp 162–232.

31. Seckel HPG: Concepts relating the pituitary growth hormone to somatic growth of the normal child. *Am J Dis Child* **99**:349, 1960.

32. Reid JD: Congenital absence of the pituitary gland. *J Pediatr* **56**:658, 1960.

33. Lovinger RD, Kaplan SL, Grumbach MM: Congenital hypopituitarism associated with neonatal hypoglycemia and microphallus: Four cases secondary to hypothalamic hormone deficiencies. *J Pediatr* **87:**11–71, 1975.

34. Honnebier WJ, Swaab DF: The influence of anencephaly upon intrauterine growth of fetus and placenta, and upon gestation length. *J Obstet Gynaecol* Br Commonw **80:**577, 1973.

35. Naeye RL, Blanc WA: Organ and body growth in anencephaly: a quantitative morphological study. *Arch Path* **91:**140, 1971.

36. Ducharme JR, Grumbach MM: Studies on the effects of human growth hormone in premature infants. *J Clin Invest* **40:**243, 1961.

37. Wiedman ER, Bala RM: Direct mitogenic effects of human somatomedin on human embryonic lung fibroblasts. *Biochem Biophys Res Commun* **92:**577, 1980.

38. Hill DJ, Holder AT, Seid J, et al: Increased thymidine incorporation into fetal rat cartilage in vitro in the presence of human somatomedin, epidermal growth factor and other growth factors. *J Endocr* **96:**489, 1983.

39. Kaplowitz PB, D'Ercole AJ, Underwood LE: Stimulation of embryonic mouse limb bud mesenchymal cell growth by peptide growth factors. *J Cell Physiol* **112:**353, 1982.

40. D'Ercole AJ, Underwood LE: Ontogeny of somatomedin during development in the mouse: serum concentrations, molecular forms, binding proteins and tissue receptors. *Devl Biol* **79:**33, 1980.

41. D'Ercole AJ, Underwood LE: Growth factors in fetal growth and development, in Novy MJ, Resko JA (eds), *Fetal Endocrinology: ORPC Symposia on Reproductive Biology*. New York, Academic Press, 1981, pp 155–182.

42. Foley TP, DePhilip R, Perricelli A, Miller A: Low somatomedin activity in cord serum from infants with intrauterine growth retardation. *J Pediat* **96:**605, 1980.

43. Bennett A, Wilson DM, Liu F, et al: Levels of insulin-like growth factors I and II in infants with idiopathic macrosomia and infants of diabetic mothers. *Pediat Res* **17:**286A, 1983.

44. Clemmons DR, Underwood LE, Van Wyk JJ: Hormonal control of immunoreactive somatomedin production by cultured human fibroblasts. *J Clin Invest* **67:**10, 1981.

45. Hurley TW, D'Ercole AJ, Handwerger S, et al: Ovine placental lactogen induces somatomedin: A possible role in fetal growth. *Endocrinology* **101:**1635, 1977.

46. Gospodarowicz D, Moran JS, Owashi ND: Effect of fibroblast growth factor and epidermal growth factor on rate of growth of amniotic fluid-derived cells. *J Clin Endocrinol Metab* **44:**651, 1977.

47. Crain SM, Peterson ER, Leibman M, Schulman H: Dependence on nerve growth factor of early human fetal dorsal root ganglion neurons in organotypic cultures. *Expl Neurol* **67:**205, 1980.

48. Walker P, Weil ML, Weichsel ME Jr, Fisher DA: Effect of thyroxine on nerve growth factor concentration in neonatal mouse brain. *Life Sci* **28:**1777, 1981.

49. Adams PA, Teramo K, Raiha N, et al: Human fetal insulin metabolism early in gestation: Response to acute elevation of the fetal glucose concentration and placentral transfer of human insulin $^{131}$I. *Diabetes* **18:**409, 1969.

50. Posner BI: Insulin receptors in human and animal placental tissue. *Diabetes* **23:**209, 1974.

51. Sperling MA: Carbohydrate metabolism: Glucagon, insulin and somatostatin, in Tulchinsky D, Ryan KJ (eds), *Maternal–Fetal Endocrinology*. Philadelphia, WB Saunders Co., 1980, pp 333–354.

52. Persson B: Insulin as a growth factor in the fetus, in Ritzen M, Aperia A, Hall K, et al, *The Biology of Normal Human Growth*. New York, Raven Press, 1981, pp 213–221.

53. Hill DE: Effect of insulin on fetal growth. *Seminars in Perinatology* **2:**319, 1978.

54. Spencer GSG, Hill DJ, Garssen GJ, et al: Somatomedin activity and growth hormone levels in body fluids of the fetal pig: Effects of chronic hyperinsulinemia. *J Endocr* **96**:107, 1983.

55. Fisher DA: Thyroid function in the fetus, in Fisher DA, Burrow GN (eds), *Perinatal Thyroid Physiology and Disease*. New York, Raven Press, 1975, p 21.

56. Chopra IJ, Crandell BF: Thyroid hormones and thyrotropin in amniotic fluid. *N Engl J Med* **293**:740, 1975.

57. MacFaul R, Grant DB: Early detection of congenital hypothyroidism. *Arc Dis Child* **52**:87, 1977.

58. Beitins IZ, Bayard F, Ances IG, et al: The metabolic clearance rate, blood production, interconversion and transplacental passage of cortisol and cortisone in pregnancy near term. *Pediatr Res* **7**:509, 1973.

59. Davies IJ: The fetal adrenal, in Tulchinsky D, Ryan KJ (eds), *Maternal–Fetal Endocrinology*. Philadelphia, WB Saunders Co., 1980, pp 242–251.

60. Thorburn GD: The role of the thyroid gland and kidneys in fetal growth, in Elliot K, Knight J (eds), *Size at Birth*, CIBA Foundation Symposium #27. Amsterdam, Elsevier, 1974, pp 185–200.

61. Gruenwald P: Growth of the human fetus: Normal growth and its variation. *Am J Obstet Gynecol* **94**:1112, 1966.

62. Lubchenco LO, Hansman C, Boyd E: Intrauterine growth in length weight and head circumference as estimated from live births at gestational ages from 26 to 42 weeks. *Pediatrics* **37**:403, 1966.

63. Usher R, McLean F: Intrauterine growth of live-born caucasian infants at sea level: Standards obtained from measurements in 7 dimensions of infants born between 25 and 44 weeks of gestation. *Pediatrics* **74**:901, 1969.

64. Brenner WE, Edleman DA, Hendricks CH: A standard of fetal growth for the United States of America. *Am J Obstet Gynecol* **126**:555, 1976.

65. Dubowitz LMS, Dubowitz V, Goldberg C: Clinical assessment of gestational age in the newborn infant. *J Pediatr* **77**:1, 1970.

# 3
# Growth in Infancy

In this chapter we will describe normal growth patterns of infancy extending from birth to 2 years of age. This is a period of rapid but decelerating growth.

## GROWTH PATTERNS IN INFANCY

If we plot growth in infancy on charts displaying velocity of growth, we see a rapidly decelerating curve of both height and weight leveling off at about 2–3 years of age (Figure 3-1). Although the infant's length and weight increase dramatically during this 2-year period, the rate of height increase experienced in centimeters per year and the rate of weight change in kilograms per year are decreasing noticeably from the very high velocity of growth achieved in utero. The velocity of growth has fallen to about 3 cm per 4 weeks by birth, still a very rapid velocity approaching 35–40 cm/yr (1). Weight gain likewise decelerates in the final weeks in utero, at least partly because of limit in uterine size (uterine restraint), to reach a level of 8–9 kg per year at the time of birth (1).

The average white American newborn weighs 3499 g and measures 50 cm, boys being slightly heavier than girls. Approximately 95% of infants weigh between 2500 and 4600 g and measure between 45–55 cm. Head circumference averages 34–35 cm at birth (2). Velocity of growth continues to decelerate after birth so that by 2–3 years of age the growth velocity (length) will be 5–10 cm/yr and weight acquisition will have dropped to 2–3 kg/yr. Except for puberty, there will never again be a period of such rapid growth (1).

### Growth during the First Year

Loss of excess fluid during the first few days accounts for a weight loss of about 5–10% of birth weight, but birth weight has usually been recovered by about 10 days of life. Thereafter, the infant gains about 20 g/day for the first 5 months, at which point the infant has doubled his birth weight.

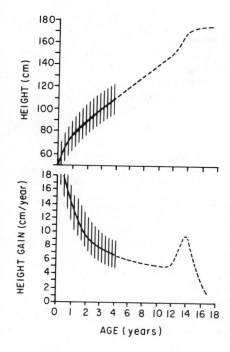

**Figure 3-1.** Shape of growth curves for height emphasizing rapid increase in height attainment (*upper figure*) during the first 2–3 years and rapid deceleration of height gain or velocity (*lower figure*). After infancy rate of growth slows until puberty. Weight change curves in infancy are similar. (Adapted with permission from Rimoin DL, Horton WA: Short stature, Part I. *J Pediatr* **92:**523, 1978.)

For the remainder of the first year, the infant gains about 15 g/day to triple his birth weight by one year. Length increases by 25–30 cm during the first year or about a 50% increase in height. Head circumference increases rapidly during the first year because of continuing rapid brain growth. The head circumference increases from 34 to 44 cm by 6 months but only 3–4 cm is added during the final 6 months of the first year (2).

## Growth during the Second Year

Further deceleration in the rate of growth occurs in the second year. There is a weight gain of only 2.5 kg and an increase in length of about 12 cm. During the second year, the child begins to thin out and become more lean and muscular. Fat has been accumulating at a rapid rate, reaching a peak at about 9 months of age, but shortly before the end of the first year of life, there is a decrease in appetite, coincident with the decelerating growth in length and weight. At that time, there is a decrease in fat acquisition with actually some loss of subcutaneous fat. As the child assumes an upright position, mild lordosis and pot belly become apparent. Brain growth continues to decelerate during the second year. By the time the infant is one year of age, the brain has achieved nearly two-thirds of its final size, and by two years, four-fifths of its final size. There is only a 2 cm increase in head circumference during the entire second year (2).

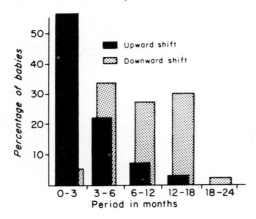

**Figure 3-2.** Percentage of ninety infants whose longitudinal growth curve crossed one or more percentile lines upward or downward on percentile growth charts between birth and 2 years of age. (Reproduced by permission Smith DW, Truog W, Rogers JE, et al: Shifting linear growth during infancy: Illustration of genetic factors in growth from fetal life through infancy. *J Pediatr* **89**:225, 1976.)

## Shifting Patterns of Growth in Infancy

Birth weight and birth length do not always provide reliable clues about subsequent growth pattern of the child nor the ultimate adult height, weight, or body build. Tanner reports a correlation coefficient of only 0.25 between birth length and ultimate height. However, by 2 years of age, the correlation between length and adult height has risen to nearly 0.80 (3). Between these two points in time, many infants shift growth channels, seeking a channel of growth consistent with their genetic background, best described by the mean stature of parents (4).

That growth patterns of infants might be quite variable, was highlighted several decades ago by Reynolds and Sonntag who observed that growth patterns during the first year of life commonly showed disparities of more than one standard deviation between height, weight, and bone age (5). They describe infants whose height and weight curves coincide with each other (proportional body type); others tall for weight or short for weight; some who shift from one body type to another; and some whose growth rate is irregularly variable or cyclic (5). Such shifts in growth pattern in otherwise normal infants was reaffirmed by Smith et al., who found that two-thirds of normal full-term infants followed during the first two years of life were observed to shift growth rates by one or more percentile lines (4) (Figure 3-2). Infants shifting upward had usually begun their shift within the first three months of life and shifting was generally complete by 12 to 18 months. "Lag-down" growth, or shifting to lower percentiles, began a little later, and some were not completed until the 18th to 24th month (4) (Figure 3-2). Miller and Merritt found less shifting across percentile lines in the first few months of postnatal life if adjustment was made for gestational age. They found that short full-term infants with normal postnatal growth velocity still remained short at 1 to 2 years of age (6). The studies of Smith et al. reaffirm what many have observed anecdotally: that infancy is a period of variable linear growth and that a child cannot be expected to indicate his or her future channel of growth until about 2 years of age.

## GROWTH OF ORGAN SYSTEMS IN INFANCY

The organ systems that change most dramatically at the time of birth or during early infancy include heart, lungs, adrenal glands, brain, the nervous system, and the skeleton. The lymphoid and gonadal tissues undergo major development later in childhood and adolescence.

### The Cardiovascular System

A number of fairly dramatic changes must occur in the cardiovascular and respiratory systems to insure survival of the infant immediately after birth. During intrauterine life, the blood of the fetus is oxygenated by the placenta and carried to the heart by the umbilical vein and the ductus venosus, which empties into the inferior vena cava not far from the right atrium. The oxygenated blood preferentially passes through the open foramen ovale into the left heart, and hence, into the ascending aorta to the brain and upper body, bypassing the fetal lungs (Figure 3-3). The blood returning to the right atrium, via the superior vena cava, preferentially passes through the right ventricle and into the descending aorta, via the ductus arteriosus, to the remainder of the body, again bypassing the nonfunctional fetal lungs. From the iliac arteries arise the umbilical arteries, which return the deoxygenated blood to the placenta (Figure 3-3).

At birth, the blood flow to and from the placenta is abruptly interrupted and the umbilical vein, the ductus venosus, and the umbilical arteries are obliterated by muscular contraction of their walls and by clotting of blood within them. This creates an immediate need for oxygenation of blood through the lungs, which will only occur efficiently if the shunts permitting the blood to bypass the pulmonary circulation are closed. Both the foramen ovale and the ductus arteriosus are usually closed shortly after birth.

Initially, there is a functional closure of the foramen ovale because of an increase in left atrial pressure, which occurs with the increased flow of blood through the newly expanded lungs. Later, there is fusion of the valvular flaps. Failure of closure and high right atrial pressure may result in a persistent right to left shunt and inadequate oxygenation of the blood, which persistently bypasses the lungs, now the only source of oxygenation. The ductus arteriosus is first closed by muscular contraction of its walls. Eventually the lumen of the ductus is obliterated and the vessel converted into a fibrous cord, the ligamentum arteriosum. The ductus may remain patent during the first days, or even weeks, of postnatal life and increasing pressure in the aorta allows a left to right shunt to occur (7). Constriction and obliteration may be prevented by prostaglandin E, which has been implicated as a possible cause of persistent ductus arteriosus (PDA) in

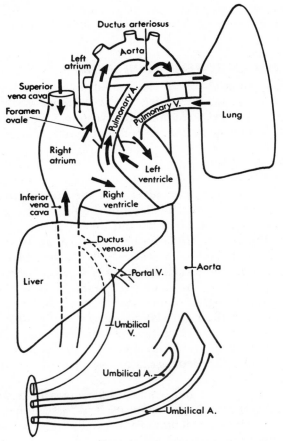

**Figure 3-3.** Fetal circulation showing placental vessels and blood flow through the fetal heart with shunting of blood through the foramen ovale and ductus arteriosus. (Reproduced by permission from Sinclair D: *Human Growth after Birth,* ed 3. London, Oxford University Press, 1978.)

prematurity or respiratory distress syndrome. PDA results in shunting of blood from the aorta to the pulmonary artery and a left to right shunt which can produce heart failure and may require surgical closure (8, 9).

The size of the heart in relation to the thorax is larger at birth than later in childhood or in adulthood. In infancy, the heart occupies about 40% of the lung field seen on X-ray compared to about 30% in the adult (9). The thickness of the right and left ventricular walls is about equal in infancy. During the first year of life, the size of the heart roughly doubles, but no further changes in complexity of function occur once the postfetal circulation is established (9). The heart rate at birth averages about 140 beats per minute. There is a gradual decline in rate throughout childhood.

By age 2, the average heart rate is 110 beats per minute, and by age 10 has declined to 90 beats per minute. Within the first week of life, a blood pressure of 80–85/45–50 might be expected (flush method). By 2 years, blood pressure will have risen to about 100/65 and by 10 years to 110/60 (8). Sinus arrhymthia is a common physiologic occurrence in infancy and childhood. Heart sounds are higher pitched, of shorter duration, and greater in intensity than later in life.

Innocent murmurs are common throughout infancy and childhood (8). The vibratory murmur is a low pitched, early systolic murmur, heard best at the lower left sternal border in the reclining position. A pulmonic ejection murmur, due to turbulence of blood in the outflow tract of the right ventricle, is loudest in the upper left intercostal spaces. A "venus hum" is continuous, generally heard best at the base of the heart, and is usually accentuated in the upright position (8). Vibratory and pulmonic ejection murmurs may be easily confused with murmurs of cardiac disease. It is, of course, important not to overlook organic heart disease, but it is equally important not to unnecessarily alarm parents over innocent murmurs. The character and intensity of the murmur may be sufficiently characteristic in many cases, especially to an experienced examiner. Innocent murmurs seldom exceed grade 2 in intensity. When heart disease is suspected, a careful and thorough evaluation is essential (8).

## The Respiratory System

The respiratory system must change from an essentially nonfunctioning to a fully functioning organ system almost instantaneously. The airways have developed extensively in the intrauterine period, but with little growth of the alveoli. Respiratory movements during fetal life lead to an accumulation of amniotic fluid within the lungs, which is rapidly replaced by air at birth (10). The lungs grow rapidly after birth, increasing about threefold in weight and sixfold in volume during the first year. Alveoli multiply rapidly after birth, most being formed within the first three months; but some alveolar budding continues through much of childhood. Later growth is mainly an enlargement of existing alveoli (9).

At birth, expansion of the alveoli for respiration results in opening of the pulmonary capillary bed and acceptance of a suddenly expanded pulmonary blood flow. Initially, the pressure within the pulmonary artery is high, but falls within the first week to a level well below that of the systemic circulation, where it remains. Surfactant, which appears in the fetal lung by 24 weeks gestation, lines the alveolar walls and helps maintain stability by decreasing surface tension (11). In prematurely born infants, diminished pulmonary vascular bed or persistent elevation of pulmonary pressure may block adequate oxygenation of the blood and lead to cyanosis. This may be aggreaved in the premature infant by inadequate surfactant formation (12), lack of adequate pulmonary elastic tissue (persistent atelectasis), feeble respiratory musculature, a soft bony thorax, and by reduced sensitivity of the respiratory centers in the brain to diminished oxygenation.

Apnea or periodic breathing are characteristically present in early infancy, though prolonged apneic spells are seldom a problem in the normal newborn. Normal respiratory function in the infant presupposes normal development of the lungs and thorax, normal muscles of respiration, and normal function of the central nervous system regulating apparatus. Low oxygen tension seems to be the stimulus responsible for initiating respiration, but many other factors can affect the rhythmic stimulation of respiration. Hyperthermia, hyperinflation of the lungs, vigorous nipple feeding, and catheter suction of the pharynx may produce reflex hypoventilation via the CNS respiratory center. Extended hypoxia, hypoglycemia, CNS depressants, and sepsis may interfere with afferent impulses, which may also lead to hypoventilation or apneic spells. In the prematurely born infant, immaturity of the central nervous system's regulation of respiration may be the basic cause of apnea. With increasing maturity, more regular respiration occurs. It should, however, be noted that respiration is diaphragmatic throughout infancy and early childhood (10).

## Development of the Nervous System in Infancy

Though growth of the brain has been phenomenal during the intrauterine period, rapid growth and critical functional maturation continue throughout infancy. At birth, the brain has reached about 25% of its adult size for weight, and by 2 years 75%, so that within the first 2 years after birth, the brain completes half of its growth. It has been suggested that all nerve cells with which the organism is to function during a lifetime are formed within the first 6 to 7 months of intrauterine life and that all subsequent growth merely transforms them into functional units by adding axones, the long process of the nerve which distributes the neural impulse to distant structures, and dendrites, the multibranched short appendages to the nerve cell which allow each neurone to make connection with as many as 3000 other nerve cells (1). Neuroglial cells, which act as supporting tissue for the nerve cells proper and form about half the cellular volume of the brain, are formed for support as required. New neuroglial cells are formed up to about two years postnatally (1).

The most primitive portions of the brain, that is, the medulla, pons, and midbrain, complete their development first and are most advanced in development and function at birth. The cerebrum follows with its rapid growth in late fetal life and the first one to two years of postnatal life. The cerebellum exhibits the latest peak growth velocity, generally having its main spurt of growth after birth. This differential timing of development and nerve cell function may determine, to some extent, the effect on brain growth and brain function of insult or injury to the developing organism. Both animal and human studies suggest that there may be critical periods of brain growth when injury may result in irreversible damage. One such period may well be during early fetal life when neurones are being formed. Irradiation or infectous agents (such as rubella) in the first trimester interrupt brain growth, resulting in brain deficiency, but such agents have little effect on the brain during the third trimester. On the other hand, malnutrition during the third trimester, or early infancy, seems capable of reducing the number of brain cells formed, leading indirectly to reduced intelligence, but not affecting the primitive brain function. The cerebellum, with its late growth spurt after birth, would predictably be particularly vulnerable to injury during infancy (13).

Functional development of the nervous system seems to be related to maturation of the structural elements of the CNS. There appears to be a correlation between maturation of function and myelinization of fibers. In general, the main sensory pathways receive their myelin sheaths before the motor pathways (9). Fibers of the acoustic system begin to myelinate by the sixth fetal month, but myelinization proceeds slowly and is not completed until the fourth year of postnatal life. By contrast, the fibers of the visual system do not begin to myelinate until shortly before birth, but then do so very rapidly. Functionally, sound is more important to the fetus, but after birth, visual function is much more rapidly developed (1).

According to Tanner, the primary motor area in the precentral gyrus is the most advanced part of the cortex at birth, followed, in turn, by the primary sensory area or postcentral gyrus, then the primary visual area in the occipital lobe, and lastly the primary auditory area in the temporal lobe (1). By 3 months of postnatal life, all primary areas of the cortex are fairly mature, the motor areas being the most advanced. Nerve cells controlling the arm and upper trunk develop ahead of those controlling the leg, and this is reflected in the function of the baby who can control arms and trunk well, but has not yet begun to use the legs. After 6 months, the rate of development is greatest in the temporal and occipital lobes and least in the parietal and frontal lobes, which have already achieved most of their development. By 2 years, the primary sensory area has caught up with the primary motor, but some associaton areas are still quite immature (1).

*Visual sensation* develops rapidly after birth. The baby keeps the eyes closed much of the time in the first weeks of life, perhaps, because of some photophobia, and perhaps, because tearing is not well established until about 2 months of age. Most newborns can see objects held before them shortly after birth, but do not follow objects deliberately until about 4 months. Binocular vision develops by about 6 months, but depth perception requires a much longer time to develop. *Auditory sensation* is present at birth, but response to noises is primarily reflex in nature until about three to four months in age. The infant can localize sound by about 3 months and by 4 months may make searching movements in response to new sounds. Toward the end of the first year, listening and language skills develop. *Taste* is present at birth, but is relatively undifferentiated. By two to three months, taste has developed quite acutely and the infant explores his world by taste. He can, at this stage, already discriminate changes in formula and may reject a formula adulterated with medications or condiments. *Tactile sensation* is not well developed by birth. Initially, the baby will respond only to strong, painful stimuli by crying or by general body movement. By 7 to 9 months, there is some localization of the point of irritation, but specific response with appropriate behavior may not be perfected until 12–17 months (8).

## The Digestive System

At birth, digestive function is reasonably mature, though during infancy there is increase in size of the system and maturity of functional activity. The pancreas is capable of function, though trypsin and lipase activity are somewhat low. Digestive enzyme levels increase gradually throughout infancy.

The liver is the largest organ of the digestive system. The liver commonly remains palpable throughout infancy and early childhood. Bile acids are low in infancy, contributing to some poor tolerance of fats in some infants. Physiologic immaturity of liver function in the newborn is shown by physiologic hyperbilirubinemia of the newborn due to low levels of glucuronyl transferase for bilirubin, low prothrombin levels, low albumin levels, tendency to fasting hypoglycemia due to slow conversion of protein to glucose (gluconeogenesis), and low serum cholesterol levels. Albumin and globulin levels, remain somewhat low even into childhood (8).

At birth, the lower intestine is filled with meconium, a viscid material composed of digestive juices and cells shed from the lumen of the gut during intrauterine life. Fecal material is normally passed by 24 hours in the normal infant. Within the first week, the stools contain some remnants of meconium but gradually change to reflect food intake by the infant. Stools from breast-fed infants are soft, sour, pasty, and yellow. Two to four stools per day can be expected from breast-fed infants, a little less from a bottle-fed infant. By 2 years of age, the stool becomes formed and darker (8).

## Urinary-Genital System

The size of the kidney doubles by 6 months and triples by the end of the year, following the general somatic pattern for growth. New glomeruli may be formed in the first few postnatal months and all glomeruli undergo considerable enlargement during infancy. Many of the tubules are formed after birth. The functional immaturity of the new born kidney is shown in a variety of ways. The glomerular filtration rate is approximately 30–50% of the adult rate by 1 year. There is a decreased ability to excrete a sodium load, poor response to antidiuretic hormone (ADH), and poor ability to excrete a water load. The infant has a relatively high extracellular fluid volume at birth and the exchange of fluid is rapid. On the average, an infant has a daily exchange of 600–700 mL of water, which represents nearly 50% of his extracellular volume (8). Immaturity of the function of the loop of Henle leads to a poor ability to concentrate urine. Maximal concentration is approximately 700 milliosmol/kg of water during infancy and early childhood. This provides the infant with a very small margin of safety to prevent acidosis, dehydration, or edema (8).

Testes, ovaries, and internal and external genitalia are formed and present at birth. There is little further growth and change in function until puberty.

## Hematopoietic System

At birth, blood elements are formed in the bone marrow, which occupies most of the medullary cavities of the skeleton. Liver and spleen, extensively used during fetal life, retain their capacity to form blood elements under appropriate stimulation. The red blood cell count and hemoglobin are relatively high at birth. A fall begins shortly after birth, reaching a nadir at about the third or fourth month after birth, then rises again reaching stable levels by about 2 years of age. Red blood cell production is regulated by erythropoetin, present after the third week of life.

At birth, 80% of the infant's hemoglobin is fetal hemoglobin (HgbF). With its higher affinity for oxygen, it protects the infant effectively against anoxia at birth or in the neonatal period. After birth, the fetal hemoglobin is replaced by adult hemoglobin (HgbA) so that by 20 weeks only about 5% of the hemoglobin is HgbF. It is replaced completely by mid-childhood.

Newborns have the same number of platelets and megakaryocytes as adults, although premature and some fullterm infants have decreased platelet function, such as decreased platelet aggregation. In spite of low levels of a number of clotting factors, including prothrombin and factors VII, IX, and X, bleeding tendencies in the neonate are rare. Injection of vitamin K, necessary for formation of certain clotting factors, has become routine to prevent hemorrhagic disease of the newborn because newborn levels are only about half to one-third the levels found in older children. Breast-fed infants seem to derive some protection from small amounts of vitamin K in breast milk (8).

## The Immune System

The immunologic defense mechanisms of the newborn are fewer than those of older children. The physical barriers of the skin and the mucosa, digestive enzymes, intestinal motility, and intestinal bacteria, as well as humoral substances in the blood, such as complement, opsonins, and interferon are available to the infant and the child, though a little less effective in some instances. Cellular immunity seems to be well developed in the newborn. In addition, the infant receives from mother additional humoral protection in the form of immunoglobulin G, which crosses the placenta freely.

Immunoglobulin G (IgG) contains most of the antibacterial immuno-globulins. IgG is transferred from the maternal to the fetal circulation during the last trimester, so prematurely born infants may not receive optimal levels. Passive immunity of the infant will reflect the mother's immune experiences with infections and vaccinations. This acquired immunity will protect the infant for 6–9 months after birth. After birth, the infant's levels of IgG fall, reaching a nadir at about 3–5 months. As the infant is exposed to infectious agents, plasma cells proliferate and antibody formation occurs, resulting in eventual rise in IgG to adult levels by 2 years of age. IgA levels are very low in the newborn, which may increase the susceptibility of the infant to gram-negative bacterial infec-tions, some viral infections, and sepsis. IgM is formed rapidly after birth, reaching adult levels by 1 year of age. The response of IgM production to antigenic stimulation is more rapid than that of the other immunoglob-ulins in infancy. Intrauterine infections call forth a response of IgM and very high serum levels are found in infants who have congenital infections with rubella, toxoplasmosis, and cytomegalic inclusion virus (8).

Immunologic defenses during the newborn period are not completely effective and the infant appears peculiarly susceptible to a number of infections; these include sepsis (infections are poorly localized in the neonate), cytomegalic inclusion virus, Coxsackie and herpes simplex viruses (causing also generalized infections), some strains of Escherichia coli and B-group streptococci. Proteus, Klebsiella and Listeria monocytogenes are pathogenic for infants and seldom cause disease thereafter (8).

## Skeletal Growth in Infancy

The primary centers of ossification are present in all long bones at birth and one or two secondary centers have appeared (Figure 3-4). The first secondary center appears at the lower end of the femur, which is present in virtually all fullterm newborns. The proximal tibial center may also be present at birth. Ossification of epiphyses and growth of long bones generally follows an orderly pattern throughout infancy and childhood. Study of the epiphyses, their progression toward maturation, and eventual fusion with the metaphysis of the bone provides a mechanism for following and estimating the progress of bone maturation. The order and tempo of the maturation of bone and of the organism is seemingly under genetic control. It exhibits normal variation as well as variations imposed by race, sex, and environmental factors which can influence the amount and tempo of growth.

Primary centers in the limb girdles are established in early fetal life. In the foot, two or three tarsal bone ossification centers are formed at birth; in the wrist, the first carpal centers appear during the first year after birth (Figure 3-4). Secondary centers appear gradually in the limb bones over

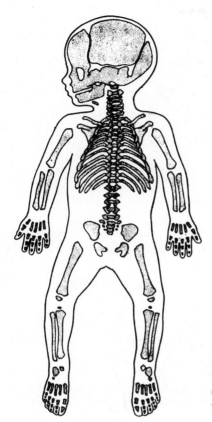

**Figure 3-4.** Ossification of the skeleton in a newborn baby. Note the absence of any centers in the wrists, the separate centers for the components of the hip bones, and the lack of any secondary centers for the long bones except the lower end of the femur and the upper end of the tibia. (Reproduced by permission from Sinclair D: *Human Growth after Birth*, ed 3. London, Oxford University Press, 1978.)

a long period of time, some as late as 14–15 years, and fusion is not complete until late adolescence or early adulthood. At birth, the pelvic bones are separate. After birth, the pelvis and lower limbs grow more rapidly than the rest of the bones of the body and with walking, the sacral curvature increases, the ilia becomes thicker and stronger, and the acetabulae deeper (9).

The skull is large at birth to accommodate the rapidly growing brain. It continues to enlarge rapidly during infancy, more than doubling its volume by age two (from 400 to 950 mL). Growth of the skull occurs by membranous apposition of bone. The bones of the skull are separated in infancy by fibrous tissue which allows compression during birth and expansion in response to rapid brain growth. The anterior fontanelle is a large, fibrous gap between skull bones which remains as a fibrous structure till well into the second year of life. Bone growth continues to occur at the fibrous junctions or joints which are called sutures. Appositional bone is applied to the outer surfaces to achieve thickness of the skull, while bone is resorbed from the inside to accommodate brain growth (9). With

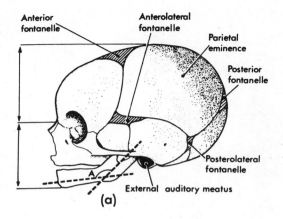

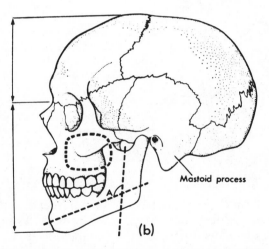

**Figure 3-5.** Growth of the skull. (A) Skull at birth. Notice the fontanelles, the smooth, nonserrated suture lines, the absence of a mastoid process, the obliquity of the angle of the mandible, and the relatively small size of the face. (B) Skull of adult. Notice absence of fontanelles, suture lines are now serrated, strong mastoid process, more upright mandible, and great increase in the vertical diameter of the face due to the eruption of teeth and the development of the jaws. The position of the maxillary sinus is indicated by the dotted line. (Reproduced by permission from Sinclair D: *Human Growth after Birth*, ed 3. London, Oxford University Press, 1978.)

growth of the skull, change in contour of the skull also occurs. The face changes with development of the nasal bridge, the facial sinuses, and especially the jaw. Jaw size and shape change as teeth are formed. Surface area for teeth is progressively increased by appositional bone growth posteriorly and resorption of bone in front of the ramus (9) (Figure 3-5).

Growth of the vertebral column is quite complex, though the major growth during infancy is through cartilaginous proliferation at the growing plates, located at the top and bottom of each vertebrae. Each vertebrae has a central and several lateral epiphyseal centers which fuse to form a boney plate that continues to grow by apposition. At birth the lumbar and sacral vertebrae are small and must grow rapidly to catch up to the better developed cervical and thoracic vertebrae (9).

## NUTRITIONAL REQUIREMENTS OF INFANCY

To assure proper growth in infancy, the infant must be assured of adequate nutrients. These nutrients include water; calories from carbohydrate, fat, and protein; minerals; and vitamins. The nutrients must not only be offered in adequate quantities, but must be of optimal quality as well. The infant must have the capacity to accept, digest, and absorb the nutrients. Within the recipient tissues, proper enzyme systems must be available to metabolize the nutrients and direct their use for optimal growth. The key role played by nutrition in infancy is emphasized by our social and emotional attention to feeding of the baby, and underscored by the grim reminder that half the population of the world is exposed to malnutrition during infancy and/or childhood (14).

### Nutritional Requirements
### Water

*Water* is the most basic nutrient required for growth in infancy. There is heavy water turnover in infancy compared to later childhood. There is a heavy water loss through the lungs and skin, and the kidneys have a reduced capacity to concentrate urine and save water. At birth, water requirements approximate 80–90 mL/kg/day, with an increase during the first month to 120 mL/kg/day. Thereafter, in the first year of life, the average newborn will require about 150 mL/kg/day of fluid to supply needs for growing tissues, and high fluid turnover, and to compensate for limited concentrating capacity of the kidney. Low birth weight infants may need up to 170 mL/kg/day, though some become edematous with high fluid intake and require less than 100 mL/kg/day (15).

### Calories

Growth of the infant depends on the provision of adequate *calories* for tissue building and energy expenditure. The average infant requires 100–120 kcal/kg/day, of which about 55 kcal/kg is needed for basal metabolism.

For growth and physical activity, 40 kcal/kg is needed and a small remainder is needed for fecal excretion and the specific dynamic action of protein. This total daily requirement falls gradually through infancy and childhood (15) (Figure 4-3).

## Carbohydrates

*Carbohydrate* is one of the infant's major sources of energy. Lactose from milk forms the major source of carbohydrate for the infant, with fructose and sucrose being introduced later with fruits, and starches being introduced with cereals and breads. Starches are digested slowly in infancy because of limited availability of intestinal amylases. Galactose in milk is generally transformed rather promptly to glucose, except when galactosemia is present. Fructose may be transformed to glucose or drawn directly into the three-carbon energy metabolism cycle. Glucose may be used directly for energy by brain, red blood cells, and gut mucosa, but most of the glucose is transformed to glycogen in the liver or muscle. There is, however, a limited storage of carbohydrate as glycogen, which provides glucose as a source of energy for only a few hours. Glucose, which is not burned immediately on ingestion or stored as glycogen, is converted to fat for storage (15).

## Fat

*Fat* represents a concentrated form of energy and, as subcutaneous tissue, may also serve the infant as insulation against cold or heat. Ingested fat requires intestinal and pancreatic lipases for digestion to fatty acids and bile salts are required for emulsification to promote absorption. Low birth weight infants lack usual amounts of bile salts and experience difficulty in fat absorption. Fatty acids are changed into triglycerides in the intestinal mucosa. Triglycerides are bound with lipoproteins to form chylomicrons, which are then carried into the circulation by the lymphatic system. Two of the fatty acids, linoleic and arachidonic, are essential fatty acids. The skin of infants deprived of these fatty acids becomes dry and thickened, desquamates, and becomes susceptible to intertrigo, an inflammation of the skin in the folds of the groin or axilla (15).

## Protein

*Protein* is the principal building material of tissues and is found in body fluids and secretions as well. Most enzymes of the body are made of protein and many specialized structures rely on a combination of lipid or carbohydrate with protein to lend them their unique structure or function. Proteins are broken down by digestive enzyme action to amino acids, the form in which protein is absorbed. The amino acids are then distributed to body tissues for production of specifically required proteins.

Although there is no firm agreement yet concerning the optimal or minimal protein requirements in infancy, certain qualitative requirements are known. The protein ingested must contain specific amounts of each of the essential amino acids. These are amino acids that cannot be formed within the organism, either by transamination of endogenous ketoacids or from fragments of other amino acids. Feedings containing less than 2 g/kg/day of protein, lead in a significant number of infants, to edema, a manifestation of hypoproteinemia. Formulas supplying 9 g/kg/day, often lead to hyperpyrexia and azotemia. Daily intakes of protein in the range of 2.25–5.0 g/kg/day are generally satisfactory for growth (16).

### Salt and Minerals

For each gram of protein retained by the infant, 0.3 g of *salt or mineral* becomes part of the tissue. Minerals are used within the body in many locations and for a multitude of functions (15). In infancy, there is a need for calcium, phosphate, and magnesium for bone growth. Calcium is also necessary for muscle contraction, nerve irritability, coagulation of blood, cardiac action, and production of milk. Lack of calcium leads to poor mineralization of teeth and bones, tetany, rickets, and impairment of growth. Fluorine is needed to lend strength and integrity to bone and teeth. Iodine is necessary for thyroxine formation; a deficiency leads to goiter and hypothyrodism. Iron and copper are essential for hemoglobin formation and both are essential elements of many enzyme systems; a deficiency of either leads to anemia. Magnesium is essential to all metabolic processes; it activates enzymes for carbohydrate metabolism and is necessary for muscle and nerve irritability. In addition to being a constituent of bones and teeth, phosphorus plays a key role in structure of cells, in energy transfer, and in metabolism of cell nutrients. Potassium is essential for muscle contraction and nerve conduction and is the major intracellular mineral regulating osmotic pressure and fluid balance. Sodium and chloride provide osmotic pressure in the extracellular fluids, are essential for acid-base and water balance, and play a role in muscle and nerve irritability. Sulfur is a constituent of proteins, mucopolysacharides, mucous, connective tissue, cartilage, and a number of enzymes. Zinc, molybdenum, cobalt, iron, manganese, and chromium are essential for enzyme functions—the list may be extended almost endlessly (15). In addition to its role in enzyme function, zinc may play at least a permissive role in growth processes.

### Vitamins

*Vitamins* are organic compounds required in minute amounts to catalyze cellular metabolism. They are generally not formed within the body and must be included in foodstuffs offered the infant to assure normal growth and tissue maintenance. Deficiencies of a number of vitamins have been shown to create health problems in infancy. *Vitamin K* deficiency, due to inadequate synthesis within the infant's gut, may result in hemorrhagic disease of the newborn. *Vitamin D* deficiency in infancy leads to rickets, tetany, and poor bone growth. *Vitamin C* deficiency may result in infantile scurvy associated with irritability, slow growth, susceptibility to infection and hemorrhagic problems. *Pyridoxine* deficiency may lead to anemia, irritability and convulsions in infants. *Folic acid* deficiency produces a megaloblastic anemia of the infant. *Niacin, riboflavin, and thiamine* deficiencies lead to pellagra, ariboflavinosis, or beri-beri, and poor growth. *Vitamin A* deficiency leads to poor growth plus eye, tooth, mucus membrane, and skin disorders (15).

## Feeding the Infant

In order to provide the necessary nutrients for growth, the infant will require from six to nine feedings per 24 hours after the first week of life. Breast-fed infants may require even shorter intervals. The initial food of infancy usually consists of milk with supplementation of a few vitamins (A, D, C) and minerals.

### Human Breast Milk

*Human breast milk* is, without dispute, the ideal vehicle for nutrients required by the newborn infant and is the only required source of nutrients for as much as 8–9 months of the first year of life, though supplementation with other nutrients is often practiced much earlier. Colostrum, the secretion from the breast in the first few days before the milk production begins, is high in protein and minerals, low in carbohydrate and fat, and contains heavy concentrations of immunoglobulins (15). Human milk provides the infant with ideal proportions of protein, carbohydrate, and fat, including all the essential amino acids and essential fats. Human milk also contains immunoglobulins for protection against bacterial and some viral illnesses and promotes colonization of the gut with lactobacilli (an aid to digestion). Breastfeeding also aids in mother–infant bonding, a feature of infant growth deserving of increased attention.

### Cow's Milk

Infants offered a *cow's milk formula* in place of human breast milk usually receive sufficient nutrients for growth, provided the amount offered and accepted by the infant fulfills the requirements for fluid and calories mentioned above. In Table 3-1, the constituents of human breast milk are compared with those of unmodified cow's milk. It may be noted that the water and calorie content are about the same, but that the calories are derived from different sources. There is more lactose in human milk and more protein in the cow's milk. The type of protein is also different, being chiefly casein in cow's milk and lactoprotein in human milk. The curd from lactoprotein is fine and flocculant; the curd of casein must be altered by heat or pH changes to render it equally digestible. Low birth weight infants, in particular, may have difficulty in digesting the casein curd. The unsaturated fat of human milk is also more digestible than the saturated fat of cow's milk. There is less mineral in human milk; both provide low levels of iron, however, the iron is better absorbed from human milk. Both may be deficient in vitamins D, K, and C, which require supplementation (15).

Formulas for infants offer a variety of modified cow's milk products, most of which reduce protein content toward that of human milk, increase the carbohydrate content, and replace some of the saturated with unsaturated fats. Vitamin and sometimes iron supplements are provided. Goat's milk, soy formulas, and milk substitutes, artificially compounded to offer protein, carbohydrate, and fat roughly resembling human or modified cow's milk formulas are available for specific nutritional needs, such as allergy to cow's milk, persistent diarrhea, or phenylketonuria. All such formulas are designed to aid the physician and family to provide the infant with adequate nutrition for growth.

## Feeding Patterns in Infancy

Social problems, such as inadequate mothering and psychosocial deprivation, are a frequent cause of underfeeding in infancy. Brief periods of diarrhea and constipation may occur during infancy in many healthy infants who grow well and show only temporary fluctuations of weight. Persistent diarrhea and constipation may lead to alterations of the growth pattern and must be investigated to discover and alleviate the cause. When a nutritional deficiency has caused cessation of growth, restitution of normal nutrition usually results in a period of catch-up growth, returning the infant to its former growth pattern.

During the second year of life there is a continuing deceleration in the rate of growth and a reduction in the caloric requirement per kg, which leads to a decrease in appetite. This phenomenon is often viewed by the parent as a lack of interest in food or a "picky appetite" and viewed as a possible aberration from a normal growth process. Attempts to force food on the infant during this period may result in even more pronounced "dawdling" or outright refusal of food, compounding the fears of the parent that the child's health is suffering because of self-imposed malnutrition. That a deceleration of growth naturally results in need for less food (calories) is sometimes difficult for parents to accept emotionally and some overfeeding or emotionally charged confrontations occur that may haunt both parent and child with poor nutritional habits later. Infants offered a variety of foods and left to choose for themselves which foods they will eat, generally receive an adequate variety of nutrients. Persistent avoidance of parrticular foods by the infant may not involve taste or conscious aversion, but may suggest allergy to the food, which may provoke discomfort each time it is ingested. Allergy to a wide variety of foods and consequent inability to use them for nutrient requirements may lead to malnutrition.

**Table 3-1. Composition of Colostrum, Human Milk, and Cow's Milk**

| Constituent | Human Milk | Human Colostrum | Cow's Milk |
|---|---|---|---|
| Water | 88 | 87 | 88 |
| Protein | 1.1 | 2.7 | 3.3 |
| Casein | 0.4 | 1.2 | 2.7 |
| Lactalbumin | 0.4 | | 0.4 |
| Lactoglobulin | 0.2 | 1.5 | 0.2 |
| Fat | 3.8 | 2.9 | 3.8 |
| % polyunsaturated | 8.0 | 7.0 | 2.0 |
| Lactose | 7.0 | 5.3 | 4.8 |
| Ash | 0.2 | 0.5 | 0.8 |
| Calcium mg/100 g | 34 | 30 | 117 |
| Phosphorus mg/100 g | 15 | 15 | 92 |
| Sodium meq/L | 7 | 48 | 22 |
| Potassium meq/L | 13 | 74 | 35 |
| Chloride meq/L | 11 | 80 | 29 |
| Magnesium mg/100 g | 4 | 4 | 12 |
| Sulfur mg/100 g | 14 | 22 | 30 |
| Chromium μg/L | | | 10 |
| Manganese μg/L | 10 | tr | 30 |
| Copper μg/L | 400 | 600 | 300 |
| Zinc mg/L | 4 | 6 | 4 |
| Iodine μg/L | 30 | 120 | 47 |
| Selenium μg/L | 30 | | 30 |
| Iron mg/L | 0.5 | 0.1 | 0.5 |
| Amino acids (mg/100 mL) | | | |
| Histidine | 22 | | 95 |
| Leucine | 68 | | 228 |
| Isoleucine | 100 | | 350 |
| Lysine | 73 | | 277 |
| Methionine | 25 | | 88 |
| Phenylalanine | 48 | | 172 |
| Threonine | 50 | | 164 |
| Tryptophan | 18 | | 49 |
| Valine | 70 | | 245 |
| Arginine | 45 | | 129 |
| Alanine | 35 | | 75 |
| Aspartic acid | 116 | | 166 |
| Cystine | 22 | | 32 |
| Glutamic acid | 230 | | 680 |
| Glycine | 0 | | 11 |
| Proline | 80 | | 250 |
| Serine | 69 | | 160 |
| Tyrosine | 61 | | 179 |
| Vitamins (liter) | | | |
| Vitamin A (IU) | 1898 | | 1025 |
| Thiamine (μg) | 160 | | 440 |

**Table 3-1. (Continued)**

| Constituent | Human Milk | Human Colostrum | Cow's Milk |
|---|---|---|---|
| Riboflavin (μg) | 360 | | 1750 |
| Niacin (μg) | 1470 | | 940 |
| Pyridoxine (μg) | 100 | | 640 |
| Pantothenate (mg) | 2 | | 3 |
| Folacin (μg) | 52 | | 55 |
| $B_{12}$ (μg) | 0.3 | | 4 |
| Vitamin C (mg) | 43 | | 11 |
| Vitamin D (IU) | 22 | | 14 |
| Vitamin E (mg) | 2 | | 0.4 |
| Vitamin K (μg) | 15 | | 60 |

Reproduced with permission from Vaughan VC, McKay RJ, Behrman RB (eds), *Nelson's Textbook of Pediatrics*. ed 11, Philadelphia, WB Saunders Co., 1979, p 198. Collated from Foman SJ: *Infant Nutrition*. ed 2, Philadelphia, WB Saunders Co., 1974, pp 360 and Macy IG, Kelly HJ, Sloan RE: The Composition of Milks. NAS-NRC Publication, 254, 1953.

The concept of critical periods of growth deserves emphasis when we speak of nutrition for the infant; especially critical periods of maturation of the brain. The rapid growth and development of the brain throughout the period of infancy has been described in an earlier section of this chapter. Winick has described the deleterious effects of malnutrition on the growth and function of brain of both animals and human. He suggests that malnutrition in infancy can both reduce brain growth and permanently reduce intellectual function (14). He points out that the earlier in infancy the malnutrition occurs, the more likely there will be permanent damage to brain growth and function. After infancy, the brain seems to become progressively more resistant to the effects of malnutrition (14).

## ENDOCRINOLOGY OF GROWTH IN INFANCY
Growth is the product of the interaction of genetic codes, cellular growth factors, and many hormones. Certain hormones might be singled out for their noticeable effect on growth in infancy.

### Growth Hormone and Somatomedin
In the previous chapter it was noted that somatomedins may play a pivotal role in the regulation of fetal growth, but the role of growth hormone is uncertain. At birth there is a change in the regulation of growth. After birth, tissues of the body appear to become progressively more sensitive to the growth regulating stimuli of human growth hormone (17). Infants deficient in pituitary growth hormone are nearly normal in size at birth but fail to grow adequately thereafter. Usually within the first year of life,

but often somewhat later, a noticeable lag in growth occurs which becomes progressively worse with time. The transition to dependency on growth hormone often seems to be delayed or prolonged (18).

Somatomedin C (IGF I) appears to be one of the principal mediators of postnatal growth, but concentrations are low at birth and remain low throughout the first year of life (19) despite extremely rapid growth during the same period. This suggests that the somatomedin levels that we measure in the serum may not represent active peptide produced by, or acting on individual tissues (18), or that growth in infancy is somatomedin-dependent, but not reflected in the low blood somatomedin concentrations (18). Normal response of tissues to somatomedin and growth hormone also depends on the normal action of insulin, corticosteroids, and thyroxine to which tissues also become more sensitive after birth. The regulation of skeletal growth is, therefore, under elaborate control of a number of interacting hormones and growth stimulating substances.

**Thyroid Hormone**

Growth is affected in a number of ways by thyroxine. It is essential for normal maturation of bone and brain and regulates general body metabolism, affecting nearly every cell of the body, most obviously, the circulatory, digestive, and nervous systems. Thyroxine is essential for growth from earliest infancy and, indeed, essential for brain and bone maturation in utero. It appears to be essential for protein synthesis in the brain and for normal development of nerve cells (1). Inadequacy of thyroxine in utero or the neonatal period results in lack of normal brain growth and permanent intellectual deficit. The intellectual deficit seems to be more profound with absolute lack of thyroxine in infancy and becomes progressively more severe the longer the infant goes without recognition and correction of the thyroxine deficiency.

Lack of skeletal development is also noted in infants with thyroid deficiency. Thyroxine deficiency hampers stimulation of cartilage proliferation by somatomedin, resulting in slow growth of bones and lack of formation of epiphyses. Delay in appearance of epiphyses, that is, delay in bone maturation, is one of the most consistent effects of thyroxine deficiency. Epiphyses, which do appear during thyroxine deficiency, are often fragmented and poorly formed (epiphyseal dysgenesis). Lack of normal bone growth in infancy due to thyroxine deficiency leads to a characteristic growth pattern with a retention of infantile body proportions. Lack of thyroid prevents the usual catch-up growth of the lower extremities after birth and the body proportions remain "infantile," that is, the legs remain short compared to the trunk.

**Vitamin D, Parathyroid Hormone, and Calcitonin**

The skeleton is dependent for its growth upon formation of cartilage and availability of calcium and phosphorus for transformation of cartilage into bone. In infancy, Vitamin D appears to play a major role in promoting mineralization of cartilage to form bone and is aided by parathyroid hormone and calcitonin in maintaining calcium and phosphorus levels in the optimal range to facilitate bone formation and mineralization. Vitamin D is a sterol hormone derived from skin ergosterol by photo-transformation. Because adequate exposure to sunlight is not always realized in infancy, it is customary to supplement the infant's diet with Vitamin D. A deficiency of Vitamin D in infancy leads to inadequate mineralization of the skeleton (rickets). Poor growth of bones and deformities of softened long bones may lead to profound growth failure in infancy (see Chapter 9—Rickets).

The action of parathyroid hormone (PTH) in infancy is critical to provision of optimal levels of calcium and phosphorus for bone formation and many other functions as well. A lack of PTH in infancy results in hypocalcemia, producing tetany of the newborn. Calcitonin balances the action of PTH on calcium levels by preventing hypercalcemia in the infant, but it appears not to have a significant role in the growth process. [For a more complete discussion of hormonal regulation of calcium and phosphorus homeostasis, see Chapter 4].

## Other "Growth" Hormones of Infancy

*Insulin* is an anabolic hormone and would be expected to contribute to growth in infancy—a period of intense anabolism. Other than a general role in supplying substrate for tissue building and energy, however, a direct effect of insulin on growth in infancy is difficult to demonstrate. A large part of somatomedin activity is termed "insulin-like" and it has been suggested that insulin and somatomedins may work in concert in the formation of muscle and adipose tissue (20). Deficiency of insulin in infancy is not common. Infants born without a pancreas, however, are small at birth and do experience slow growth through infancy, at least in part, perhaps as a result of inadequate insulin.

At birth, the function of the *adrenal gland* changes dramatically from that of providing dehydroepiandrosterone sulfate (DHEAS) for placental estrogen synthesis to production of gluco- and mineralo-corticoids for homeostasis of carbohydrate and fluid-electrolyte metabolism. A late third trimester surge of fetal cortisol may induce lung maturation and signal readiness for parturition. The "fetal" zone of the adrenal cortex, which makes up the bulk of the fetal adrenal, undergoes rapid involution after birth, disappearing entirely by 1 year of age, by which time the adrenal assumes adult form with three morphologic zones derived from the outer layer of the cortex.

*Glucocorticoids* probably do not play an important role in growth in infancy unless they are administered in excess, or produced in excess by an adrenal tumor or hyperplasia. Excess steroids impair linear growth of the infant and, through deposition of excess adipose tissue, may produce obesity. Cortisol excess interferes both with somatomedin production and its action on cartilage, preventing cartilage proliferation and delaying bone growth and maturation. Cortisol also blocks protein production in other tissues and interferes with the anabolic effects of growth hormone. The result of cortisol excess in infancy is a stunted, obese, weak infant with Cushing syndrome. Removal of the source of excess glucocorticoid allows resumption of the infant's growth and rapid catch-up growth usually occurs. The catch-up may be poor and permanent stunting can occur if use of corticosteroids is prolonged (21). An enzymatic block in cortisol synthesis may lead to excessive adrenal androgen production resulting in virilization of the external genitalia of the fetus (newborn) and rapid growth, progressive virilization, and accelerated bone maturation through infancy and childhood. (See Congential Adrenal Hyperplasia, Chapter 9)

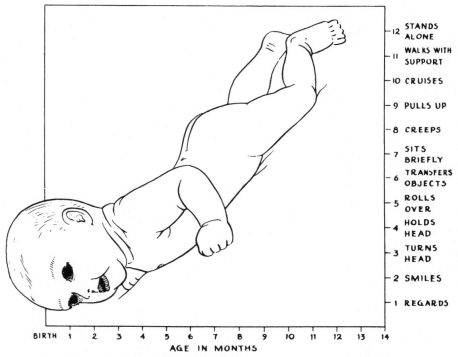

**Figure 3-6.** Progression of skill achievements cephalad to caudad. Skills developed during the first year of life are listed on the right side of the figure with the age of the infant across the bottom. Earlier skills concern mastery of head or trunk; later arms and finally legs. (Reproduced by permission from Lowrey G: Behavior and personality, *Growth and Development in Children,* ed 7. Copyright © 1978 by Year Book Medical Publishers, Inc, Chicago, after Aldrich CA and Hewitt ES: Outlines for well baby clinics: Development for the first twelve months. *Am J Dis Child* **71:**131, 1946.)

# BEHAVIOR AND PERSONALITY DEVELOPMENT IN INFANCY

In this section, only those features of neurologic or behavioral development will be highlighted that seem to be closely related to the growth of the infant, or that might be affected by disturbances in growth. For a more complete discussion of development patterns in infancy, the reader is referred to appropriate texts or monographs listed among the references. The appearance of behavioral traits of an infant are dependent upon general health, integrity of the nervous system, and an interplay of the infant with the environment. Earliest development involves use of the head with later skills involving trunk, arms, and finally legs. This progression of skill achievement, cephalad to caudad, is dramatically depicted in Figure 3-6.

The neonatal developmental status is generally judged by the presence or absence of neurologic reflexes which reflect the status of development of the brain and the nervous system. At birth, the infant has good muscular tone and a good grasp reflex. In either the prone or supine position, the infant can turn the head and thus defend itself from suffocation. The newborn infant usually has a vigorous sucking reflex present at birth, and when the cheek is grazed, the infant will turn his head toward the stimulus and purse his lips (rooting reflex). The tonic neck reflex is generally well

### Table 3-2. Developmental Screening Inventory

| | **4 Weeks** |
|---|---|
| Gross motor | Asymmetrical tonic neck reflex positions predominate. |
| | Head sags forward in sitting. |
| Fine motor | Hands fisted. |
| | Hands clench on contact. |
| Adaptive | Regards object in line of vision only. |
| | Follows to midline. |
| | Drops toy immediately. |
| Language | Vague indirect regard. |
| | Small throaty noises. |
| Personal–social | Stares indefinitely at surroundings. |
| | Regards observer's face and diminishes activity. |
| | **16 Weeks** |
| Gross motor | Symmetrical postures predominate. |
| | Head steady in sitting. |
| | Head lifted 90 degrees when prone; on forearms. |
| Fine motor | Hands engage. |
| | Reaches, grasps objects, brings to mouth. |
| Adaptive | Eyes follow slowly moving object well. |
| | Arms activate on sight of dangling toy. |
| | Regards toy in hand and takes to mouth. |
| | Regard goes from hand to object when sitting. |

Table 3-2. (Continued)

| Language | Laughs aloud. |
| | Excites and breathes heavily. |
| Personal–social | Spontaneous social smile. |
| | Hand play with mutual fingering. |
| | Pulls dress over face. |
| | Anticipates food on sight. |

**28 Weeks**

| Gross motor | Sits briefly leaning forward on hands. |
| | Supports large fraction of weight in standing. |
| | Bounces actively in supported standing. |
| | Rolls over. |
| Fine motor | Has radial palmar grasp of toy. |
| | Rakes at small pellet with whole hand. |
| Adaptive | One-hand approach and grasp of toy. |
| | Bangs and shakes rattle. |
| | Transfers toy from one hand to the other. |
| Language | Vocalizes "m-m-m" when crying. |
| | Talks to toys. |
| Personal–social | Takes feet to mouth. |
| | Reaches for and pats mirror image. |

**40 Weeks**

| Gross motor | Sits indefinitely steady. |
| | Creeps and pulls self to feet at rail. |
| Fine motor | Crude release of toy. |
| | Plucks pellet easily with thumb and index finger. |
| | Exploring poke with forefinger. |
| Adaptive | Matches 2 objects in hands. |
| | Index finger approach. |
| | Spontaneously rings bell. |
| Language | Says "mama" and "dada" with meaning. |
| | One other "word". |
| Personal–social | Waves "bye-bye" and pat-a-cakes (or other nursery trick). |
| | Feeds self cracker and holds own bottle. |

**52 Weeks**

| Gross motor | Walks with 1 hand held. |
| | Stands momentarily alone. |
| | Cruises. |
| Fine motor | Neat Pincer grasp of pellet. |
| Adaptive | Tries to build tower of 2 cubes. |
| | Releases cube in cup (after demonstration). |
| | Serial play with objects. |
| Language | Two words besides "mama" and "dada". |
| | Gives toy on request or gesture. |
| Personal–social | Offers toy to image in mirror. |
| | Cooperates in dressing. |

## Table 3-2. (Continued)

### 15 Months

| | |
|---|---|
| Gross motor | Toddles independently.<br>Creeps upstairs. |
| Fine motor | Puts pellet into bottle. |
| Adaptive | Builds tower of 2 cubes.<br>Puts 6 cubes in and out of cup.<br>Incipient imitation of stroke. |
| Language | Jargons.<br>Four to 6 words, including names.<br>Follows simple commands. |
| Personal–social | Says "thank you" or equivalent.<br>Points or vocalizes wants.<br>Indicates wet pants.<br>Casts objects in play or refusal. |

### 18 Months

| | |
|---|---|
| Gross motor | Walks, seldom falling.<br>Seats self in small chair and climbs into adult chair.<br>Hurls ball in standing position. |
| Fine motor | Turns pages of book 2–3 at once. |
| Adaptive | Builds tower of 3–4 cubes.<br>Imitates stroke with a crayon and scribbles spontaneously.<br>Dumps pellet from bottle. |
| Language | Has 10 words.<br>Looks selectively at pictures and identifies 1.<br>Names ball and carries out 2 directions ("on the table", "to mother"). |
| Personal–social | Pulls toy on string.<br>Carries and hugs doll.<br>Feeds self in part with spilling. |

### 24 Months

| | |
|---|---|
| Gross motor | Runs well, no falling.<br>Walks up and down stairs alone.<br>Kicks large ball on request. |
| Fine motor | Turns pages of book singly. |
| Adaptive | Builds tower of 6–7 cubes.<br>Aligns cubes for train.<br>Imitates vertical and circular strokes. |
| Language | Uses pronouns.<br>Three-word sentences; jargon discarded.<br>Carries out 4 directions with ball ("on the table", "on the chair", "to mother", "to me"). |
| Personal–social | Verbalizes toilet needs consistently.<br>Pulls on simple garment. |

Reproduced with permission from Lowrey GH: Behavior and Personality in *Growth and Development of Children*. ed 7, copyright 1978 by Year Book Medical Publishers, Inc, Chicago.

# DENVER DEVELOPMENTAL SCREENING TEST

STO. = STOMACH
SIT = SITTING

PERCENT OF CHILDREN PASSING
25  50  75  90

May pass by report →
Footnote No. →
see back of form

Test Item

Date
Name
Birthdate
Hosp. No.

| PERSONAL-SOCIAL | FINE MOTOR-ADAPTIVE | LANGUAGE | GROSS MOTOR |
|---|---|---|---|

**PERSONAL-SOCIAL**

- REGARDS FACE
- SMILES RESPONSIVELY
- SMILES SPONTANEOUSLY
- INITIALLY SHY WITH STRANGERS
- PLAYS PAT-A-CAKE
- FEEDS SELF CRACKERS
- RESISTS TOY PULL
- PLAYS PEEK-A-BOO
- WORKS FOR TOY OUT OF REACH
- IMITATES HOUSEWORK
- PUTS ON CLOTHING
- USES SPOON, SPILLING LITTLE
- WASHES & DRIES HANDS
- BUTTONS UP
- PLAYS BALL WITH EXAMINER
- INDICATES WANTS (NOT CRY)
- DRINKS FROM CUP
- HELPS IN HOUSE – SIMPLE TASKS
- DRESSES WITH SUPERVISION
- SEPARATES FROM MOTHER EASILY
- PLAYS INTERACTIVE GAMES e.g., TAG
- REMOVES GARMENT
- DRESSES WITHOUT SUPERVISION
- * 100% pass at birth

**FINE MOTOR-ADAPTIVE**

- FOLLOWS TO MIDLINE
- EQUAL MOVEMENTS
- FOLLOWS PAST MIDLINE
- HANDS TOGETHER
- GRASPS RATTLE
- REGARDS RAISIN
- FOLLOWS 180°
- REACHES FOR OBJECT
- SIT, LOOKS FOR YARN
- SIT, TAKES 2 CUBES
- RAKES RAISIN ATTAINS
- PASSES CUBE HAND TO HAND
- THUMB-FINGER GRASP
- BANGS 2 CUBES HELD IN HANDS
- NEAT PINCER GRASP OF RAISIN
- SCRIBBLES SPONTANEOUSLY
- TOWER OF 2 CUBES
- TOWER OF 4 CUBES
- TOWER OF 8 CUBES
- IMITATES VERTICAL LINE WITHIN 30°
- COPES ○
- IMITATES BRIDGE
- COPES +
- COPIES □
- IMITATES □ DEMONSTR
- DRAWS MAN 3 PARTS
- PICKS LONGER LINE 3 OF 3
- DRAWS MAN 6 PARTS

**LANGUAGE**

- RESPONDS TO BELL
- VOCALIZES - NOT CRYING
- LAUGHS
- SQUEALS
- TURNS TO VOICE
- IMITATES SPEECH SOUNDS
- DADA OR MAMA, NONSPECIFIC
- DADA OR MAMA, SPECIFIC
- 3 WORDS OTHER THAN MAMA, DADA
- COMBINES 2 DIFFERENT WORDS
- POINTS TO 1 NAMED BODY PART
- NAMES 1 PICTURE
- FOLLOWS DIRECTIONS/2 of 3
- USES PLURALS
- GIVES 1ST & LAST NAME
- COMPREHENDS COLD, TIRED, HUNGRY/2 of 3
- COMPREHENDS PREPOSITIONS/3 of 4
- RECOGNIZES COLORS/3 of 4
- OPPOSITE ANALOGIES 2 of 3
- DEFINES WORDS/6 of 9    87%
- COMPOSITION OF/3 of 3    87%

**GROSS MOTOR**

- STO LIFTS HEAD
- STO HEAD UP 45°
- STO HEAD UP 90°
- BEAR SOME WEIGHT ON LEGS
- PULL TO SIT NO HEAD LAG
- STO CHEST UP ARM SUPPORT
- SIT-HEAD STEADY
- ROLLS OVER
- SITS WITHOUT SUPPORT
- STANDS HOLDING ON
- PULLS SELF TO STAND
- GETS TO SITTING
- WALKS HOLDING ON FURNITURE
- STANDS MOMENTARILY
- STANDS ALONE WELL
- STOOPS & RECOVERS
- WALKS WELL
- WALKS BACKWARDS
- KICKS BALL FORWARD
- THROWS BALL OVERHAND
- WALKS UP STEPS
- JUMPS IN PLACE
- PEDALS TRICYCLE
- BALANCE ON 1 FOOT 1 SECOND
- BROAD JUMP
- BALANCE ON 1 FOOT 5 SECONDS/2 of 3
- HOPS ON 1 FOOT
- BALANCE ON 1 FOOT 10 SECONDS/2 of 3
- CATCHES BOUNCED BALL/2 of 3
- HEEL TO TOE WALK/2 of 3
- BACKWARD HEEL-TOE/2 of 3

MONTHS: 1 2 3 4 5 6 7 8 9 10 11 12 13 14 15 16 17 18 19 20 21 22 23 24
YEARS: 2½ 3 3½ 4 4½ 5 5½ 6

©1969 William K. Frankenburg, M.D. and Jacob B. Dodds, Ph.D. University of Colorado Medical Center.

developed by one month of age and persists until about 4 to 6 months of age. A startle response (Moro reflex) characterized by extension of all extremities and momentary increase in muscle tone, incomplete before 35 weeks gestation, persists for about 5 months (8).

The Babinski reflex, elicited by stroking the lateral plantar surface of the foot, is present in the majority of newborns at birth and may persist through most of the first year. The behavior of the neonate may be assessed by observing the baby's consciousness or alertness and response to stimuli including bright lights, pin prick, visual objects, human voice, pull-to-sit position, and covering the face with a cloth (22).

Beyond the neonatal period, developmental progress is assessed in terms of acquisition of gross and fine motor skills and social and adaptive or language skills (Table 3-2). The mean age for appearance of skills or behavior patterns and early or late limits may be depicted on an age scale such as the Denver Developmental Screening Test (DDST) (23) (Figure 3-7). To make it easier for the clinician to administer the test during routine health maintenance visits, an abbreviation in method of administration of the DDST has recently been introduced together with a revised form that allows graphic portrayal of the child's rate of development (24).

## GROWTH CHARACTERISTICS
## OF LOW BIRTH WEIGHT INFANTS

Newborn infants may be classified according to their size and gestational age at birth as large, appropriate, or small for gestational age (25). The norms for appropriate size are determined by the average weights of normal infants at various gestational ages (Figure 2-7). Growth patterns for infants large or small for gestational age will be discussed in Chapter 8, entitled "Growth Problems in Infancy". Low birth weight infants appropriate for gestational age are prematurely born infants and exhibit growth patterns appropriate for their gestational age.

Infants born before 28 weeks are generally not viable. Infants born after 28 weeks of gestation but before 38 weeks are said to be born prematurely. The appearance, growth pattern, and behavioral characteristics of prematurely born infants are similar to a fetus of similar age (Table 2-1). Vaughan reports that infants weighing 1000–1500 g tend to be immobile. The skin is thin, the head large, in comparison to the body,

←
**Figure 3-7.** Sample from Denver Developmental Screening Test (DDST) cross sectional norms. Development skills or behavior from each of four groups (gross motor, language, fine motor-adaptive, personal–social) are depicted graphically by age of expected mastery by the child. The bars indicate percent of children passing a given skill by the corresponding age. (Reproduced by permission from Frankenburg WK, Dodds JB: The Denver Developmental Screening Test: *J Pediatr* **71**:181, 1967, University of Colorado Medical Center, copyright 1969.)

and rounded; reflexes and muscles are both weak. The infant sleeps much of the time, the suck reflex is weak, and the infant must be gavage fed to provide adequate calories for growth. Infants weighing 1500–2000 g have a little more subcutaneous fat and better muscle tone and reflexes. They have a fairly well-developed sleep/wake pattern and are willing to feed, some can even feed at the breast sufficiently well to get enough calories for growth. Infants 2000–2500 g resemble full-term infants, though with less subcutaneous fat tissue. They have a good cry and muscle tone, and though they exhibit some developmental immaturity, the major feature distinguishing them from the full-term infants is their thinness (2).

Prematurely born infants tend to have some health handicaps because of their immaturity, which may interfere initially with growth. They have respiratory immaturity and are prone to repiratory distress syndrome. They have faulty temperature control and decreased resistance to infection. Their stores of glycogen and substrate storage for gluconeogenesis are often inadequate, leading to hypoglycemia. Immature kidneys predispose them to nutritional edema and dehydration. Anemia and hemorrhagic disease of the newborn readily occur from lack of iron stores or lack of vitamin K.

If the premature infant can overcome these handicaps, growth may be expected to occur similar to that expected for an infant in utero of the same conceptual age (26). There may be some catch-up growth during infancy and, by one year of age, development is a little slow but appropriate if adjusted for the amount of prematurity. By the end of the second year, growth has generally been corrected and the genetically determined pattern of growth is sought and maintained thereafter (27).

## REFERENCES

1. Tanner JM: *Fetus Into Man: Physical Growth From Conception To Maturity*. Cambridge, Harvard University Press, 1978, pp 37–51, 87–102, 103–116.

2. Vaughan VC III: Growth and development, in Vaughan VC, McKay RJ, Behrman RE (eds), *Nelson's Textbook of Pediatrics*. Philadelphia, WB Saunders Co., 1979, pp 10–46.

3. Tanner JM, Healy MJR, Lockhart RD, et al: Aberdeen growth study: I. The prediction of adult body measurement from measurements taken each year from birth to five years. *Arch Dis Child* **31**:372, 1956.

4. Smith DW, Truog W, Rogers JE, et al: Shifting linear growth during infancy: Illustration of genetic factors in growth from fetal life through infancy. *J Pediatr* **89**:225, 1976.

5. Reynolds EL, Sontag LW: The Fels composite sheet: II. Variations in growth patterns in health and disease. *J Pediatr* **26**:336, 1945.

6. Miller HC, Merritt TA: Prenatal and postnatal growth: Is there a continuum? in *Fetal Growth in Humans*. Year Book Medical Publishers Inc., 1979, pp 149–154.

7. Lind J, Stern L, Wegelius C: *Human Fetal and Neonatal Circulation*. Springfield, Charles C Thomas Publisher, 1964.

8. Lowrey GH: *Growth and Development of Children*, ed 7. Chicago, Year Book Medical Publishers Inc., 1979, pp 113–160, 205–278.

9. Sinclair D: Growth of Tissues, in *Human Growth After Birth*, ed 3. London, Oxford University Press, 1978, pp 46–67.

10. Avery ME, Fletcher BD: *The Lung and its Disorders in the Newborn Infant*, ed 4. Philadelphia, WB Saunders Co., 1981.

11. Charnock EL, Doershuk CF: Developmental aspects of the human lung. *Pediatr Clin North Am* **20:**275–292, 1973.

12. Gluck L, Kulovich MV: Fetal lung development, current concepts. *Pediatr Clin North Am* **10:**367–379, 1973.

13. Patel AJ, Balazs R, Altman J, et al: Effect of X-irradiation on the biochemical maturation of rat cerebellum: Postnatal cell formation. *Radiat Res* **62:**470, 1975.

14. Winick M: Malnutrition and brain development. *J Pediatr* **74:**667, 1969.

15. Barness LA: Nutrition and nutritional disorders, in Vaughan VC, McKay RJ, Behrman RE (eds), *Nelson's Textbook of Pediatrics*. Philadelphia, WB Saunders Co., 1979, pp 173–237.

16. Cox WM JR, Filer LJ: Protein intake for low-birth-weight infants. *J Pediatr* **74:**1016, 1969.

17. Kaplan SL, Grumbach MM, Shepard TH: The ontogenesis of human fetal hormones: Growth hormone and insulin. *J Clin Invest* **51:**3080, 1972.

18. Underwood LE, D'Ercole AJ: Insulin and insulin-like growth factors/somatomedins in fetal and neonatal development. *Clin Endocrinol Metab* **13:**69, 1984.

19. Kaptowitz PB, D'Ercole AJ, Van Wyk JJ, Underwood LE: Plasma somatomedin-C during the first year of life. *J Pediatr* **100:**932, 1982.

20. Sizonenko PC: Endocrinological control of growth. *Postgrad Med J* **54**(1):91, 1978.

21. Mosier HD Jr, Smith FG Jr, Schultz MA: Failure of catch-up growth after Cushing's syndrome in childhood. *Am J Dis Child* **124:**251, 1972.

22. Brazelton TB: Assessment of the infant at risk. *Clin Obstet Gynecol* **16:**361–375, March, 1973.

23. Frankenburg WK, Dodds J: The Denver Developmental Screening Test. *J Pediatr* **71:**181, 1967.

24. Frankenburg WK, Fandal AW, Sciarillo W, et al.: The newly abbreviated and revised Denver Development Screening Test. *J Pediatr* **99:**995, 1981.

25. Battaglia FC, Lubchenco LO: A practical classification of newborn infants by weight and gestational age. *J Pediatr* **71:**159, 1967.

26. Cruise MO: A longitudinal study of growth of low birth weight infants: Velocity and distance growth, birth to three years. *Pediatrics* **51:**620, 1973.

27. Manser JI: Growth in the high-risk infant. *Clinics in Perinatology* **11**(Feb):19, 1984.

# 4

# Normal Growth in Children

Childhood is a period of stable growth, sandwiched in between periods of rapid growth in infancy and adolescence. As the rapid growth of infancy decelerates into the slow and steady growth of childhood there is a noticeable decrease in growth and food intake, prompting many parents to wonder if there might be a growth problem in the child who is eating much less than previously and seems to have stopped growing.

## CHARACTERISTICS OF GROWTH IN CHILDHOOD

By 2 years of age, the child's growth has usually undergone shifts in order to attain the pattern which will be followed throughout childhood. This pattern seems to be genetically determined and quite constant throughout childhood. Height achievement through childhood is correlated with mid-parent height. Mother–child correlations of height and weight are slightly higher than father–child correlations (1). There is considerable height variation among parents and their offspring but mid-parent height remains the most useful tool in describing the genetic relationship of growth between parents and children (2).

### Growth Velocity Versus Achievement

The child registers small but steady increments in height throughout childhood. If growth is plotted on a growth attainment chart, the growth curve describes essentially a straight line between the ages of 2 and 11 (Figure 4-1). Height velocity falls slowly throughout childhood, although not as dramatically as during the infancy period. Immediately before puberty, the height velocity reaches its lowest point in childhood. This is followed by the accelerated growth of puberty with its final deceleration and termination of growth (Figure 4-1). Weight gain, on the other hand, reaches a point of lowest velocity at about 2 years of age and then slowly

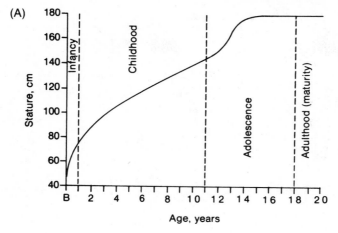

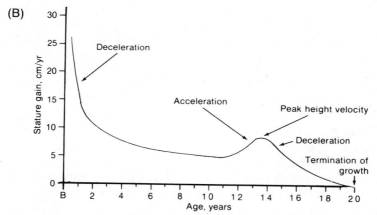

**Figure 4-1.** (A) A distance curve for stature (growth achievement curve) showing the different periods of postnatal growth. Note the steady growth pattern in childhood from 2–11 years. (B) A velocity curve showing different phases of growth for stature. Note the slow fall of height velocity through the childhood period (ages 2–11) sandwiched in between decelerating growth of infancy and the acceleration of puberty. (Reproduced by permission from Malina RM: *Growth and Development: The First 20 Years in Man.* Minneapolis, Burgess Publishing Company, 1975.)

increases throughout childhood. Acceleration of weight gain accompanies the pubertal growth spurt. After the second year of life, growth in height proceeds at a rate of at least 5 cm/yr and the weight increase is about 2.5 kg/yr. Although the growth during childhood is generally steady, some children exhibit a mild increase in growth velocity at about age 6 or 7, the so-called "mid-growth" spurt. This growth acceleration is inconstant and

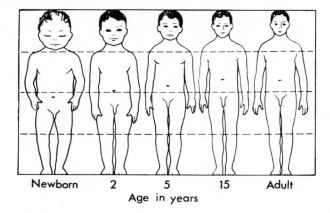

Newborn    2    5    15    Adult

Age in years

**Figure 4-2.** Changes in bodily proportion with age. The figures are divided into quarters by horizontal lines to emphasize relative sizes. Note the dramatic changes in relative size of head and lower limbs with increasing age and the change in the upper segment/lower segment ratio. (Reproduced by permission from Sinclair D: *Human Growth After Birth*, ed 3. London, Oxford University Press, 1978.)

of small magnitude. The cause of this phenomenon, when it does occur, is not known (3).

### Growth Patterns of Boys versus Girls

The growth patterns of boys and girls are very similar throughout childhood. In the last trimester of fetal growth and in early infancy boys grow a little faster than girls and are typically a little taller than girls; this growth differential is thought to be an androgen effect from the infant boy's testes. Growth velocities become equal by about 7 months and then the girls grow slightly faster until about age 4 (3). From then on until adolescence no difference in velocity can be detected (3). Girls become taller than boys at the beginning of adolescence because of earlier sexual maturation (and an earlier adolescent growth spurt).

### Changes in Shape and Body Proportion

The head of the infant is large compared to the remainder of the body because of the rapid growth of the brain in utero and in infancy. At birth, the ratio of head to body is about 1:4, but differential growth of the body and head reduces this proportion to 1:7.5 by adulthood (4) (Figure 4-2). Failure to appreciate this body–head disproportion in infancy led early European painters to depict the Christ child with adult proportions, lending an unreal aura to paintings of Madonna and child.

The lower limbs develop more slowly than the upper limbs or trunk, giving rise to what are termed "infatile body proportions." Expressed as a ratio of upper segment (crown to pubis) to lower segment (pubis to floor) the US/LS ratio is 1.7 at birth, that is, the head and trunk are nearly double the length of the lower extremities. By age 10, the lower limbs have grown at a sufficiently rapid rate to reduce this ratio to approximately 1. During adolescence there is a brief reversal of the ratio, which returns again to about one in adulthood (Figure 4-2). These changes in body proportion demonstrate a descending pattern of growth priority. The head matures before the trunk, and trunk before the limbs. The more peripheral parts of limbs mature earlier than the proximal parts, for example, the foot matures earlier than the thigh (4).

Changes occur in the spine and pelvis when the child assumes an upright posture (4). The spine of the infant is concave until the baby begins to hold its head up, producing a cervical convexity. The lumbar curvature develops when the baby sits at 6 to 8 months of age. When the baby stands, the lumbar curvature is increased. Because of a relatively large liver, his center of gravity is far forward and exaggeration of the lumbar curvature is necessary to maintain the vertical position. The infant assumes a bowlegged stance with legs wide apart; this slowly corrects itself so that by age 3 most children have a mildly knock-knee stance. By 6 years, the upright position can be easily maintained with legs straight. As the legs straighten and the weight is transmitted through the pelvis to the femora, the pelvis is remodelled. The sub-pubic angle is increased, the acetabula of the pelvis become deeper and the hip joints more stable (4).

## ORGAN AND TISSUE DEVELOPMENT IN CHILDHOOD

Most of the growth during childhood can be accounted for by muscle, fat, and bone growth. Most organ systems follow a growth pattern similar to overall body growth during childhood, but there are a few notable exceptions. The growth of neural tissue takes place early in infancy and childhood and, by late childhood, has achieved a nearly mature state. Lymphoid tissue, such as tonsils, thymus, and lymph nodes grow rapidly in early childhood, reaching their maximum size around puberty. After puberty, their size declines. The gonadal tissues undergo initial differentiation and maturation in utero and remain relatively unchanged throughout infancy and childhood.

### Muscle and Bone Growth

Nearly half of all tissue growth in childhood is growth of musculature. There is a steady increase in muscle mass paralleling the overall weight growth curve of the child. Bone growth, especially long bone growth, is responsible for the steady increase in height during childhood. Centers of ossification appear and mature in a predictable sequence throughout childhood. Epiphyseal growth centers during childhood can be used to determine the rate of physiologic maturation of the child. (See Chapter 6).

The skull continues to grow throughout childhood and it has nearly reached adult size by puberty. Sutures, the areas between bones of the skull, remain open, although closely meshed together. Facial growth is determined by growth of teeth, tongue and muscles of mastication. As teeth develop, the upper jaw increases in size and the mandible grows to maintain the bite between upper and lower teeth. Growth of the mandible and teeth are largely responsible for the changes in the appearance of the face during adolescence (4) (Figure 3-5).

By approximately 2 to 3 years of age, the twenty deciduous teeth have erupted. During early childhood, the face grows and the jaw widens to accommodate the developing permanent teeth. By age 6 the first permanent teeth, the "6-year" molars, have erupted and they are followed by sequential replacement of the deciduous teeth, usually in the same order as their appearance, beginning with the lower central incisors (5) (Tables 4-1 and 4-2).

## Growth of Fat

The growth of the fat deposits is somewhat unique. Fat deposits increase until around the end of the first year, then decrease until age 6 to 8 when they begin to increase again. "Girls have a little more total fat than boys at birth and the difference becomes gradually more marked during childhood" (3). After 8 years, the difference in subcutaneous tissue thickness between boys and girls diverges more widely.

## Growth of Internal Organs

Though there is growth in size of each organ to accommodate the needs of the enlarging child, differentiation and function accomplished in utero and during infancy are continued relatively unchanged throughout childhood. The *skin* becomes more cornified and is a more effective protective covering. *The senses* of touch, sight, hearing, and taste are well developed by childhood. The *circulatory system* is fully developed. The average pulse rate continues to fall gradually as the blood pressure rises. *Bone marrow* becomes restricted gradually to ribs, vertebrae, sternum, skull, and pelvis—the main locations of marrow in the adult. Childhood white blood counts are higher than adults; red blood cell counts and hemoglobin levels slightly lower. Fetal hemoglobin is completely replaced by adult hemoglobin by 6 years of age. *Immunologic competence* increases gradually throughout childhood. Vaccinations are used extensively in infancy and childhood to promote active protection against infection (6).

The lining of the *digestive system* is constantly replaced. Alveolar growth in the *respiratory system* continues until about age 8, leading to growth and arborization of the bronchioles. Maturation of the *urinary system* results in the improvement of concentrating and diluting capacity (6). *Brain* growth,

**Table 4-1. Chronology of Human Dentition**

*Primary or Deciduous Teeth*

| | Calcification | | Eruption | | Shedding | |
|---|---|---|---|---|---|---|
| | Begins at | Complete at | Maxillary | Mandibular | Maxillary | Mandibular |
| Central incisors | 5th fetal month | 18–24 months | 6–8 months | 5–7 months | 7–8 years | 6–7 years |
| Lateral incisors | 5th fetal month | 18–24 months | 8–11 months | 7–10 months | 8–9 years | 7–8 years |
| Cuspids (canines) | 6th fetal month | 30–36 months | 16–20 months | 16–20 months | 11–12 years | 9–11 years |
| First molars | 5th fetal month | 24–30 months | 10–16 months | 10–16 months | 10–11 years | 10–12 years |
| Second molars | 6th fetal month | 36 months | 20–30 months | 20–30 months | 10–12 years | 11–13 years |

Adapted from chart prepared by PK Losch, who carried out roentgenographic assays of the jaws of 1,000 children in metropolitan Boston in 1942 at the Harvard School of Dental Medicine and provided the data for this chart.

Reproduced with permission from Vaughan VC, McKay RJ, Behrman RE (eds), *Nelson's Textbook of Pediatrics*, ed 11. Philadelphia, WB Saunders Co, 1979, p 32.

## Table 4-2. Chronology of Human Dentition

| | Secondary or Permanent Teeth | | | |
| | Calcification | | Eruption | |
| | Begins at | Complete at | Maxillary | Mandibular |
|---|---|---|---|---|
| Central incisors | 3–4 months | 9–10 years | 7–8 years | 6–7 years |
| Lateral incisors | Max., 10–12 months Mand., 3–4 months | 10–11 years | 8–9 years | 7–8 years |
| Cuspids (canines) | 4–5 months | 12–15 years | 11–12 years | 9–11 years |
| First premolars (bicuspids) | 18–21 months | 12–13 years | 10–11 years | 10–12 years |
| Second premolars (bicuspids) | 24–30 months | 12–14 years | 10–12 years | 11–13 years |
| First molars | Birth | 9–10 years | 6–7 years | 6–7 years |
| Second molars | 30–36 months | 14–16 years | 12–13 years | 12–13 years |
| Third molars | Max., 7–9 years Mand., 8–10 years | 18–25 years | 17–22 years | 17–22 years |

Adapted from chart prepared by PK Losch, who carried out roentgeonographic assays of the jaws of 1000 children in metropolitan Boston in 1942 at the Harvard School of Dental Medicine and provided the data for this chart.

Reproduced with permission from Vaughan VC, McKay RJ, Behrman RE (eds). *Nelson's Textbook of Pediatrics*, ed 11. Philadelphia, WB Saunders Co, 1979, p 32.

still rapid during early childhood, decelerates so that by age 7, 90% and by 10, 95% of the adult brain weight has been achieved. Differentiation of most centers of the brain has been achieved by childhood, but there continues to be an increase in the complexity of functions and associations. Myelinization of nerve cells and growth of dendritic connections occur concomitantly with the increase in functional sophistication (3).

## DEVELOPMENTAL MILESTONES IN CHILDHOOD
### Preschool Years
In contrast to the self-centered behavior patterns of infancy and its immediate demands, the 2 to 6 year old is exploring his world, becoming aware of others, and becoming a social being. The following resumé of developmental milestones during childhood is taken from a behavior inventory appearing in "*Growth and Development of Children*", by Lowrey (6). Behavior characteristics described are those generally seen at various

age levels but should be applied with caution to the individual child. (He, his, etc. should also be read as she, hers, etc.)

At 30 months the child jumps up and down and walks backward, holds a crayon in his fist, copies a crude circle or closed figure, and names drawings of a house, shoe, ball, or dog. He refers to himself as "I", knows his full name, helps put things away, and unbuttons large buttons.

At 3 years, the child alternates feet going upstairs, rides a tricycle, holds a crayon with fingers, builds a tower of nine to ten cubes, and imitates a three-cube bridge. He copies a circle and imitates a cross, uses plurals, gives his sex and full name, obeys two prepositional commands, feeds himself well, and puts on his own shoes.

At 4 years, the child walks downstairs alternating feet, does a broad jump, throws a ball overhand, and hops on one foot. He can draw a man with two parts, copy a cross, count three objects correctly, imitate a five-cube gate, name one or more colors correctly, and obey five prepositional commands. He washes and dries his face and hands, brushes his teeth, distinguishes the front from the back of clothes, laces shoes, and goes on errands.

At 5 years, the child skips alternating feet, stands on one foot, catches a bounced ball, draws a man with body, head, and most complete parts, copies a triangle, and counts ten objects correctly. He knows four colors, makes descriptive comments on pictures, can carry out three assigned jobs, dresses and undresses without assistance, and prints a few letters.

At 6 years, the child throws well, stands on each foot alternately with eyes closed, walks backward, can walk heel to toe, draws a man with neck, hands, and clothes, and copies a diamond. He defines words by function or composition (e.g., a house is to live in), ties shoelaces, differentiates a.m. and p.m., knows the right from the left, and counts up to 30 (6).

The Denver Developmental Screening Test (DDST) can be used to assess developmental milestones up to the age of 6 (7). The DDST shows the average age at which gross motor, language, fine motor-adaptive and personal-social skills are generally achieved (Figure 3-7).

## Mid-Childhood Years

During early school years the child becomes increasingly independent of his/her parents, exploring the world outside his/her home and forming close friendships which may take the form of clubs and groups. The child develops a feeling of individuality and sometimes his/her attempts at independence are irritating to parents and cause behavior problems at school. This is a period of increasing contact with others and of development of the concept of cooperation. It is characterized by concrete thinking. The following characteristics from a behavior inventory by Lowrey display the increasingly sophisticated behavior of the child during the mid-childhood years (6).

The 6-year-old is restless and has difficulty making decisions. Activity is almost constant. He is good at starting things, but poor at finishing them. Accidents at the table are common. Rudeness and temper tantrums are also frequent. Behavior patterns are explosive and unpredictable. Jealousy toward siblings is the rule. Play is imaginative. Favorite radio or TV programs are followed religiously. Most 6-year-olds like school and want to learn. Parental love and praise are very important (6).

The 7-year-old is more apt to be thoughtful and pensive. He has likes and dislikes, but is less vehement in expressing them. He is adept at dressing and undressing and becomes conscious of his own sex and avoids self exposure in front of the opposite sex. He is introspective and needs approbation from his peers and parents. He is cooperative but, at the same time, tends to dawdle and be sloppy. He can tell time, copy a diamond, grasp the basic idea of addition and subtraction, and repeat five numbers in a series (6).

The 8-year-old has smoothness and poise. Play becomes very rowdy. He plays with others, but prefers those of his own sex. He is aware of social approval and behaves better away from home or with strangers. He is developing special interests and hobbies and reads or watches much TV. The eight-year-old generally enjoys school. He knows the days of the week. He can make correct change for money. He appreciates the difference between real and fictitious characters (6).

The 9-year-old has the capacity to complete tasks, even if interrupted. He plans ahead for work and play. He is truthful and honest and self-sufficient. He can dress himself without help and is anxious to please. He tends to have better manners. He plays or associates only with those of his own sex. He can tell time and date and do simple multiplication and division and tends to be critical, especially of himself (6).

## Prepubertal Years

At age 10, the girl becomes more poised and socially mature than the boy and sexual maturation may begin (girls). Both boys and girls are aware of social problems. Most events and people are categorized as good or bad and the desires of the 10-year-old are ambiguous. Team work becomes possible. Friendships are very important and lasting friendships are frequently formed.

By age 11, girls are apt to be taller than boys because of an earlier adolescent growth spurt, but they are apt to be behind boys in physical strength and endurance. Membership in groups and clubs is increasingly important. The child becomes more critical of his own labors, and there is an urge for financial independence. The 11-year-old can define some abstract terms, such as justice, honesty, and revenge, which leads quite naturally into the abstract thinking characteristic of adolescence. The 11-year-old tends to be shy and has a diversity of interests and skills. Both

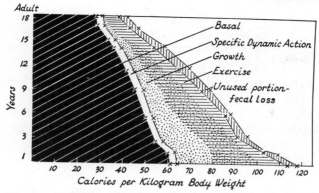

**Figure 4-3.** Total daily expenditure of calories per kilogram of body weight at different ages with approximate distribution among requirements for basal growth, exercise, and other factors. (Calorie = kilocalorie = kcal). (Reproduced by permission from Vaughan VC, McKay RJ, Berhman RE (eds), in *Nelson Textbook of Pediatrics*, ed 11. Philadelphia, WB Saunders Co, 1979.)

boys and girls are on the threshold of adolescence, both physically and mentally, though girls usually precede boys by 1 or 2 years (6).

## NUTRITION IN CHILDHOOD

Growth of the child depends upon provision of adequate nutrients. The high caloric requirements of infancy decrease as the rate of growth decelerates, so that by age 3, the requirement for calories has decreased to about 90 kcal/kg per day, and by age 12, has decreased further to about 70 kcal/kg (Figure 4-3). There is considerable variation in the distribution of calories used for growth and for activity or exercise, as can be appreciated from the distribution pattern shown in Figure 4-3. Since growth during childhood is slow and steady, the food required for basal metabolism and growth will be fairly constant. Variability in caloric requirements will depend primarily upon the amount of activity in which the child engages (8).

### Basic Nutritional Requirements

There is a need in childhood for all the basic nutrients described in the previous chapter. The young child is learning to feed himself and developing tastes for a variety of foods. He may at times seem to be eating poorly because of an exaggerated interest in a specific food or foods, but if allowed to choose from a variety of foods, he will eventually choose foods representing a fairly balanced meal plan.

Adequate nutrients can be supplied by offering a variety of foods from the four basic groups: (1) milk, (2) meat and eggs, (3) fruits and vegetables, and (4) breads and cereals. If variety is offered, even if not always consumed, most children will not suffer from deficiencies of protein, calories, minerals, or vitamins. It is, nonetheless, customary to offer supplements of Vitamins A, D, and C through at least early childhood, and fluoride throughout childhood, to reduce tooth decay and provide adequate enamel hardening.

The 5-year-old usually has a good appetite, although he may have no time for breakfast. He may be slow in eating but usually gets sufficient calories despite his tendency to dawdle. The 6-year-old is very active and frequently requests food, but usually starts a meal and snack better than he finishes it. The 7-year-old is developing likes and dislikes in food and a host of other things. Patience, and a good example from parents and older children, will pay off in helping the child to develop good eating habits and an interest in wholesome food. By 9 years, the child can eat carefully and neatly. He is quite self-sufficient and can usually choose his own food with a minimum of supervision. The athletically active child is becoming muscular and eats to supply energy for his activities, while the more sedentary child handles food somewhat more circumspectly (6).

## Nutritional Deficiencies of Childhood

Except among children of low income families and certain cults and religious sects with dietary proscriptions, protein-calorie malnutrition is uncommon in this country. Families on a very limited budget may be unable to provide optimal diversity of food, and this may contribute to specific nutrient deficiencies such as iron deficiency anemia, or Vitamin D deficiency rickets. The ten state nutrition survey targeted iron deficiency as the most prevalent nutritional problem among children in the United States (9), though there has been some interest recently in the relationship of growth to trace metal deficiencies such as zinc. Although zinc has been implicated in growth failure in animals and in man, it is difficult to establish the connection between clinical signs and laboratory measurements of trace metals in tissues and fluids. Walravens and Hambidge claim that zinc intake is low in two-thirds of low income children with short stature and suggest that inadequate zinc may be contributing to the growth failure in preschool children from low income families (10). Families deprived of meat as a source of protein may well encounter zinc deficiency, but at the moment there are no laboratory assays which can unequivocally demonstrate zinc deficiency, though hair and plasma zinc levels are often low when zinc intake is inadequate.

Low levels of trace minerals or vitamins are commonly found in disorders of maldigestion (cystic fibrosis) or malabsorption (celiac disease), but it is difficult to separate specific nutrient deficiencies from the overall protein-calorie malnutrition. Supplements of vitamins and minerals are often used together with therapeutic measures aimed at reducing the malabsorption to improve the nutritional status and prevent or correct deficiencies of vitamins or minerals.

## ENDOCRINE REGULATION OF GROWTH IN CHILDHOOD

Among the hormones which are required for adequate growth in childhood are human growth hormone, somatomedin, thyroid hormone, and insulin. Vitamin D, calcitonin, and parathormone are required for regulation of calcium and phosphorus for bone growth and bone remodelling. Glucocorticoids and adrenal androgens may influence growth under special circumstances. Androgens, estrogens, and gonadotropins play a minor role in regulation of growth during childhood but assume a major role in growth stimulation during adolescence.

Many of the growth-promoting hormones have highly developed and complex regulatory systems involving target tissues, primary hormones, trophic hormones from the pituitary, hypothalamic humoral factors, and higher centers of the central nervous system with elaborate feedback stimulation or suppression systems (Figure 4-4). The specificity of each hormone for its target tissue resides in receptors which are located on or within cells of the target tissue and upon the competancy of the tissue to respond to the hormonal signal. Each hormone reacts with specific receptors to bring about the chain of events leading to the action for which the hormone was designed. In Figure 4-4, the interdependence of hormones is depicted to illustrate that growth of bone is dependent upon a series of hormones, each in turn regulated by other hormones. In the illustration, somatomedins are shown to be formed in the liver, a prototype of the endocrine somatomedin production; as paracrine hormones, these growth promoting peptides are also produced in a number of other target tissues (11).

### Human Growth Hormone System

When human growth hormone (hGH) from the pituitary gland was initially discovered, it was generally assumed that it affected target tissues directly to promote growth. However, intensive continuing research has brought to light a group of intermediate hormones, the somatomedins, which seem now to be the primary hormones which stimulate cellular growth. Although growth hormone affects fat and carbohydrate metabolism directly, most of its growth-promoting properties are mediated via somatomedins. Since the growth hormone–somatomedin system is pivotal to regulation of growth in childhood, we shall describe in some detail the actions and regulation of the components of this system of growth regulation as currently understood.

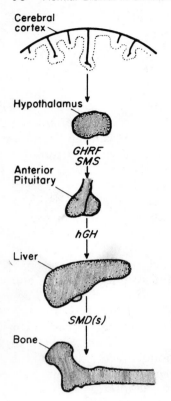

**Figure 4-4.** Growth hormone regulating system (axis). GHRF = growth hormone releasing factor, SMS = somatostatin, hGH = human growth hormone (pituitary), SMD(s) = somatomedin(s). (Reproduced by permission from Rimoin DL, Horton WA: Short stature, Part I. *J Pediatr* **92**:523, 1978.)

## Human Growth Hormone

*Human growth hormone* is a single chain peptide of 191 amino acids with two disulphide bridges. It is formed in the pituitary gland, in the cells which stain with acidophilic stains, and is the most abundant polypeptide hormone in the pituitary. From 5 to 10 milligrams of human growth hormone can be extracted from a single pituitary gland (12). Growth hormones are found in most mammals, but they are generally species specific; the only growth hormones active in humans are those from human or simian pituitaries. Growth hormone is measured in the serum by means of a radioimmunoassay. It is secreted in bursts, resulting in random levels of 0 to 20 ng/mL and from 7 to 60 ng/mL with stimulation (13).

The actions of growth hormone can be divided into two main groups; the growth promoting actions and the anti-insulin actions (Figure 4-5). Growth hormone stimulates growth of cartilage and deposition of calcium for bone formation. In the muscle, growth hormone stimulates protein synthesis and an increase in muscle mass (hyperplasia), and is essential for the adaptive growth of kidney tissue after the loss of one kidney.

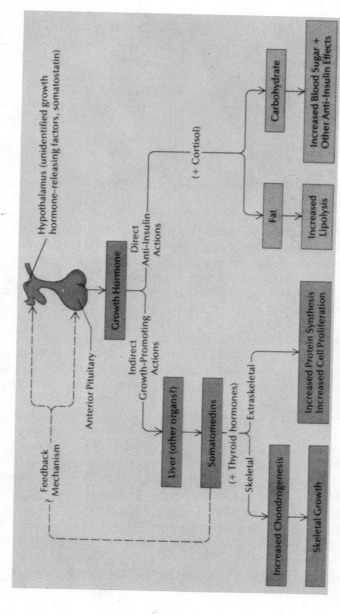

**Figure 4-5.** Actions of human growth hormone. Growth promoting actions on skeletal cells and protein synthesis are mediated by somatomedins and influenced positively by thyroid hormones. Anti-insulin action on fat and carbohydrate is direct and is similar to anti-insulin action of cortisol. (Reproduced by permission from Van Wyk JJ, Underwood LE: Growth hormone, somatomedins, and growth failure. *Hosp Pract* **13**(August):57, 1978, illustration by A. Miller.)

These growth promoting actions of growth hormone, that is, increased chondrogenesis and skeletal growth and increased protein synthesis and cell proliferation, appear to be mediated by the actions of somatomedins, the small peptides formed in organs such as the liver and kidney and in target tissues under stimulation by growth hormone (13) (Figure 4-5).

Growth hormone also promotes lipolysis and a decrease in fat deposits. In the liver, the released fat is transformed into β-hydroxy-butyrate and acetoacetate and there is an increase in serum ketones. This action on fat tissues is similar to that produced by glucocorticoids. A low blood sugar promotes release of growth hormone which acts synergistically with glucocorticoids, epinephrine, and glucagon to normalize the blood sugar. These actions of growth hormone are termed anti-insulin actions. Excess growth hormone, such as is seen in acromegaly, may lead to persistent elevation of blood sugar, that is, growth hormone is "diabetogenic". The anti-insulin effects of growth hormone appear to be either a direct action of growth hormone or the action of "closely related diabetogenic peptides acting in concert with cortisol" (13).

The secretion of growth hormone seems to be chiefly regulated by humoral substances from the hypothalamus. The hypothalamic releasing and inhibiting substances are themselves stimulated or inhibited by a variety of stimuli (low blood glucose, peptide hormones, amino acids), the most important being the levels of growth hormone or of somatomedin in the blood stream (14, 15) (Figures 4-4 and 4-5).

### Growth Hormone Releasing Factor

*Growth hormone releasing factor* (GHRF) is formed in the medial basal area of the hypothalamus; lesions in this area result in growth failure and lack of release of growth hormone in response to stress or insulin-induced hypoglycemia. Growth hormone is secreted in bursts and levels vary widely, but a single burst of growth hormone stimulates production of somatomedins sufficiently to raise somatomedin levels for at least 24 hours, insuring continuous stimulation of growth (16). Spontaneous bursts are common, as are bursts after strenuous exercise or stress. The most consistent bursts of growth hormone occur during sleep. An increase in the number of bursts occurs during the growth spurt of adolescence, although average levels in the blood do not seem to be elevated. Pharmacologic agents which may stimulate secretion include insulin, L-arginine, glucagon, L-dopa, norepinephrine, and serotonin. The stimulating effects of some of these agents provide a basis for provocative tests of growth hormone secretory capacity.

### Somatostatin

*Somatostatin*, also known as somatotrophin release inhibiting factor or SRIF, is a fourteen amino acid compound found in the central nervous system, the pancreas and the stomach. SRIF inhibits the release of growth hormone to all known stimuli. It also inhibits insulin and glucagon secretion from the pancreas and suppresses gastrin, secretin and other G.I. hormones. The precise physiologic role of somatostatin is unknown, but it appears to be an inhibitor of growth hormone secretion and possibly other pituitary hormones as well (13, 15, 17).

## Somatomedin

The growth promoting actions of growth hormone appear to be mediated by a group of small peptides called *insulin-like growth factors* (IGF) or *somatomedins* (Sm) (12). An insulin-like growth factor can be defined as a structural analogue of insulin that exerts insulin-like biological effects, while "somatomedin" implies that the IGF level is regulated by growth hormone (18). Two main types of IGF have been characterized by their immunological and structural properties and by their receptor reactivity (18): IGF I, which is also called somatomedin C (Sm C) (19), and IGF II, analogous to "multiplication stimulating activity" (MSA) in the rat (20). The identification and characterization of somatomedins (and that of tissue growth factors) is a field of intense interest and rapid change. The descriptions given here will undoubtedly be revised as our understanding of peptide growth factors increases. The major growth promoting actions of the somatomedins include cartilage stimulating activity, insulin-like activity, and mitogenic activity. When compared with insulin, "somatomedins appear to have a greater potency in stimulating cartilage growth, comparable potency for insulin-like activity in muscle but less in fat, and more potency for mitogenic activity" (21).

The IGF peptides resemble insulin in size, sequence of amino acids and, to some extent, molecular structure. Therefore, it is not surprising that IGF I and II elicit biological responses similar to those of insulin (18). IGF stimulates glycogen accumulation in muscle and transfer of amino acids into cells for protein synthesis. Effects of IGF on lipid storage are much less striking than those of insulin (22). Levels of IGF in serum are much higher than those of pancreatic insulin; it follows then that much of the circulatory IGF must be inactive to prevent permanent hypoglycemia (23). The binding of IGF to its carrier protein inhibits its access to cell membrane receptors, rendering it metabolically inactive. The somatomedin-carrier protein complex has a long life and may play a role in tissue selectivity and delivery of somatomedin to target tissues (16). In promoting chondrogenesis, somatomedins stimulate synthesis of RNA, DNA, and protein and incorporation of sulfate into proteoglycan and of proline into collagen (24). Long term growth effects include cell multiplication and cell differentiation (18).

Somatomedin production is stimulated by pituitary growth hormone, but a number of other stimulating and inhibitory factors affect the final action of somatomedins (Figure 4-6). In the figure, the liver is depicted as the source of somatomedins. It should be remembered that other

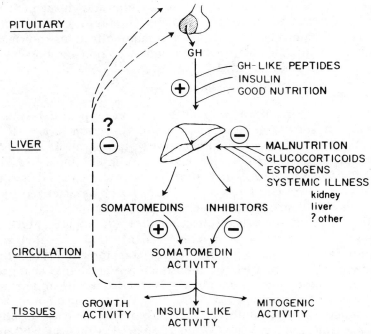

**Figure 4-6.** Regulation of somatomedin activity. Factors regulating somatomedin production and activity include positive factors such as growth hormone, insulin, nutrition, and growth hormone-like peptides, as well as negative factors such as malnutrition, systemic illness, some hormones, and a negative feedback system. (Reproduced by permission from Phillips LS, Vassilopoulou-Sellin R: Somatomedins. *New Engl J Med* **302:**439, 1980.)

organs (lung, heart) and target tissues (muscle, bone) may also be sites of somatomedin production (11). Somatomedin production may be enhanced by good nutrition, by insulin, and by growth hormone-like peptides (21). Human prolactin and human chorionic somatomammotropin (placental lactogen) have amino acid structures similar to that of growth hormone and have weak but demonstrable growth-promoting activity, thought to be the result of stimulation of somatomedin production. Chorionic somatomammotropin (hCS) may be responsible for normal levels of somatomedin in pregnancy and may play a pivotal role in regulation of embryonic or fetal growth (25). In some children, after removal of hypothalamic tumors, there is a period of normal or catch-up growth accompanied by normal somatomedin levels, even though growth hormone is absent or low (26, 27). Such youngsters often become obese from overeating and the somatomedin production is thought to be modulated by the increased insulin accompanying the obesity (28).

Somatomedin production is inhibited by under-nutrition and chronic disease. Children with protein-calorie malnutrition (kwashiorkor) have low somatomedin activity and poor growth despite normal growth hormone levels. Animal studies have suggested that when protein deficiency is present, somatomedins, even when present, cannot stimulate normal cartilage production. These data suggest that the effects of nutrition on somatomedin activity and production may be of equal, or even greater importance than that of growth hormone (29) (Figure 4-6). Not surprisingly, in liver disease there is a decrease in somatomedin production which appears to be related to effects of liver failure on protein production. In kidney failure, somatomedin levels are normal but there is a decrease in somatomedin activity attributed to low molecular weight inhibitors which blunt the ability of somatomedins to stimulate protein synthesis and cellular growth (29). Inhibition of somatomedin production and/or activity has been suggested to be present also in malnutrition (esp. anorexia nervosa) and in diabetes (21). Insulin deficiency with development of hyperglycemia and ketonemia is associated with a fall in somatomedin activity and decreased cartilage growth. This cannot be reversed by human growth hormone administration without simultaneous restoration of good control of diabetes with intensive insulin therapy (29). Both insulin and good nutritional status seem to be necessary for growth hormone to exert its effect on somatomedin production (29). The growth-promoting effects of insulin and of nutrition can best be understood by their interrelationship with somatomedins.

Somatomedin production is blunted by glucocorticoid excess and by pharmacologic dosages of estrogens (28) (Figure 4-6). The impairment of growth by glucocorticoids is caused by inhibition of cartilage growth and blunting of the growth stimulating effect of growth hormone. This antagonism of growth by glucocorticoids occurs with supraphysiologic amounts of cortisol and appears to be due to impairment of somatomedin activity by somatomedin inhibitors (29) or a direct inhibitory effect of cortisol on the target tissue (11). In most children, growth delay is seen only when the dosage of cortisol exceeds 45 mg/m$^2$/day, though there is abundant evidence that, at least in younger children, lower dosages can suppress growth. The metabolic and growth-promoting effects of growth hormone are also blunted by pharmacological dosages of estrogens. These actions are attributed to a decrease in somatomedin production (28). Androgens appear to have no direct affect on cartilage or on somatomedin production (28). Direct effects of thyroid on somatomedin production or activity have not been shown, though thyroid does appear to potentiate the stimulation of growth by growth hormone. Conversely, the growth-promoting effects of growth hormone are blunted by thyroid deficiency, which is associated with low plasma levels of Sm C/IGF I (28).

Both human growth hormone and somatomedin play a vital role in insuring adequate growth throughout childhood. The child with growth hormone deficiency grows very slowly throughout childhood and never achieves normal adult size unless supplementary hormone can be provided. In children with growth hormone deficiency, administration of human growth hormone produces a noticeable increase in growth rate. There is stimulation of protein synthesis with increase in lean body mass and relative loss of body fat. The changes in muscle and fat reach a peak after about 1 month of treatment whereas peak linear growth is usually not seen until about 3 to 6 months (3).

In normal children somatomedin levels are correlated with age. Low values are found in early childhood with highest values at puberty (11). Somatomedin levels are lower in infants than in children and adults, yet the rate of growth in infants is much higher than that of children. The rapid growth of infancy would be more understandable if infant cartilage were more sensitive to somatomedin growth-promoting activity. Cartilage of young animals seems more sensitive to somatomedin than that of older animals and this may also be true of human infants and children. Rapid fetal growth poses an even greater problem of interpretation. Somatomedin levels are detectable in the fetus throughout pregnancy but are lower than maternal levels. Somatomedin levels do correlate with the fetal length and weight, suggesting that they play a role in intrauterine growth (25). The Laron dwarf, however, with low somatomedin levels unresponsive to growth hormone, appears to be only modestly small at birth, suggesting that other growth factors may be operative in utero as well.

From the discussion of factors affecting somatomedin activity above, it is clear that regulation of the growth process is complex and that hormones, peptides, and paracrine growth factors all affect and are affected by many factors including sensitivity of the target tissue to the humoral messengers. With the recent rapid development of our understanding of IGF peptides and tissue growth factors, it is quite possible that other levels of regulation may soon be discovered.

### Insulin

Insulin is one of the body's chief anabolic hormones. It facilitates entry of glucose and amino acids into cells and promotes lipogenesis, glycogenesis, and protein synthesis. Similarities between the action of insulin and somatomedins suggest that they may act in concert to bring about growth at the cellular level (Figure 4-7). Insulin may play a permissive role in growth hormone stimulation of somatomedin production. Insulin is required for the full anabolic effect of growth hormone, although its major action is probably to provide substrate for cellular metabolism (25).

### Thyroid Hormone

The role of thyroid hormone in growth of children has been recognized for many years. Deficiency of thyroid leads to decreased growth and delay in skeletal maturation. In the fetus and infant, thyroid is essential for

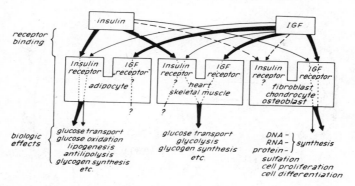

**Figure 4-7.** Complementary anabolic action of insulin and IGF. (Reproduced with permission from Zapf J, Schmid Ch, Froesch ER: Biological and immunological properties of insulin-like growth factors (IGF) I and II. *Clin Endocrinol Metab* **13**:3, 1984.)

brain maturation. Failure of development of the thyroid may lead to variable degrees of mental impairment after birth. Recognition in the immediate neonatal period and early replacement therapy may reduce the amount of brain damage (30).

Both thyroxine ($T_4$) and triiodothyronine ($T_3$) are produced by the thyroid gland, though much of the $T_4$ is transformed to $T_3$ at the tissue level. $T_3$ is three to four times as active biologically as $T_4$ and is generally considered to be the active thyroid principle at the tissue level. The precise role of thyroid hormones in stimulating growth has not been defined, though thyroxine stimulates hypertrophy of chondrocytes in synergism with growth hormone and promotes mineralization of the skeleton by accelerating bone resorption and formation (30). Progressive development and growth at the epiphyseal growth plates (skeletal maturation) seems to depend on thyroxine, and a lack of thyroid hormone at any time results in profound delay in skeletal maturation and/or epiphyseal dysgenesis (fragmented ossification and deformity of the epiphyses).

Thyroxine, like insulin, must be present for growth hormone to exert its full effect on growth. Furthermore, a normal thyroid state is essential for growth hormone secretion to occur optimally. The basis for this "permissive" action of thyroid is not known. The widespread influence of thyroxine on body metabolism and growth processes has led to the presumption that thyroxine's chief role in growth is a permissive one. Normal thyroxine levels may be necessary for other tissues, including those forming other hormones, to function normally (3).

Thyroxine production and release from the thyroid is stimulated by TSH (thyroid stimulating hormone) from the pituitary gland which, in

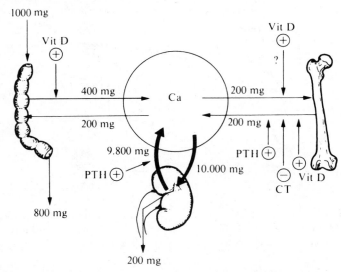

**Figure 4-8.**  Major sites of action of Vitamin D, parathyroid hormone (PTH), and calcitonin (CT) showing stimulation (+) or inhibition (−) of hormonal action on *calcium* at bone, kidney, and gut. (Reproduced by permission from Russell RG: Regulation of calcium metabolism. *Ann Clin Biochem* **13:**518, 1976.)

turn, is released in response to thyrotropin releasing hormone (TRH) from the hypothalamus. TSH levels rise whenever thyroxine becomes deficient and falls again when the thyroxine level is sufficient. This finely tuned negative feedback system is highly responsive to circulating hormone levels.

### Calcium–Phosphorus Homeostasis

The growth of bones and hence, height of an individual, may be determined primarily through actions of growth hormone, somatomedin and thyroid, but the mineralization of bone clearly contributes to the normal growth process and deficiency of bone mineralization produces deformities and disordered growth. Bone formation and mineralization are intimately related to calcium and phosphorus homeostasis, which in turn, is regulated by Vitamin D, parathyroid hormone (PTH), and calcitonin (Figure 4-8).

Deposition of calcium salts in cartilage to form bone is stimulated by Vitamin D, a hormone formed from a sterol derived from the skin by phototransformation of cholesterol. Vitamin D (cholecalciferol) is hydroxylated in the liver and kidney to produce 1,25-dihydroxy-cholecalciferol, the active form of Vitamin D. Vitamin D promotes calcium absorption from the gut, regulates calcium deposition and absorption from bone, and regulates calcium and phosphate resorption from the kidney (in concert with PTH) (Figure 4-8).

Parathyroid hormone (PTH) affects serum calcium level by promoting resorption of calcium from bone, stimulating resorption of calcium and excretion of phosphorus by the kidney, and indirectly promoting calcium absorption from the gut by promoting formation of dihydroxy-Vitamin D by stimulation of 1-alpha-hydroxylation in the kidney (Figure 4-8). Calcitonin, formed in the parafollicular cells of the thyroid, acts to prevent excessive calcium levels in the serum by inhibiting calcium absorption from bone and blocking calcium resorption by the kidney tubule. PTH and calcitonin participate in bone resorption and remodeling by stimulating or inhibiting the actions of osteoblasts and osteoclasts. Together Vitamin D, PTH, and calcitonin present a finely balanced mechanism which keeps the calcium and phosphate levels within a physiologic range to provide minerals required for bone formation.

## Glucocorticoids

Glucocorticoids, primarily cortisol from the adrenal cortex, do not seem to have a major role in regulation of normal growth processes, but in pathologic or pharmacologic amounts, they may exert a profound effect on growth (31). Growth retardation is one of the prominent signs in Cushing syndrome and in children treated with pharmacologic doses of corticosteroids. Glucocorticoids may interfere with growth by suppression of growth hormone secretion, blockage of growth hormone action, or by direct inhibition of cartilage proliferation (30). Excess cortisol interferences with growth in hypopituitary dwarfs receiving treatment with growth hormone (32). Low somatomedin levels in children treated with cortisone suggests that cortisol may interfere with growth hormone action by blocking somatomedin production (33). In addition, glucocorticoids may interfere with somatomedin stimulation of chondrocyte growth per se (34). Growing cartilage is very sensitive to glucocorticoids. Amounts just minimally above normal may block DNA synthesis and interfere with normal somatic growth (30).

## FACTORS AFFECTING GROWTH IN CHILDHOOD

Growth in childhood appears to be determined first and foremost by the genetic template inherited from the child's parents and by growth patterns already established and modified by genetic influences in intrauterine and infancy periods. Nutrition which is adequate to provide substrate for energy and growth and appropriate amounts of growth-promoting hormones for regulation and guidance of growth are of paramount importance.

Developmental defects, enzyme deficiencies, hormonal deficiencies or tissue unresponsiveness (lack of specific receptors for endogenous growth stimulators) represent some of the intrinsic factors that might influence growth. In addition, numerous environmental factors such as disease, toxins, malnutrition, psycho-social deprivation, tumors, or destruction of hormone-producing glands may interfere with expected growth achievements. The effects of such factors on growth will be the subject of Chapter 9, entitled "Growth Disorders in Childhood."

## REFERENCES

1. Mueller WH: Parent–child correlations for stature and height. *Hum Biol* **48:**379, 1976.
2. Tanner JM, Israelsohn WJ: Parent–child correlations for body measurements of children between ages of one month and seven years. *Ann Hum Genet* **26:**245, 1963.
3. Tanner JM: *Fetus Into Man: Physical Growth from Conception to Maturity.* Cambridge, Harvard University Press, 1978, pp 7–23, 87–102, 103–116.
4. Sinclair D: *Human Growth After Birth,* ed 3. London, Oxford University Press, 1978, pp 21–45, 68–97, 117–139.
5. Taranger J, Lichtenstein H, Svennberg-Redegren I: Dental development from birth to 16 years. *Acta Paediatr Scand* [Suppl], **258:**83–96, 1976.
6. Lowrey GH: *Growth and Development of Children,* ed. 7. Year Book Medical Publishers, 1978, pp 133–198, 205–278.
7. Frankenberg WK, Dodds JB: The Denver Developmental Screening Test. *J Pediatr* **71:**181, 1967.
8. Barness LA: Nutrition and nutritional disorders, in Vaughan VC, McKay RJ, Behrman RE (eds), *Nelson's Textbook of Pediatrics.* Philadelphia, WB Saunders Co., 1979, pp 173–189.
9. Ten State Nutritional Survey: 1968–1970, U.S. Department of Health, Education, and Welfare, HEW Publication No. (HSM)72-8130.
10. Walravens PA, Hambridge KM: Growth of infants fed zinc supplemented formulas. *Am J Clin Nutr* **29:**1114, 1976.
11. Hall K, Sara VR: Somatomedin levels in childhood, adolescence and adult life. *Clin Endocrinol Metab* **13:**91, 1984.
12. Van Wyk JJ, Underwood LE, Hintz RL, et al: Somatomedins: A family of insulin-like hormones under growth hormone control. *Recent Prog Horm Res* **30:**259, 1974.
13. Van Wyk JJ, Underwood LE: Growth hormone, somatomedins, and growth failure, *Hosp Pract* **13**(August):57–67, 1978.
14. Martin JB: Brain regulation of growth hormone secretion, in Martin L, Ganong WF (eds), *Frontiers in Neuro-Endocrinology.* New York, Raven Press, Vol. 4, 1976, p 129.
15. Martin JB: Neural regulation of growth hormone secretion. *Med Clin North Am* **62:**327, 1978.
16. Hintz RL: Plasma forms of somatomedin and the binding protein phenomenon. *Clin Endocrinol Metab* **13:**31, 1984.
17. Gerich JE, Patton GS: Somatostatin: Physiology and clinical applications. *Med Clin North Am* **62:**375–392, 1978.
18. Zapf J, Schmid Ch, Froesch ER: Biological and immunological properties of insulin-like growth factors (IGF) I and II, *Clin Endocrinol Metab* **13:**3, 1984.
19. Klapper DC, Svoboda ME, Van Wyk JJ: Sequence analysis of somatomedin-C: Confirmation of identity with insulin-like growth factor I. *Endocrinology* **112:**2215, 1983.
20. Rechler MM, Nissley SP, King GL, et al: Multiplication stimulating activity (MSA) from the BRL 3A rat liver cell line: Relation to human somatomedin and insulin. *J Supramol Struct and Cell Biochem* **15:**253, 1981.

21. Phillips LS, Vassilopoulou-Sellin R: Somatomedins. *N Engl J Med* **302:**371–380, 438–446, 1980.

22. Poggi C, LeMarchand-Brustel Y, Zapf J, et al: Effects and binding of insulin-like growth factor I (IGF I) in the isolated soleus muscle of lean and obese mice: Comparison with insulin. *Endocrinology* **105:**723, 1979.

23. Zapf J, Walter H, Froesch ER: Radioimmunological determination of insulin-like growth factors I and II in normal subjects and in patients with growth disorders and extra hepatic tumor hypoglycemia. *J Clin Invest* **68:**1321, 1981.

24. Zapf J, Froesch ER, Humbel RE: The insulin-like growth factors (IGF) of human serum: Chemical and biological characterization and aspects of their possible physiologic role. *Curr Topics in Cell Reg* **19:**257, 1981.

25. Underwood LE, D'Ercole AJ: Insulin and insulin-like growth factors/somatomedins in fetal and neonatal development. *Clin Endocrinol Metab* **13:**69, 1984.

26. Kenny FM, Guyda HJ, Wright JC, et al: Prolactin and somatomedin in hypopituitary patients with "catch-up" growth following operations for craniopharyngioma. *J Clin Endocrinol Metab* **36:**378, 180, 1973.

27. Costin G, Kogut MD, Phillips LS, et al: Craniopharyngioma: The role of insulin in promoting post-operative growth. *Clin Endocrinol Metabl* **42:**370, 1976.

28. Clemmons DR, Van Wyk JJ: Factors controlling blood concentration of somatomedin-C. *Clin Endocrinol Metab* **13:**113, 1984.

29. Phillips LS, Unterman TG: Somatomedin activity in disorders of nutrition and metabolism. *Clin Endocrinol Metab* **13:**145, 1984.

30. Sizonenko PC: Endocrinological control of growth. *Postgrad Med J* **54**(1):91, 1978.

31. Mosier HD Jr, Smith FG Jr, Schultz MA: Failure of catch-up growth after Cushing's syndrome in childhood. *Am J Dis Child* **124:**251, 1972.

32. Soyka LF, Crawford JD: Antagonism of cortisone of the linear growth in hypopituitary patients and hypophysectimized rats with human growth hormone. *J Clin Endocrinol Metab* **25:**469, 1965.

33. Elders MJ, Wingfield BS, McNatt ML, et al: Glucocorticoid therapy in children. *Am J Dis Child* **129:**1393, 1975.

34. Rappaport R: Hormonal control of skeletal growth and maturation. *Acta Endocrinol* **199**(Suppl):71, 1975.

# 5
# Growth and Maturation in Adolescence

*Puberty* is "the stage of maturation in which an individual becomes physiologically capable of sexual reproduction" (1) and is characterized by maturation of the organs of reproduction, development of secondary sexual characteristics, and acceleration of somatic growth (the adolescent growth spurt). *Adolescence* is the period in life of an individual in which pubertal maturation takes place and encompasses the sexual maturation, growth, and psychological and behavioral changes which take place simultaneously. The two terms may be used interchangeably when speaking of the physiological events surrounding puberty. For girls, this period roughly encompasses the ages 10½–15 years and for boys, 11½–16 years.

## THE ADOLESCENT GROWTH SPURT

At puberty there is a rapid growth spurt accompanied by characteristic changes in body shape and composition, emphasizing specific physical differences between boys and girls. The acceleration of growth at puberty represents a brief return to the rapid growth rate of infancy. It is, however, short-lived, and soon after reaching the peak growth rate, growth decelerates rapidly until growth ceases (Figure 5-1). Although a spurt of growth is expected at the time of puberty, the onset, duration, and amount of growth are quite variable. "No two youngsters start together, finish together, or follow the same pattern" (2).

### Adolescent Growth in Girls

Velocity of growth just before the adolescent growth spurt is about 5 cm/ yr for both boys and girls. The rate of growth has been falling gradually throughout childhood and reaches its lowest point just before puberty (Figure 5-1). Girls usually begin their growth spurt earlier than boys but generally do not reach as high a peak height velocity. In the Harpenden

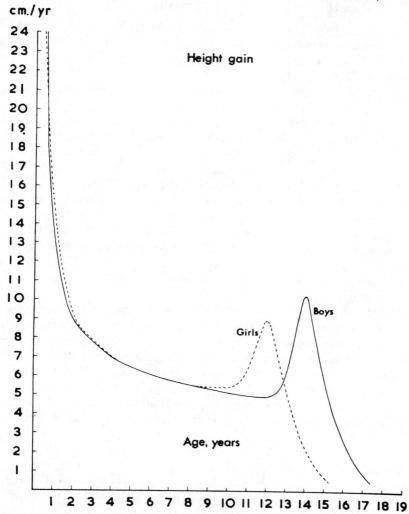

**Figure 5-1.** Typical individual velocity curves for *height* in English boys and girls. (Reproduced by permission from Tanner JM, Whitehouse RH, Takaishi M: Standards from birth to maturity for height, weight, height velocity, and weight velocity for British children 1965, Parts I and II. *Arch Dis Child* **41**:454, 613, 1966.)

Growth Study reported by Marshall and Tanner, girls measured at 3-month intervals throughout the adolescent years averaged a peak height velocity (PHV) of 9 cm/yr with a standard deviation of 1.03 cm/yr (3). The PHV represents a growth rate approximately double that of the preadolescent rate. The mean age for reaching PHV for girls was 12 years with a standard deviation of 0.88 years. Maximum growth rates for most adolescent girls will occur between 10 and 14 years of age. During the year of fastest growth, the girl may gain 6–11 cm in height and over the 3-year period of adolescent growth will increase an average of 20 cm (3).

## Adolescent Growth in Boys

Boys begin their adolescent growth spurt about 2 years later than girls but have a higher peak height velocity (PHV). In the Harpenden study there was an average PHV of 10.3 cm/yr with a standard deviation of 1.53 cm/yr. Growth during the year centered on the PHV ranged from 7 to 12 cm (4). The mean age for PHV in boys was 14 years with a standard deviation of 0.92 years. Most adolescent boys reach their PHV between the twelfth and sixteenth birthdays and they can be expected to add an average of 23 cm to their height during the 3 years of most rapid adolescent growth (5). Since girls begin their growth spurt earlier than boys, there is a brief period, around age 11–13, when girls are taller than boys. However, as the girl's growth begins to slow down the boy's growth will be accelerating and the combination of longer period of preadolescent growth, plus a higher PHV, allows boys in the end to become taller than girls by an average of about 13 cm (5).

Changes in growth that occur during adolescence should be recorded on velocity curves showing the rate of growth rather than conventional height achievement curves. Though there is a change of the achievement curve slope at adolescence, the average change is so slight that it is difficult to discern when the increased rate of growth begins or even peaks and only the slowing down, shown by a flattening of the curve, is readily evident. By contrast, the change in growth at adolescence can be readily appreciated on a velocity curve such as those constructed by Tanner (Figure 5-1).

## Variations in Adolescent Growth

Since every child follows his or her own growth pattern, there are almost limitless variations in patterns of growth, illustrating the effects of both genetic patterns and the timing of the adolescent growth spurt. In Figure 5-2, subject 1 represents a boy or girl of average height who begins puberty at the usual time and ends up in the average height range as an adult. Subject 2 represents a boy or girl who experiences an early adolescent growth spurt and at that point is taller than his or her peers, but early completion of the growth spurt often results in less than average height achievement and shorter than average adult height. The growth curve for subject 3 shows the pattern of growth of the late maturing boy or girl who grows more slowly than his or her peers through much of childhood and early teens. Late puberty and acceleration of growth often propel such youngsters eventually into the average or even above-average range. Subjects 4 and 5 represent genetically small and tall subjects who follow

## NORMAL GROWTH PATTERNS

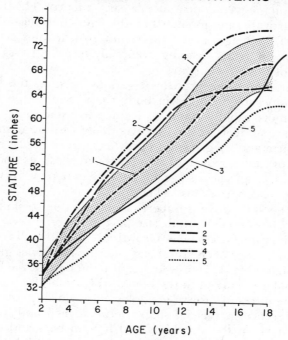

**Figure 5-2.** Growth in stature of five normal boys. (1) Average stature and rate of maturation. (2) Early maturing boy with early adolescent growth spurt and low average adult height. (3) Late maturing boy with delayed growth spurt. (4) Tall stature (familial) with normal timing of maturation. (5) Short stature (familial) with normal timing of maturation. (Redrawn by permission from Marshall WA: Growth and sexual maturation in normal puberty. *Clin Endocrinol Metab* **4**:3, 1975.)

a persistent pattern, above or below the average, with puberty occurring at about the average time.

It is clear from such illustrations that a child who is taller than average may represent either one who is genetically designated to be tall or one who is maturing early, and conversely, a child who is shorter than average may be so because he or she is a late maturer or a child from small parents who has a genetically small adult target height.

## Changes in Body Proportion and Differential Growth Rates

The adolescent growth spurt does not begin at the same time in all parts of the body nor proceed at the same rate, so there are constant changes in body proportion during the growth spurt. Lengthening of the legs is the first event to affect general height. During this period, the ratio of the upper (trunk) to lower (legs) segments may drop to less than 1.0 describing the long-legged appearance of early puberty. The trunk reaches its maximum growth rate about 6 months later, but because it persists longer, much of the height in the adolescent growth spurt actually comes from growth of the trunk, leading eventually to a US/LS ratio of about 1.0 at the end of the growth spurt.

The order in which the growth of various parts of the body occurs brings about noticeable changes in body shape and proportion. Hands and feet grow more rapidly than legs, leading to a temporary appearance of large hands and feet which will eventually assume a more normal proportion as arm and leg growth occurs. Leg growth occurs before trunk growth, which precedes growth of shoulders and chest, so a boy may grow out of his shoes at an early stage of puberty and may grow out of his trousers before he outgrows his jacket (5).

Growth of the skull during puberty is mainly due to skull thickening since the brain is essentially adult size by this time. However, the facial bones undergo noticeable changes. Growth of the skull and frontal sinuses produces a prominence of the forehead, and the jaw bones grow forward, especially the mandible. This produces a straightening of the facial profile, which is particularly marked in the boy (5) (Figure 3-5B).

One of the features of growth in adolescence, which produces the most noticeable difference in skeletal shape between men and women, is the differential growth of the shoulders and hips in boys and girls. During adolescence, the hips of girls widen considerably, while in boys, the shoulder width undergoes a similar growth spurt. This is not a universal phenomenon, however; many boys and girls become tall and long-legged and retain narrow hips and shoulders. Tanner suggests that differential growth patterns occur because cartilage cells in girls' hips or boys' shoulders are specialized to respond to estrogens or androgens, respectively (5). Girls at birth already have a wider pelvic outlet so the design for childbearing is present from very early growth in the girl.

## Changes in Body Composition

It is common to think of boys becoming muscular (mesomorphic) and of girls becoming fatter (endomorphic) during adolescence, and there is some physiologic basis for this generalization. Increase in muscular tissue during adolescence is greater in the boy than in the girl, but girls also add considerable muscle tissue, and since their growth spurt antedates that of the boy, during the early phase of their growth spurt girls may actually have more muscle than boys (Figure 5-3). The increase in muscle mass of boys leads to greater strength in boys than in girls. This is not evident before puberty, but the differential growth at puberty produces a noticeable difference in strength between boys and girls. "Boys develop larger hearts as well as larger skeletal muscles, larger lungs, higher systolic blood

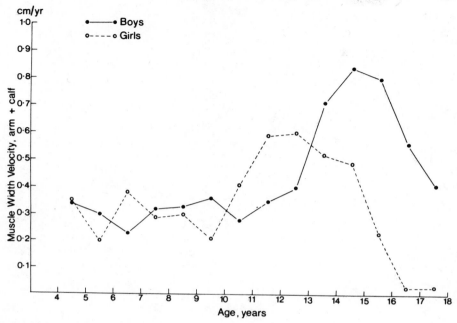

**Figure 5-3.** Muscle growth at adolescence for boys and girls. (Reproduced by permission from Tanner JM: *Fetus into Man.* Cambridge, MA, Harvard University Press, 1978.)

pressure, lower resting heart rate, and a greater capacity for carrying oxygen in the blood" (5). Adolescent boys have higher numbers of red blood cells and a higher hemoglobin than girls: an effect of higher androgen levels in boys. All of this seems to adapt the male for heavier work and is, at least partially, responsible for the noticeable increase in athletic prowess of boys at adolescence.

Fat accumulation decelerates in both boys and girls as they approach peak height velocity. As measured by x-ray, there is actually a loss of fat in boys. In girls there is a corresponding decrease in fat accumulation but not an actual loss. With deceleration of height velocity, there is a resumption of rapid fat accumulation that is approximately twice as high in girls as in boys. The end result is a decrease in proportion of fat to lean body mass in the boy and an increase in the girl, leading to the generalization about body built alluded to above.

Skeletal mass and the size of most organs, including heart, lungs, liver, spleen, kidney, pancreas, thyroid, adrenals, and genital organs double during puberty. The central nervous system changes very little, and the thymus, tonsils, and adenoids decrease in size (6).

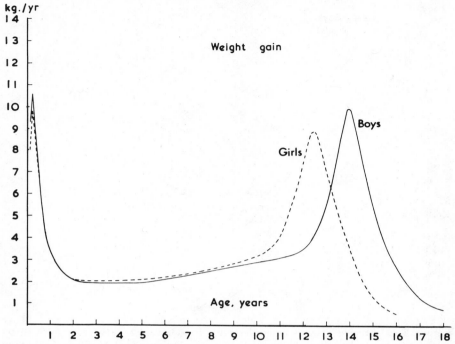

**Figure 5-4.** Individual velocity curves for *weight* in English boys and girls. (Reproduced by permission from Tanner JM, Whitehouse RH, Takaishi M: Standards from birth to maturity for height, weight, height velocity, and weight velocity for British children 1965, Parts I and II. *Arch Dis Child* **41**:454, 613, 1966.)

## Changes in Weight during Puberty

About 50% of adult body weight is gained during puberty (6). In boys, rapid gain in weight reaches a peak weight velocity at about the same time as peak height velocity is reached. In girls, peak weight velocity lags behind peak height velocity by about 6 months (6) (Figure 5-4). In girls, the peak weight velocity averages 8.3 kg/yr (ranging from 5.5 to 10.6 kg/yr) at an average age of 12½ years. In boys, weight gain reaches an average peak weight velocity of 9 kg/yr (ranging from 6.1 to 12.8 kg/yr) at about age 14 (7) (Figure 5-4). Deceleration of weight gain occurs in a pattern similar to that described for height during puberty. Serious deviation from normal weight gain should raise the question of incipient obesity or illness associated with failure to thrive.

## SEXUAL DEVELOPMENT IN ADOLESCENCE

The growth spurt occurring at the time of adolescence is closely related to events of sexual maturation or puberty.

## Sexual Maturation in Boys

Maturation of the reproductive system in boys includes growth and maturation of the testes (seminiferous tubules and testosterone-secreting cells), penis, and accessory sex organs (epididymis, seminal vesicles, and prostate) and appearance of secondary sex characters (growth of the genitalia and appearance of pubic hair). Androgen production from the adrenal gland increases very early in pubertal development and may be a "trigger" to subsequent virilization from testicular androgen (9). Testosterone exerts specific effects also on axillary and facial hair, larynx, and sweat and sebaceous glands during pubertal development.

The volume of the testes in prepubertal boys is usually 3 mL or less. At onset of puberty, the testes enlarge to a volume of 4 mL or more (Figure 5-5). A distinct lumen appears in the seminiferous tubules and they enlarge rapidly and become tortuous. Spermatogonia begin to divide and Sertoli cells appear. At about the time spermatogonia are being formed in the germinal epithelium, Leydig cells appear and begin testosterone production. By the time the Leydig cells are fully mature, spermatids and spermatozoa are being formed. In the fully developed testes, about two-thirds of the seminiferous tubule is made up of germinal epithelium and the remainder of Sertoli cells which serve primarily as support cells (8).

Early testicular enlargement is usually accompanied by a reddening and thinning of the scrotal sac. The scrotum and penis have changed very little throughout childhood except for some gradual increase in overall size. Within a year after the testes begin to enlarge, the penis follows suit and pubic hair appears. The testes increase about tenfold in volume from a prepubertal volume of 1–3 mL to an adult size of 15–25 mL (8) (Figure 5-5). The epididymis and prostate increase about sevenfold or more in size, while the penis doubles in length from a prepubertal mean of 6.2 cm to an adult length of 13.2 centimeters (ranging from 7.5 to 15.5 cm) (8).

### Sequence of Sexual Maturation in Boys

The relationships of the major events of puberty in the boy are shown in Figure 5-6. The sequence and timing of events of puberty are average values for European and North American boys (5). Testicular growth antedates penile growth by 6 months to a year. Acceleration of testicular growth generally begins by about 11.5 years, but may be seen as early as 9.5 years and as late at 13.5 years. Penile growth normally begins at about 12.5 years at about the same time that the pubertal growth spurt begins. Pubic hair generally antedates the penile enlargement by about 6 months and is generally at about stage 4 at the time the peak height velocity is reached in the growth spurt. In a recent review of normal ages of pubertal events among American boys and girls, Lee (10) found pubertal events to correspond reasonably closely to the published data from Great Britain

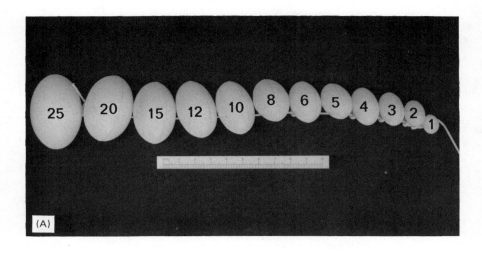

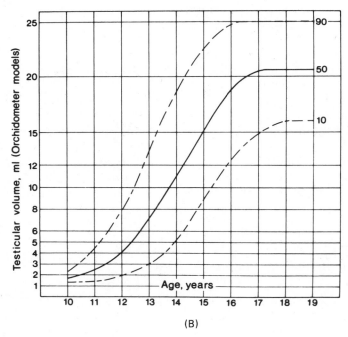

**Figure 5-5.** (A) Orchidometer (Prader); the numbers indicate volume in mL. (B) Growth curve of testis size. Estimated 10th, 50th, and 90th percentiles by age from prepubertal to adult development, based on measurements made by orchidometer (Prader) on Dutch, Swiss, and Swedish males. (Reproduced by permission from Tanner JM: *Fetus into Man,* Cambridge, MA, Harvard University Press, 1978, based on data from van Wieringen, et al, 1971, Zachmann, et al, 1974, and Taranger, et al, 1976.)

110

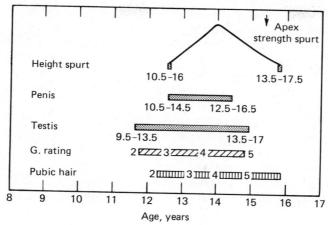

**Figure 5-6.** Sequence of development of physical changes of puberty in boys with reference to Tanner's stages of pubic hair (PH) and genital (G) rating. (Reproduced by permission from Marshall WA, Tanner JM: Variation in pattern of pubertal changes in boys. *Arch Dis Child* **45**:13, 1970.)

(3, 4). Onset (G2, PH2) and completion (G5, PH5) of genital and pubic hair maturation were a little later than the English data, but not significantly different (10).

Secretions from the prostate and seminal vesicles form seminal fluid which may be ejaculated spontaneously, beginning about a year after acceleration of penile growth. Spontaneous ejaculation commonly occurs during sleep, accompanied by dreaming, the so-called "wet dream" of adolescence. At first, the seminal fluid contains relatively few sperm, suggesting the probability of a period of relative infertility, but this is neither absolute nor definable as a risk.

The sequence of events, though not perfectly followed by every boy, is less variable than the time of onset. The spurt in height begins about a year after first testicular enlargement and reaches its maximum (PHV) after about 1½ years (average age of PHV is 14 years). At the time PHV is reached, the penis has been growing rapidly for over a year and the pubic hair is in stage 3 to 4 development (Figure 5-6). Axillary hair appears after pubic hair reaches stage 4; facial hair appears somewhat later (5). Body hair appears gradually thereafter and is not specifically related to events of puberty. The deepening of the voice occurs relatively late in puberty and is due to enlargement of the larynx and increase in length of the vocal cords. This usually occurs after the testes are fully developed and adult levels of testosterone are being produced (5, 6).

### Breast Development in Boys
Some changes in the male breast normally occur during puberty. There is enlargement of the areola in all adolescent boys, and in some, there will

also be noticeable glandular tissue enlargement beneath the areola. This may be tender and may be only unilateral, but in the majority it is bilateral and nontender. In most adolescents this benign gynecomastia appears during mid-adolescence and spontaneously regresses over the next 6–18 months. The exact number of adolescent boys who will develop noticeable breast enlargement varies with the degree of enlargement termed "gynecomastia" by observers. On the average, 30% or more of adolescents will develop noticeable breast tissue between the ages of 12 and 15 (6), but many authors report palpable tissue in up to 65% of pubertal boys (11, 12). Although the usual pubertal breast changes regress spontaneously within 12–18 months, marked pubertal gynecomastia does not. For those who are sufficiently disturbed by the breast tissue and insist on active treatment, surgery is usually advocated, although Danazol (an antigonadotropin) (13) and clomiphene (an antiestrogen) (14) have also been reported to be effective.

### Assessment of Stages in Sexual Development of Boys

It is often desirable to assess how far a child has progressed through puberty. For this purpose, Tanner has introduced a set of rating scales describing the successive stages of growth of the genitalia and pubic hair for boys. (Similar scales for breast and pubic hair development for girls are discussed below.) The scales range from prepubescence [stage 1] to adult development [stage 5]. In addition, testicular size, as tested by the Prader orchidometer (Figure 5-5), may be measured and related by age to the other events of pubertal development in boys (5). Table 5-1A lists the stages of development of the genitalia in boys and Figure 5-7 provides visual confirmation of the progression of penile and scrotal growth. Stage G-1 represents the prepubertal state and G-5 describes genitalia which are adult in size and shape.

Description of pubic hair stages in boys provided by Tanner are listed in Table 5-1C and depicted in Figure 5-8A. The stages of development are denoted PH-1 to PH-5, representing prepubertal to adult pubic hair development. In about 80% of men and 10% of women, the pubic hair spreads up over the abdomen or laterally over the thighs (stage 6), but this hair growth is seldom reached before age 20 and need not be considered in pubertal development (8).

The age of onset of secondary sexual development, the duration of successive stages, and even the sequence of events of puberty are quite variable. This "normal" variability must be appreciated to effectively use the information derived from the staging of pubertal progress. Means and normal variation in the timing of adolescent secondary sexual development are shown in Table 5-2. From the table it may be noted that a boy may begin genital enlargement (Stage G-2) by 9.5 years or he may wait until he is nearly 14. Early maturing boys may be fully developed by

## Table 5-1. Stages of Puberty

### a. Boys: Genital Development

Stage 1. (G-1)
Preadolescent. Testes, scrotum and penis are of about the same size and proportion as in early childhood.

Stage 2. (G-2)
Enlargement of scrotum and testes. Skin of scrotum reddens and changes in texture. Little or no enlargement of penis at this time.

Stage 3. (G-3)
Enlargement of penis which occurs at first mainly in length. Further growth of testes and scrotum.

Stage 4. (G-4)
Increased size of penis with growth in breadth and development of glans. Testes and scrotum larger; scrotal skin darkened.

Stage 5. (G-5)
Genitalia adult in size and shape.

### b. Girls: Breast Development

Stage 1. (B-1)
Preadolescent; elevation of papilla only.

Stage 2. (B-2)
Breast bud stage: elevation of breast and papilla as small mound. Enlargement of areola diameter.

Stage 3. (B-3)
Further enlargement and elevation of breast and areola with no separation of their contours.

Stage 4. (B-4)
Projection of areola and papilla to form a secondary mound above level of the breast.

Stage 5. (B-5)
Mature stage: projection of papilla only, due to recession of the areola to the general contour of the breast.

### c. Both Sexes: Pubic Hair

Stage 1. (PH-1)
Preadolescent. The vellus over the pubis is not further developed than that over the abdominal wall, that is, no pubic hair.

Stage 2. (PH-2)
Sparse growth of long, slightly pigmented downy hair. straight or slightly curled, chiefly at base of the penis or along labia.

Stage 3. (PH-3)
Considerably darker, coarser, and more curled. The hair spreads sparsely over the symphysis of the pubes.

Stage 4. (PH-4)
Hair now adult in type, but area covered is still considerably smaller than in the adult. No spread to medial surface of thighs.

Stage 5. (PH-5)
Adult in quantity and type with distribution of the horizontal (or classically "feminine" pattern). Spread to medial surface of thighs or elsewhere above base of the inverse triangle (spread up linea alba) occurs late, rated stage 6.

Reproduced by permission from Tanner JM: Growth and endocrinology of the adolescent, in Gardner L (ed), *Endocrine and Genetic Diseases of Childhood and Adolescence*, ed 2. Philadelphia, WB Saunders Co, 1975.

age 13 before some late maturing boys have even started sexual development, and there are some boys who do not complete their sexual development until they are over 18 years.

Variation in the time required to advance from one stage of development to another deserves emphasis. Some boys may spend up to 2½ years in stage G-2 while others may go through their complete genital development

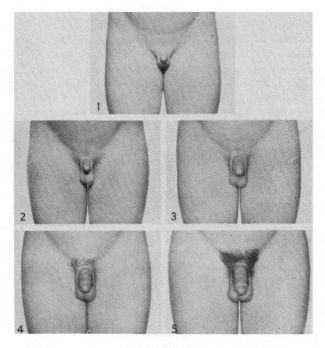

**Figure 5-7.** Standards for genital maturity in boys from preadolescent level, Stage 1, to adult genitalia, Stage 5 (see Table 5-1A for description of genitalia at each stage). (Reproduced by permission from Tanner JM: Growth and endocrinology of the adolescent, in Gardner L, (ed), *Endocrine and Genetic Diseases of Childhood,* ed 2. Philadelphia, WB Saunders Co, 1975, pp 14–64.)

in less time. Some boys require 5 years or more to complete genital development (8). The rate of progression through stages of development is variable, but those maturing slowly in early stages are more apt to be slow throughout the process. Genital growth and pubic hair development do not always develop in tandem either, although it is unusual for an individual to reach stage 2, pubic hair development, without showing any genital changes (6).

About 75% of normal boys reach their peak height and weight velocity while in stage G-4, the remainder at a later stage (G-5). This fact can be very reassuring for a boy who is looking for a growth spurt of adolescence, but is just beginning sexual development. He can look forward to the growth spurt as he moves further into pubertal development. The wide age range of normal entry into and progression through puberty displayed by these data provide physicians with reassuring information for counseling troubled adolescents who think they are too early, too late, too fast, or too slow in their pubertal growth and maturation (3, 4) (Figure 5-9).

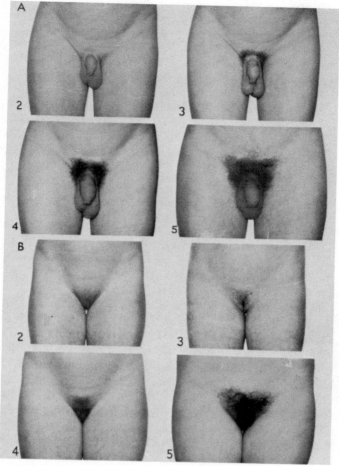

**Figure 5-8.** Standards for pubic hair ratings in boys (A) and girls (B) (see Table 5-1C for descriptions of development at each stage). (Reproduced by permission from Tanner JM: Growth and endocrinology of the adolescent, in Gardner L, (ed), *Endocrine and Genetic Diseases of Childhood*, ed 2. Philadelphia, WB Saunders Co, 1975, pp 14–64.)

## Sexual Maturation in Girls

Maturation of the reproductive system in girls involves enlargement of the ovaries and maturation of germinal tissue to form ovarian follicles, enlargement of the uterus and fallopian tubes, development of the uterine endometrium, lengthening of the vagina, and enlargement of the labia. One of the first signs of approaching puberty is an increase in superficial cells in the vaginal smear which may antedate noticeable signs of estrogen stimulation, either of breasts or vaginal mucosa. Secondary sex characters

**Table 5-2. Means and Normal Variation in the Timing of Adolescent Secondary Sexual Development**

| Stage | Mean Age of Onset ±2 SD (yr) | Stage | Time between Stages (yr) | | |
| | | | Mean | Percentile | |
| | | | | 5th | 95th |
|---|---|---|---|---|---|
| | | **Males** | | | |
| G-2 | 11.6 ± 2.1 | G2–G3 | 1.1 | 0.4 | 2.2 |
| G-3 | 12.9 ± 2.1 | PH2–PH3 | 0.5 | 0.1 | 1.0 |
| PH-2 | 13.4 ± 2.2 | G3–G4 | 0.8 | 0.2 | 1.6 |
| G-4 | 13.8 ± 2.0 | PH3–PH4 | 0.4 | 0.3 | 0.5 |
| PH-3 | 13.9 ± 2.1 | G4–G5 | 1.0 | 0.4 | 1.9 |
| PH-4 | 14.4 ± 2.2 | PH4–PH5 | 0.7 | 0.2 | 1.5 |
| G-5 | 14.9 ± 2.2 | G2–G5 | 3.0 | 1.9 | 4.7 |
| PH-5 | 15.2 ± 2.1 | PH2–PH5 | 1.6 | 0.8 | 2.7 |
| | | **Females** | | | |
| B-2 | 11.2 ± 2.2 | B2–B3 | 0.9 | 0.2 | 1.0 |
| PH-2 | 11.7 ± 2.4 | PH2–PH3 | 0.6 | 0.2 | 1.3 |
| B-3 | 12.2 ± 2.1 | B3–B4 | 0.9 | 0.1 | 2.2 |
| PH-3 | 12.4 ± 2.2 | PH3–PH4 | 0.5 | 0.2 | 0.9 |
| PH-4 | 12.9 ± 2.1 | B4–B5 | 2.0 | 0.1 | 6.8 |
| B-4 | 13.1 ± 2.3 | PH4–PH5 | 1.3 | 0.6 | 2.4 |
| PH-5 | 14.4 ± 2.2 | B2–B5 | 4.0 | 1.5 | 9.0 |
| B-5 | 15.3 ± 3.5 | PH2–PH5 | 2.5 | 1.4 | 3.1 |

Reproduced by permission from Barnes HV: Physical growth and development during puberty. *Med Clin North Am* **59**:1305, 1975.

Reproduced by permission and data derived from: Marshall WA, Tanner JM: Variation in patterns of pubertal changes in girls. *Arch Dis Child* **44**:291, 1969; and Marshall WA, Tanner JM: Variation in patterns of pubertal changes in boys. *Arch Dis Child* **45**:13, 1970.

appear coincidentally with changes in gonads and internal genitalia, most prominently development of breasts and pubic hair and redistribution of body fat. As in boys, there is a characteristic growth spurt and skeletal maturation and there may be changes in sweat and sebaceous glands.

### Sequence of Events of Puberty in Girls

The sequence of noticeable events in puberty of girls is shown in Figure 5-10 from data on pubertal sequences in girls (3). The first noticeable sign of puberty in girls is usually the appearance of a "breast bud". A growth spurt in height takes place early in the sequence of sexual maturation and often has already started by the time breast development begins. There is a great deal of variation in the time of onset of puberty in girls as well as rate of progression through the various stages of pubertal development. Breast development may begin as early as 8 or as late as 13, with an average of about 11 years (5, 10). Usually pubic hair begins to appear after "breast budding" has occurred, but in as many as one-third of girls, pubic hair appears before breast development. Most girls will have achieved adult breast form by 15 years of age, but some achieve full breast development by age 12 (before some have even begun), and others do not achieve full breast development until age 18 or later (Figure 5-9).

Menarche, the first menstrual period, occurs fairly late in the sequence of sexual development—about $2-2\frac{1}{2}$ years after first breast development. Menarche occurs after the height velocity has passed its peak, during the period of decelerating growth. The average age of menarche in North American girls of European descent is 12.8 to 13.3 years and of those of African descent, 12.5 years (5, 10, 15). In the early 1970s there were reports of earlier menarche in American girls (15), but a recent report (10) suggests that American and European girls are quite comparable in timing of pubertal events. Menarche in Central and Northern Europe ranges from 12.5 to 13.5 and the age of menarche world-wide, is within the range of 12.5–14.2 years (5). There has been a gradual decrease in the average age of menarche (earlier age of onset of puberty) in European and North American girls over the past 2 hundred years. (See Chapter 1.) This now seems to be leveling off; however, there is still a great deal of individual variation. Menarche occurring as early as 10 years or as late as 15 years may be considered within the normal range. Most girls have well-developed breasts (B-4) when menarche occurs, but about one-fourth are in earlier stages of development. Menses generally occur in girls with well-developed pubic hair (PH-3 or PH-4), but in a few, menses occur later or before any pubic hair has appeared. Menses may be irregular for twelve to eighteen months or longer after menarche. Even though the positive feedback loop (surge of GnRH associated with ovulation) may be established as early as mid-puberty, cycles are anovulatory in well over half of adolescent girls for as long as 2 years after menarche (16).

### Stages of Breast and Pubic Hair Development in Girls

As for boys, Tanner has introduced a rating scale for progression through puberty for girls. The scale describes changes occurring in the breasts from prepubertal to adult stages (Table 5-1B and Figure 5-11). Stage 4 development of the areolar mound does not occur in some girls and some never progress beyond stage 4 development (3). The size of the breast is not related to the stage of maturation. The factors determining size of the breast are not known, but heredity seems to play an important role. Nutrition plays a surprisingly small role except for the heavy breasts of obesity.

Pubic hair development is described in five stages and is identical for boys and girls (Table 5-1C and Figure 5-8B). Adult hair distribution is obtained between the ages of 12 and 17. In about 10% of women the hair spreads beyond the horizontal "feminine" pattern to the abdomen. This

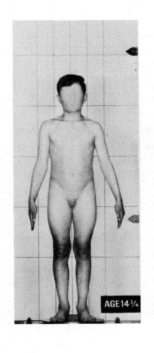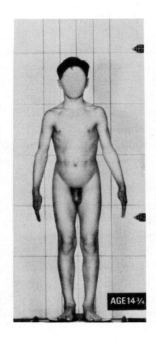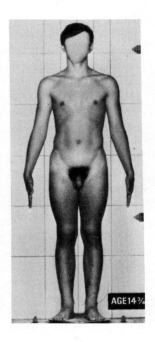

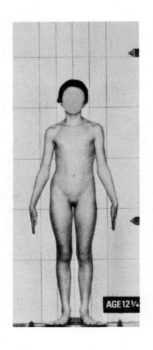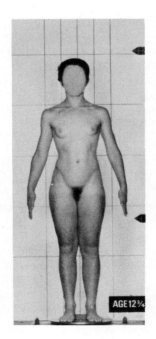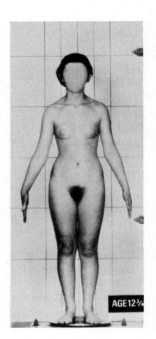

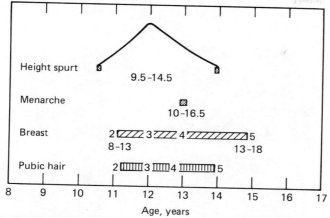

**Figure 5-10.** Sequence of development of physical changes in puberty in girls with reference to Tanner's stages of pubic hair and breast development. (Reproduced by permission from Marshall WA, Tanner, JM: Variation in patterns of pubertal changes in girls. *Arch Dis Child* **44:**291, 1969.)

may be designated stage 6, but is a late phemomenon and is not related to events of puberty or growth.

Progression through the sequence of pubertal development is usual, but wide variation in time of entry into successive stages and duration of stages is seen in normal individuals (Figure 5-9). An understanding of the wide range of normal variation is necessary in arriving at a decision to pursue pathologic causes of precocious or delayed puberty. In Table 5-2, the mean age of onset of stages of breast and pubic hair are given (6), together with the average duration of stages and the 5th and 95th percentiles for times within stages. The age of arriving at stage 2 breast development might range from 9 to 13.4 years in girls. On the average, a girl might be expected to remain in stage 2 breast development about 1 year before arriving at stage 3 with a variation between 0.6 and 1.2 years. The table also allows one to judge coincidental development of pubic hair and breast development according to means and standard deviations of expected times within stages.

←

**Figure 5-9.** Variability and timing of pubertal development and growth. Upper panel shows 3 normal boys, all age 14¾ with pubertal development ranging from Stage 1 to Stage 5. Lower panel shows three normal girls, all age 12½, with variable pubertal development ranging from prepubertal to nearly complete development. (Reproduced by permission from Tanner JM: Growth and endocrinology of the adolescent, in Gardner L, (ed), *Endocrine and Genetic Diseases of Childhood,* ed 2. Philadelphia, WB Saunders Co, 1975, pp 14–64.)

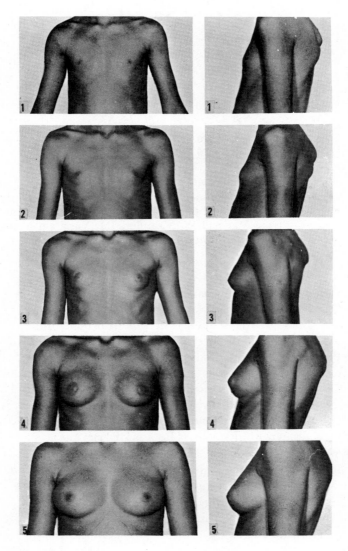

**Figure 5-11.** Standards for breast development from preadolescent, Stage 1, to mature breasts, Stage 5 (see Table 5-1B for description of stages of development). (Reproduced by permission from Tanner JM: Growth and endocrinology of the adolescent, in Gardner L, (ed), *Endocrine and Genetic Diseases of Childhood*, ed 2. Philadelphia, WB Saunders Co, 1975, pp 14–64.)

## Developmental Age and Events of Puberty

The events of puberty, although they occur at diverse chronologic ages, are generally related to the physiologic or developmental age. The developmental age is most accurately reflected in the stage of maturity of the skeleton (bone age). Although a girl or boy may be anywhere from 9 to 14 years chronologically when puberty begins, we expect the bone age will be very close to 10 to 11 for the girl or 11 to 12 for the boy. However, Marshall failed to find the expected close correlation between bone age and onset of puberty (8). Menarche in the girl was more closely related to bone age than to chronologic age, but neither stages of breast development in girls nor genital development in boys was found to be closely correlated to the bone age. Pubic hair development and, to some extent, adult genital development in boys (stage G-5) were somewhat better related to bone age but surprisingly peak height velocity was not (8). It appears, therefore, that the development of sex characteristics is independent from the mechanisms which regulate the maturation of the skeleton, at least until after mid-puberty.

The difference in timing of maturation between sexes gives rise to some of the differences in boys and girls at the time of adolescence, aside from the obvious differences in sexual differentiation. The maturation of bones, expressed as "bone age", is about 2 years earlier in girls than in boys by the time of puberty. The adolescent growth spurt begins about 2 years earlier in girls than in boys, but the onset of puberty in boys (early testicular enlargement) begins only about 6 months after the average girl begins breast development. Puberty appears to occur earlier in girls because of the early growth spurt and the obvious appearance of breast tissue. Testicular enlargement in boys may remain undetected and, until pubic hair appears or until the growth spurt and other changes of puberty occur, it is not obvious to observers that puberty has begun (8).

## ENDOCRINOLOGY OF PUBERTY

In the male, the growth spurt and sexual development of puberty is associated with increased production of *androgens*, primarily from the testicle, but also from the adrenal gland (9). At puberty, androgens stimulate growth of the penis and scrotum, initiate appearance of pubic, axillary, facial, and body hair, accelerate growth and maturation of the skeleton, and produce an increase in muscle mass.

In the female, *estrogens* from the ovary stimulate growth of the breasts, uterus, fallopian tubes, and vagina. In the vagina the epithelial lining becomes cornified and lubricated and the vaginal pH changes. There is fat deposition especially on hips, shoulders, and breasts. Skeletal maturation is accelerated. *Adrenal androgens* stimulate growth of pubic and axillary hair in the female (adrenarche) and stimulate linear growth and skeletal maturation. The adolescent growth spurt in the female may depend primarily upon the anabolic activity of the adrenal androgens (13).

## Reproductive Endocrinology in Infancy

The hypothalamic–pituitary–gonadal axis begins to function early in fetal life (17). Gonadotropin levels in both sexes (FSH and LH) and serum testosterone levels in the male fetus peak in the second trimester (17). After birth, there is a neonatal surge of gonadotropins, (primarily FSH in the female infant and LH in the male infant) accompanied by elevation of plasma estrogen (female) and testosterone (male) (18). Gonadotropins remain elevated for the first 2 years of life, declining thereafter and remaining low until the onset of adolescence (19, 20). In infants with gonadal dysgenesis, high levels of FSH may persist during the first 4 years of life (21). In male infants, testosterone levels drop temporarily after birth (perhaps due to the withdrawal of placental human chorionic gonadotropin), but there is a secondary rise in plasma testosterone to mid-pubertal levels (200–250 ng/dL) by 2–3 months of age followed by gradual decline to prepubertal levels by 6–12 months of age (18, 19). Tanner has suggested that this may contribute to the rapid growth of the male infant in the neonatal period (5).

## Reproductive Endocrinology in Childhood

During childhood, before the onset of puberty, plasma levels of gonado-tropins are low and the gonads are at rest (22). There is, however, maturation of the zone of the adrenal cortex in which androgens are produced, in preparation for the "adrenarche" phase of pubertal matur-ation (17, 23).

About 2 years before physical manifestations of puberty appear, there is a gradual increase in levels of adrenal androgens in plasma and urine in both sexes (22). Dehydroepiandrosterone (DHEA) and dehydroepian-drosterone sulphate (DHEAS) are the principal products of the adrenal with smaller amounts of androstenediol and very small amounts of testosterone. Adrenal androgens are excreted in urine where they may be measured at 17-ketosteroids. Levels remain the same for boys and girls until about age 12. Thereafter, boys excrete more 17-ketosteroids, which include testicular androgen as well (22). During puberty, adrenal androgen contributes to development of sexual hair, skeletal maturation, and the growth spurt.

The maturation of the adrenal seems to be under the influence of a separate pituitary trophic factor than that of the gonad or of ACTH. Parker and Odell have presented evidence for a separate trophic hormone from the pituitary which specifically stimulates androgen production by the adrenal cortex (cortical androgen stimulating hormone) (24).

## Endocrine Changes at Puberty

At puberty, there is a rise in plasma and urinary gonadotropins and sex steroids, as well as continued elevations of adrenal androgens (17, 18). There is ample evidence that the increase in activity of the hypothalamic–pituitary–gonadal axis correlates well with skeletal maturation and stages of puberty (17, 18, 22, 25). The prepubertal increase in adrenal androgens, described in the previous section, appears to be the earliest event announcing maturation of the pubertal endocrine system and may serve as a "trigger" to stimulate the onset of pubertal function of the hypothalamic–pituitary–gonadal axis (9, 18).

The first observed activity of the hypothalamic–pituitary–gonadal axis is an increase in sleep-associated episodic pulses of LH (and of FSH to a lesser degree) (16, 26, 27). As maturation of the system proceeds, the pulses of LH (and FSH) become more uniform throughout the 24 hour period and levels of LH and FSH gradually increase as signs of puberty appear (17). The release of gonadotropins is assumed to be linked to pulsatile release of GnRH, hypothalamic gonadotropin releasing hormone, though clear and definite elevation of GnRH has been difficult to demonstrate during pubertal development (16, 28).

In the *female*, elevation of LH and FSH is usually seen by 10 or 11 years. Thereafter, there are gradual increases in gonadotropins throughout puberty until menarche when levels become stable (Figure 5-12). LH responsiveness to GnRH increases with sexual maturation, while FSH response is variable (9, 18). Estrogen levels rise progressively during puberty, reaching adult levels by pubertal stage 4 or 5 or at the time of menarche (9) (Figure 5-12). Testosterone levels remain low throughout female pubertal development though there is a progressive rise of adrenal androgens (Figure 5-12). Sexual hair development and the adolescent growth spurt in the female appear to be dependent upon adrenal androgens, most prominently DHEA, DHEAS, and androstenedione. The ovary produces small amounts of androstenedione and testosterone, although most of the circulating testosterone in females is produced by perpheral conversion of other androgens to testosterone and its potent metabolite dihydrotestosterone (DHT) (18).

The gonadal steroid levels are closely related to pubertal developmental levels (22). Estradiol increase begins during stage 2 pubertal development (average age of 11.5), and there is a concomitant increase in the size of ovary and uterus. The rapid rise in plasma and urinary estrogens and in adrenal androgens (Figure 5-12) is associated with growth of reproductive organs and the appearance of secondary sexual characteristics (22). As the gonadal steroid levels rise, there is further maturation of the hypothalamic centers to develop a positive feedback response resulting in a cyclic preovulatory LH surge resulting in ovulation and menarche (16, 29).

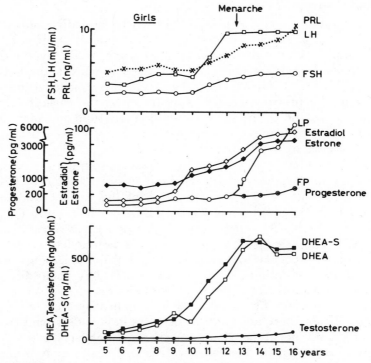

**Figure 5-12.** Hormonal changes in girls during puberty. Changes in plasma prolactin (PRL), luteinizing hormone (LH), follicle-stimulating hormone (FSH), estradiol, estrone, progesterone (before puberty and after menarche), dehydro-epiandrosterone (DHEA), dehydroepiandrosterone sulfate (DHEA-S), and testosterone before, during, and after puberty in normal girls. LP and FP represent progesterone levels during the luteal phase (open circles) and follicular phase (dotted circles) after menarche. (Reproduced by permission from Sizonenko PC: Endrocinology in pre-adolescence and adolescence, I. Hormonal changes during normal puberty. *Am J Dis Child* **132:**708, 1978, copyright 1978 American Medical Association.)

In the *male*, an increase in LH and FSH levels is seen by 11–12 years, and there are gradual increases to adult levels by late puberty (Figure 5-13). LH and FSH levels are essentially identical in males and females. At the onset of puberty there is enlargement of the testes in response to elevation of gonadotropins. With elevation of gonadotropins there is an increase in circulating plasma androgens (Figure 5-13). Testosterone is the most important male androgen, and it is derived primarily from the testes. DHEA and DHEAS from the adrenal also increase noticeably during puberty (Figure 5-13). Androstenedione may be derived from testes or adrenal and may be converted by peripheral tissues to testosterone.

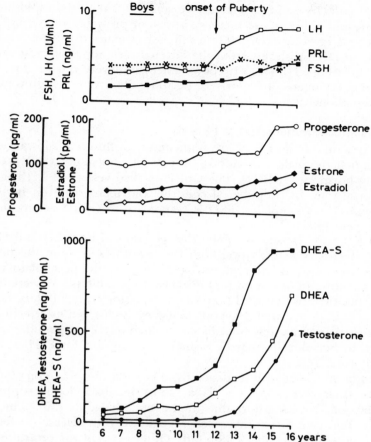

**Figure 5-13.** Hormonal changes in boys during puberty. Changes in plasma prolactin (PRL), luteinizing hormone (LH), follicle stimulating hormone (FSH), progesterone, estrone, estradiol, dehydroepiandrosterone (DHEA), dehydroepiandrosterone sulfate (DHEA-S), and testosterone before, during, and at end of puberty in normal boys. (Reproduced by permission from Sizonenko PC: Endocrinology in pre-adolescence and adolescence, I. Hormonal changes during normal puberty. *Am J Dis Child* **132:**708, 1978, copyright 1978 American Medical Association.

Smaller amounts of androstanediol, DHT, and androsterone are produced. A transient rise in activity of 5-alpha-reductase enzyme during early pubertal development stimulates formation of DHT and androstanediol from testosterone (22).

Testosterone excretion rises sharply after about 50% of skeletal maturity has been achieved; this corresponds to approximately stage 4 sexual development (9). Between 10 and 17 years (skeletal maturation) there is a twentyfold increase in plasma testosterone (30). With the rapid increase in testosterone there is also increase in size of prostate, testes, and penis. Testosterone levels are 5 to 10 times higher in males than in females and DHEA and DHEAS levels from the adrenals are approximately twice as high (Figures 5-12, 5-13). In boys, estrogen levels remain low. Most circulating estrogens are derived peripherally from testosterone and androstenedione (22).

## Hypothalamic–Pituitary Axis at Puberty

The release of LH and FSH are regulated by a humoral substance from the hypothalamus called gonadotropin-releasing hormone (GnRH) or LH-releasing hormone (LHRH). The GnRH evoked release of LH is greater in pubertal than in prepubertal children and increases even further in adulthood (17). In females, FSH is responsive to GnRH at any stage of development (30).

In the female, estrogens inhibit the secretion of both LH and FSH by negative feedback acting upon both the hypothalamus and the pituitary (25) (Figure 5-14). In addition, estrogens provoke the preovulatory surge of LH resulting in ovulation (31). Progesterone inhibits LH secretion but has no specific effect on FSH (32). In males, testosterone inhibits secretion of LH at both pituitary and hypothalamic levels (33), but its effect on FSH is obscure. A separate testicular factor, termed inhibin, a peptide probably secreted by Sertoli cells, may be primarily responsible for FSH regulation (34) (Figure 5-14).

In addition to negative feedback from gonadal steroids, gonadotropins regulate their own secretion via a "short feedback loop" suppressing gonadotropin-releasing-hormone in the hypothalamus (35). The hypothalamic releasing factor may itself regulate its own release—a feedback termed ultra-short feedback loop (36). Other areas of the central nervous system may also participate in control of gonadotropin secretion. Via such mechanisms it is possible for physical and emotional stress to influence gonadotropin secretion and hence, sexual maturation and functions. Sensory input, such as light, may also influence sexual maturation. Menarche occurs earlier in blind girls than in those with normal vision (29).

The cyclic changes in serum LH, FSH, estradiol, and progesterone which occur during an established menstrual cycle are shown in Figure 5-15. FSH release stimulates growth of the ovarian follicle which secretes estradiol. When the concentration of estradiol reaches a critical level, there is a LH–FSH surge which results in ovulation and formation of a corpus luteum. Progesterone levels rise rapidly and remain high during the luteal phase. The elevated gonadal steroids inhibit secretions of LH and FSH and as the corpus luteum undergoes involution, progesterone and estrogen levels fall and menstruation occurs. The mid-cycle LH surge appears to require maturation of hypothalamic centers. A positive or stimulatory

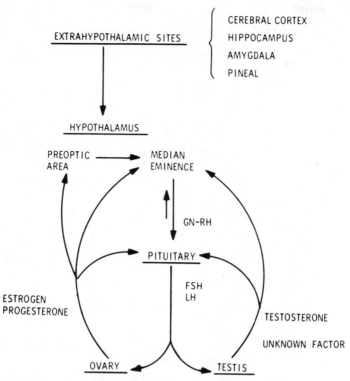

**Figure 5-14.** Regulation of secretion of LH (luteinizing hormone) and FSH (follicle-stimulating hormone). Gn-RH is gonadotropin-releasing hormone. (Reproduced by permission from Root AW: Endocrinology of puberty, I. Normal sexual maturation. *J Pediatr* **83:**1, 1973.)

feedback system is established when the hypothalamus has matured to a point of susceptibility, usually mid to late puberty (37).

## Initiation of Puberty

Although much recent work has added considerably to our understanding of the neural–hormonal interactions which occur at puberty, the precise mechanism by which pubertal development is initiated is not clearly understood. At one time, it was assumed that pituitary and gonads were entirely quiescent throughout infancy and childhood and only became active or capable of sexual maturation at the time of puberty, but with radioimmunoassay measurements of gonadal, pituitary, and hypothalamic hormones, it rapidly became evident that infantile and, in fact, fetal gonads and pituitary were capable of hormonal production. Complete sexual maturation, occurring as early as the first year of life in some children with precocious puberty, emphasizes the fact that the gonadal–pituitary–

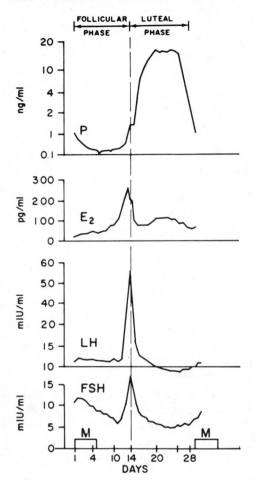

**Figure 5-15.** Cyclic hormonal changes in female subjects showing daily levels of serum LH, FSH, estradiol (E2), and progesterone (P) in a normally cycling female subject. (Reproduced by permission from Swerdloff RS: Physiological control of puberty. *Med Clin North Am* **62**:351, 1978. Copyright 1978 American Medical Association.)

hypothalamic axis is capable of integrated function well before the usual age of adolescence. Puberty does not represent the sudden activation of a dormant system, but rather represents change in the level of function of a system already endowed with total functional capacity (17).

A number of different mechanisms have been suggested to explain the lack of sexual maturation in the infant and child and the initiation of puberty in an orderly fashion at a suitable time. The concept of changing sensitivity of the hypothalamic–pituitary centers to the feedback regulation by gonadal steroids has been most widely accepted (38). According to this hypothesis, the prepubertal hypothalamus is very sensitive to the inhibitory actions of small amounts of estrogens or testosterone (26). Gonadal steroids in very small amounts succeed in preventing elevation of FSH or LH and all remain low throughout childhood. Low levels of gonadotropins and

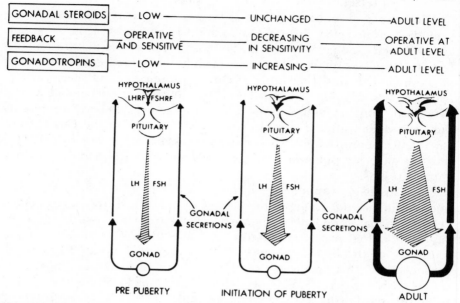

| GONADAL STEROIDS | — LOW — | UNCHANGED | ADULT LEVEL |
| FEEDBACK | OPERATIVE AND SENSITIVE | DECREASING IN SENSITIVITY | OPERATIVE AT ADULT LEVEL |
| GONADOTROPINS | — LOW — | INCREASING | ADULT LEVEL |

HYPOTHALAMUS
LHRF FSHRF
PITUITARY
LH FSH
GONADAL SECRETIONS
GONAD
PRE PUBERTY

HYPOTHALAMUS
PITUITARY
LH FSH
GONADAL SECRETIONS
GONAD
INITIATION OF PUBERTY

HYPOTHALAMUS
PITUITARY
LH FSH
GONAD
ADULT

**Figure 5-16.** Initiation of puberty. Schematic diagram of progressive change in gonadotropin secretion which results from a decrease in hypothalamic sensitivity to gonadal steroids. (Reproduced by permission from Reiter EO, Root AW: Hormonal changes of adolescence. *Med Clin North Am* **59:**1289, 1975.)

gonadal steroids are observed from about age 2 until just before puberty. Higher levels of gonadal steroids seen during infancy may be the consequence of lack of complete development of this sensitivity until late infancy.

The changes which appear to occur in the hypothalamic–pituitary–gonadal system at puberty are schematically portrayed in Figure 5-16. The prepubertal hypothalamus responds to small amounts of gonadal steroid with low levels of gonadotropin releasing hormone and only small amounts of FSH and LH are released from the pituitary. Gradually, in late childhood the "sensitivity" of the hypothalamic centers to the negative feedback inhibition of gonadal steroids decreases so that the small amounts of gonadal hormone, which previously inhibited GnRH secretion, no longer suffice (30, 39). The secretion of GnRH increases, pituitary FSH and LH rise, and gonadal secretion is stimulated until a new equilibrium is achieved at a higher level. When gonadal secretions rise to adequate levels, sex organ growth occurs and puberty is said to have begun. Continued maturation of the hypothalamic centers results eventually in equilibrium between gonad, pituitary, and hypothalamus at adult levels of sex steroids and gonadotropins.

The events of pubertal maturation can be viewed as a continuum extending from sexual differentiation and the ontogeny of the hypothalamic–pituitary–gonadal system in the fetus to full sexual maturation and fertility (38). The regulatory systems include the neurosecretory neurons of the hypothalamus (regulators of GnRH production and release, modulated by sex steroids and possibly neurotransmitters and opioid neural networks), pituitary gonadotropins, and the gonads. Puberty represents the reactivation, after a period of quiescent activity, of the GnRH neurosecretory neurons and their endogenous oscillatory secretion (38). This sets the stage for pubertal pulsatile secretion of GnRH and of pituitary gonadotropins.

Odell discusses a number of different mechanisms (16 in total) which might influence the timing of the process of sexual maturation (40). Odell believes changing gonadal response to gonadotropins may offer a better explanation for maturation of the prepubertal process than changing sensitivity of the hypothalamus. Using the rat as a model, Odell et al. demonstrated that the testes of the newborn male rat are essentially unresponsive to LH or FSH secretion (41). Gonadotropins induce LH receptors on Leydig cells, so that testicular secretion of testosterone gradually increases and negative feedback suppression of FSH and LH secretion occurs (40). Such a mechanism has not been demonstrated yet in man, but Sizonenko has shown that the rise in testosterone after administration of hCG to cryptorchid boys correlates well with FSH levels (42). Intrinsic responsiveness to gonadotropins may therefore play a role in the process of pubertal initiation.

Odell cites evidence to suggest an intrinsic "dampening" effect on the hypothalamic–pituitary system, noting that "even in agonadal children FSH and LH did not rise to high levels until the time of puberty" (40). Odell also mentions a changing pituitary responsiveness to gonadotropin-releasing hormone. FSH secretion in response to GnRH is greater in a prepubertal child than in an adult. Whether this is an intrinsic change or secondary to increasing blood levels of gonadal steroids is not known.

Mention is also made by Odell of the hypothesis of "critical weight" as a determiner of events of puberty (40). Frisch and McArthur suggested that the onset and maintenance of regular menstrual function were dependent on a minimum weight for height representing a critical fat storage (43) (Figure 5-17). As a corollary to this, early maturing girls are often heavy for age and late maturing girls light for age, and delayed menarche and amenorrhea are seen with some frequency in ballet dancers and athletes (44, 45). Variability in actual weight associated with the initiation of puberty limits the usefulness of the critical weight hypothesis, but the correlation of puberty with critical lean/fat ratio of body composition has some support from animal data (46). It is possible that the neuroendocrine systems responsible for initiation of puberty mature in

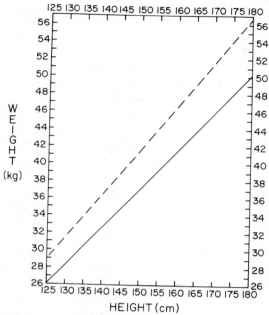

**Figure 5-17.**   Weight for height at which menarche is likely to occur (solid line) and at which regular menses are likely to be maintained (broken line). (Reproduced by permission from Barnes HV: Physical growth and development during puberty. *Med Clin North Am* **59:**1305, 1975, adapted from Frisch RF, McArthur JW: *Science* **185:**949, 1974.)

conjunction with other maturational events of the body, such as body compositional changes.

The explanations of sexual maturation mentioned by Odell are not necessarily mutually exclusive. Several of the mechanisms may be operative and still produce a harmonious progression of sexual maturation. Changing gonadal sensitivity may well determine responsiveness to FSH and LH, but changing pituitary sensitivity may simultaneously determine response to GnRH and there may still be some CNS inhibiting factor(s) preventing GnRH secretion until critical maturation of other tissues has been achieved. The initiation of puberty and the suppression of pubertal maturation during infancy and childhood is clearly complex and not yet understood. It is not a sudden or unexpected event, but rather one of progressive maturation toward full growth and capability of reproduction.

## Relation of Sex Hormones to Growth at Puberty

The adolescent growth spurt is produced by the combined actions of growth hormone and androgens. In the male, growth hormone and testosterone act synergistically to produce the growth spurt. Each alone is capable of producing only a portion of the expected growth at puberty (47). Subjects with pituitary deficiency, treated with testosterone and other pituitary replacement therapy, grow best when both growth hormone and testosterone are given together, though testosterone without human growth hormone is responsible for a greater velocity of growth than growth hormone without testosterone (48). Boys with isolated growth hormone deficiency double their velocity of growth (from 4.4 to 8.7 cm/yr) when treated with growth hormone as they enter puberty spontaneously. Boys lacking both testosterone and growth hormone when treated with testosterone alone had a growth spurt (5–6 cm/yr), but it failed to approach the expected 9cm/yr of the average normal adolescent (48). It seems clear, therefore, that both growth hormone and androgens are required to produce the adolescent growth spurt. Growth hormone levels increase progressively with pubertal maturation (49) and there is a dramatic rise in Sm C/IGF I during the adolescent growth spurt (50). There is a close correlation between Sm C concentrations and linear growth velocity during puberty (51). Human growth hormone appears to stimulate growth of about 4 cm/yr throughout puberty, and testosterone and adrenal androgens simply add an additional growth spurt of about 5 cm/yr (48). In girls, it is presumed that the growth spurt is produced by human growth hormone and adrenal androgens (48), though lack of rise in free androgens during the growth spurt suggests greater sensitivity of girls to androgen or a synergistic action of estrogen and growth hormone (52).

Thyroid seems to play a permissive role in growth stimulation during adolescence. Without thyroxine, skeletal maturation and growth do not occur optimally and sexual development may be delayed as well. In the normal adolescent there is an increase in thyroxine turnover associated with a relative increase in basal metabolic rate. The thyroid uptake of iodine is increased and iodine turnover is more rapid in adolescents than in adults (53). There may be an increased need for thyroxine during the adolescent growth spurt. TSH temporarily increases at puberty. This may lead to a transient thyromegaly which must be distinguished from pathologic enlargement due to lymphocytic thyroiditis, a common thyroidal problem during the pubertal or prepubertal years (54).

The increase in muscle mass and loss of fat in the limbs at adolescence is presumably a response to adrenal androgens in both boys and girls. The greater muscle mass in the boy is probably due to testicular testosterone (48). The differential sexual hair patterns between boys and girls may be explained by a differential target tissue sensitivity to testosterone versus adrenal androgens, perhaps related to receptors for specific androgens at the hair follicles. Differential maturation of sensitivity to androgens at different sites may produce not only the differences between boys and girls, but also the time sequence in their appearance. Testosterone given in large doses to boys whose testes fail to develop at puberty causes growth of pubic hair and penis but does not directly produce facial hair growth

(48). Facial hair growth requires 5-alpha-reductase activity for local formation of DHT, which appears not to develop adequately in cryptorchid boys.

The last stages of skeletal maturation, including closure of the epiphyses of bones, appear to be dependent upon the sex hormones, androgens or estrogens, both being effective. In a subject who produces no sex hormones (gonadal or adrenal), the skeletal maturation progresses slowly until it reaches about the 13 year bone age level. Without sex hormones, progress beyond this stage occurs slowly, if at all (48). The response to sex hormone seems to depend upon the stage of maturation of the skeleton. Androgen or estrogen given in large amounts before the age of puberty (before bone age of 13), results in rapid maturation of the skeleton, as is commonly seen in congenital virilizing adrenal hyperplasia and precocious puberty, but large doses of sex steroids after bone age 13 seem only capable of restoring the rate of maturation to normal (48).

The time of menarche in girls has been related to the growth spurt in a variety of ways. Frisch and Revelle noted a correlation between weight and/or body fat composition and time of menarche and postulated that menstruation occurs at a "critical weight" or critical lean body weight to fat ratio (55). Once peak height velocity is reached, there is an increase in velocity of fat accumulation and menarche can be expected during deceleration of linear velocity (56). Attractive as this hypothesis might be in relating events of puberty to height and weight achievements, there are too many exceptions and too much variability of the circumstances surrounding menarche to cite "critical weight" or even critical lean mass to fat ratio as a determining factor in timing of menarche (57). That changes in height, weight, and body composition are occurring at the time of menarche is evident, but they appear to be manifestations of harmonious interrelated processes rather than determinants.

## NUTRITION IN ADOLESCENCE

During adolescence nutrition assumes an important role to provide adequate substrate for a rapidly growing and active person. The complexity of the problem is compounded by the great variability in timing of the adolescent growth spurt as well as the extremely varied growth patterns of individuals passing through puberty.

### Nutritional Requirements for Growth at Adolescence

The nutritional requirements for the adolescent are strongly influenced by the velocity of growth. Until the ninth or tenth birthday the child has had a fairly steady increment of weight, averaging 2.3–2.7 kg/yr (Figure 5-4). The average girl begins her adolescent weight gain at about 10–11 years and reaches a peak at about 12½ years. The year before menses are established is usually the year of maximal growth for both height and weight. For boys, the onset of the growth spurt is about 2 years later and peak weight (and height) velocity is reached at about age 14 (7, 58) (Figure 5-4).

The adolescent growth spurt contributes only about 15% to final adult height, but there is almost a doubling of body weight during adolescence (59). Nutritional requirements are related to rapid increase in body mass, so it comes as no surprise that adolescence represents a time of peak nutritional requirement, a fact observed anecdotally by "teen watchers" everywhere: "My teenage son eats only one meal per day, beginning at 7:00 A.M. and capped off with a snack just before bedtime." Because calorie and protein requirements reach an all-time high during the adolescent growth spurt, and the adolescent is sensitive to caloric restriction, unless the increased needs for accelerated growth are met, alterations in the growth pattern and growth potential may occur (59).

## Energy Requirements of Adolescence

Any estimate of caloric requirements for adolescents must take into account the vast differences in energy requirements which occur between individuals for no apparent reason. In general, those teenagers who are largest or who are most physically active require more calories, but neither of these requirements has been shown to be absolute (58). Everyone has seen the small boy who eats more than the larger boy and the moderately active teenager who consumes more than the very active friend. Dukes, quoted by Widdowson, expresses this observation of individuality as follows: "Some children are capable of consuming and do not seem to thrive without a large quantity of food, while the same amount in others would prove a positive poison and cause ill health and disease" (60). Added to this individuality of need, the growth status of the teenager and current nutritional status must be considered before we can estimate energy requirements (61).

There is also a clear sex difference in energy requirements from about 6 years on. Boys at 6 consume approximately 100 cal/day more than girls. By age 10, the difference is 200 calories, by 14, 400 calories, and by 18, boys consume on an average 830 cal/day more than girls (59). Taking these differences into account, the World Health Organization (FAO/WHO) average energy requirements of adolescents by age, sex and weight are displayed in Table 5-3.

## Protein Requirements in Adolescence

Protein is required for formation of new tissue, and for replacement of already formed tissue. In adolescence the requirements for new tissue formation may be considerable. Added to these considerations, one must assure adequacy of calories and other nutrients needed for energy requirements. Protein intake is generally higher in boys and reaches a

**Table 5-3. Energy Requirements of Adolescents by Year**[a]

| | | Males | | | Females | |
|---|---|---|---|---|---|---|
| Age (yr) | Weight (kg) | Energy per kg per day (kcal) | Energy per person per day (kcal) | Weight (kg) | Energy per kg per day (kcal) | Energy per person per day (kcal) |
| 10 | 33.9 | 74 | 2500 | 33.8 | 68 | 2300 |
| 11 | 36.7 | 71 | 2600 | 37.7 | 62 | 2350 |
| 12 | 40.2 | 67 | 2700 | 42.4 | 57 | 2400 |
| 13 | 45.5 | 61 | 2800 | 47.0 | 52 | 2450 |
| 14 | 51.7 | 56 | 2900 | 50.3 | 50 | 2500 |
| 15 | 56.6 | 53 | 3000 | 52.3 | 48 | 2500 |
| 16 | 60.3 | 51 | 3050 | 53.6 | 45 | 2420 |
| 17 | 62.4 | 50 | 3100 | 54.2 | 43 | 2340 |
| 18 | 63.7 | 49 | 3100 | 54.6 | 42 | 2270 |
| 19 | 65.0 | 47 | 3020 | 55.0 | 40 | 2200 |

Reproduced by permission from Heald F: Adolescent nutrition. *Med Clin North Am* **59:**1329, 1975.

[a] FAO/WHO, 1973.

maximum at age 12 years in girls and at age 16 years in boys (58). In choosing the appropriate source for protein one must consider the amino acid composition of the protein. "Quality" of protein is often used to denote its content of essential amino acids; that is, those which cannot be synthesized within the body. Most animal protein sources contain all essential amino acids in approximate amounts required by other animals, including man, but vegetable proteins often contain amino acids in differing amounts and some amino acids are not present at all. This becomes a problem only when the variety of protein sources is severely restricted for economic reasons or for personal food preferences.

Protein requirements of male and female adolescents recommended by FAO/WHO are shown in Tables 5-4A and 5-4B. The table shows nitrogen requirements for an adolescent of average weight for age listing both obligatory nitrogen loss and nitrogen requirement for growth in mg/kg/day. The recommended protein intake is adjusted to reflect needs shown by balance data and an increase of 30% to cover individual variability and is expressed in grams of protein/kg/day (59).

## Vitamins and Minerals

There is remarkably little information on vitamin and mineral requirements of the growing adolescent (59). Based on (a) amounts required to prevent deficiency disease, (b) levels in populations suffering from vitamin and mineral deficiencies, or (c) controlled studies to produce or cure

**Table 5-4A.  Protein Requirements of Female Adolescents**[a]

| Age (yr) | Body weight (kg) | Obligatory N loss (mg/kg/day) | N need for growth (mg/kg/day) | Total | Safe level of intake[b] (g protein/kg/day) |
|---|---|---|---|---|---|
| 10 | 33.79 | 68 | 9 | 72 | 0.81 |
| 11 | 37.74 | 64 | 8 | 72 | 0.76 |
| 12 | 42.37 | 60 | 10 | 70 | 0.74 |
| 13 | 47.04 | 57 | 7 | 64 | 0.68 |
| 14 | 50.35 | 55 | 4 | 59 | 0.62 |
| 15 | 52.30 | 54 | 2 | 56 | 0.59 |
| 16 | 53.57 | 54 | 1 | 55 | 0.58 |
| 17 | 54.20 | 53 | 1 | 54 | 0.57 |

Reproduced by permission from Heald F: Adolescent nutrition. *Med Clin North Am* **59**:1329, 1975.

[a] FAO/WHO, 1973.

[b] Estimated total N requirement increased by 30% to coincide with balance data and further increased by 30% to cover individual variability.

deficiencies, the World Health Organization (62) and the National Research Council (63) have published tables of specific minimal allowances for all known vitamins and most minerals. The dietary need for vitamins is increased during the adolescent years because of greater energy demand and increased rate of tissue and skeletal growth. Provided basic energy needs are met by a well-balanced and diverse diet, vitamin and mineral

**Table 5-4B.  Protein Requirements of Male Adolescents**[a]

| Age (yr) | Body weight (kg) | Obligatory N loss (mg/kg/day) | N need for growth (mg/kg/day) | Total | Safe level of intake[b] (g protein/kg/day) |
|---|---|---|---|---|---|
| 10 | 33.93 | 72 | 6 | 78 | 0.82 |
| 11 | 36.74 | 70 | 7 | 77 | 0.81 |
| 12 | 40.23 | 66 | 8 | 74 | 0.78 |
| 13 | 45.50 | 62 | 11 | 73 | 0.77 |
| 14 | 51.66 | 59 | 9 | 68 | 0.72 |
| 15 | 56.65 | 57 | 6 | 63 | 0.67 |
| 16 | 60.33 | 57 | 4 | 61 | 0.64 |
| 17 | 62.41 | 56 | 2 | 58 | 0.61 |

Reproduced by permission from Heald F: Adolescent nutrition. *Med Clin North Am* **59**:1329, 1975.

[a] FAO/WHO, 1973.

[b] Estimated total N requirement increased by 30% to coincide with balance data and further increased by 30% to cover individual variability.

requirements of adolescents are readily met (58). Minerals most likely to be in inadequate supply in the diet are calcium, iron, and zinc (61).

## Vitamin Requirements of Adolescence

Though Vitamin A consumption by teenagers is often reported to be below levels recommended by the National Research Council (NRC) for teenagers, no widespread functional disability seems to occur because of this deficiency. It is likely that the recommended levels are sufficiently high that modest decreases in consumption are not truly deficiencies (63).

The need for Vitamin D in promoting bone mineralization is acknowledged, and with rapid bone formation and turnover in adolescence, increased need for Vitamin D could be predicted. A rise in 1,25 $(OH)_2$ $D_3$ is seen with the pubertal growth spurt, peak levels corresponding to peak growth rates (64). Despite this, there are no data on Vitamin D needs in adolescence (59, 62). Unless an adolescent is confined by illness away from sunlight for long periods of time, noticeable effects from Vitamin D deficiency are not seen during adolescence. Adequate amounts seem to be available through sunlight and a varied diet which includes milk fortified with Vitamin D (63).

Precise needs for Vitamin C in adolescence are not known, though amounts generally recommended for adolescents include the amount known to be necessary to prevent scurvy in adults, plus extra to cover unknown needs of growth (59, 62).

Folic acid would appear to be a critical vitamin during adolescence because of its role in DNA synthesis, but widespread deficiency among adolescents is unknown (59). Levels required by adults to provide hematologic response in deficiency states provide the model for calculating adolescent needs (62). Vitamin B-12 is needed with folic acid for DNA synthesis and hematologic integrity and might be expected to be required preferentially by the adolescent, but studies documenting the need in adolescence have not been made (59). Recommended amounts are similar to those for adults (62).

Niacin, riboflavin, and thiamin are all known to participate in energy metabolism. Therefore, recommendations for these vitamins are based on caloric requirements. There is a lack of data on actual requirements of these vitamins in adolescence (59). Vitamin B-6 is involved in a number of enzyme systems associated with nitrogen metabolism. The recommended levels (interpolated from information available for adults and infants) are easily attained by most teenagers (59, 62).

## Mineral Requirements in Adolescence

There is rapid turnover and formation of bone tissue throughout adolescence coincident with the pubertal growth spurt and accelerated bone mineralization toward the end of the pubertal growth spurt (65). This clearly represents an increased need for calcium during adolescence.

Dietary requirements during adolescence will be influenced by efficiency of absorption and the rapid growth of the skeleton (58). FAO/WHO recommendations suggest 700 milligrams of calcium per day for adolescents 11–15 years, and 500–600 mg/day for adolescents age 16–19 (62). Up to 1100 mg Ca/day has been recommended for adolescent boys (59). After adult stature is achieved, rates of bone accretion and resorption drop sharply (65).

Loss of iron occurs in feces, urine, skin, and in girls through menstruation. During adolescence iron intake must equal these losses, plus enough to supply iron for growth of red blood cells and other tissues. The current recommendations of FAO/WHO (62) and NRC (63) are 18 mg Fe/day for female and 10–12 mg/day for male adolescents. In the Ten State Nutrition Survey, iron deficiency was the most prevalent nutritional deficiency of children and adolescents (66).

Zinc is known to be essential for normal growth and may be more important than we have realized. Zinc is an essential part of the insulin molecule and is required for many enzymatic actions dealing with nucleic acid and protein synthesis. It seems to play a role in wound healing and gonadal development. In animals, deficiency of zinc produces growth failure and isolated reports suggest the same may be true for man.

## NUTRITIONAL DEFICIENCY AND SEXUAL MATURATION

In addition to its global role in growth, adequate nutrition is important for normal progression of physiologic maturation in puberty. Dreizen et al. report that substandard childhood nutrition slows the rate of skeletal maturation, delays the onset of menarche, and retards epiphyseal fusion in the long bones (67). Menarche occurred, on an average, 24 months earlier in well-nourished girls compared to under-nourished girls. Undernutrition delayed the time of the adolescent growth spurt but, because of the concomitant delay in skeletal maturation, there was a lengthening of time available for growth and ultimate height seemed not to be noticeably affected.

## PSYCHOLOGICAL ADJUSTMENTS IN ADOLESCENCE

The dramatic physical and hormonal changes occurring at the time of adolescence, together with the social expectations of society, place rather severe demands on the adolescent. At the conclusion of adolescence, adult height will be reached and sexual maturation will have prepared the individual for reproduction and maintenance of the species. Social and mental maturation must occur simultaneously to allow the adolescent to adjust smoothly and naturally to the demands of society. Because the timing and rate of progression through puberty is quite variable, some adolescents will find themselves growing rapidly and maturing sexually at an early age, while others will watch nearly all their peers shoot up in height and weight and become sexually mature while they remain child-like in their growth and maturation. Both extremes, natural though they may be, may test the ability of the adolescent to adapt gracefully to the inevitable.

Early or late physical maturation may have striking and long-term effects on adolescent behavior (68). Early maturing boys are more poised, relaxed, and good-natured than late maturing boys. They are perceived as more attractive and popular and tend to be outstanding athletes and student body officers. The late maturing boys are seen as less grown-up, less good-looking, bossy, restless, more attention-seeking, and talkative (68, 69). Early maturing girls by contrast were viewed as less attractive than late maturers. Early maturers were taller and heavier during adolescence and were below average in popularity, sociability, leadership, poise, and expressiveness, whereas late maturers excelled in each of these characteristics and in personal appearance and attractiveness. Late maturing girls had less need for recognition and exhibited fewer negative psychological characteristics (68, 70).

The boy who is shorter than his peers and whose "little brothers" pass him by and enter puberty before he does can suffer a severe desire to withdraw from fellowship with larger, more mature peers or may feel the need to attract attention by becoming quarrelsome and pugnacious. Either way, adjustment to social demands is impaired and psychological problems may arise. The girl who is taller than her peers has similar problems in adjusting to the temporary differential existing between herself and her peers. Psychological stresses may interfere with enjoyment of the adolescent period and perhaps prevent a smooth adjustment to her adult role as well.

Premature thelarche (early appearance of breast tissue), premature adrenarche (the premature appearance of pubic hair), asymmetric breast development, and benign adolescent gynecomastia are other "naturally" occurring features of adolescence which can cause a great deal of concern on the part of the adolescent. Their greatest fear is that of being different or abnormal, and they often view any pattern of growth or maturation which does not appear average as being "abnormal." For mild excursions from normal, that is, puberty occurring a little earlier or later than average, mild gynecomastia in the pubertal boy or mild asymmetry in breast development, simple reassurance of normal variations and the benign nature of the occurrence will suffice to restore the adolescent's acceptance of him or herself. If the perception of self is severely warped by the physiological disturbance of puberty, psychiatric counseling may be necessary to restore psychic equilibrium. Extreme deviations from normal adolescent growth and sexual development patterns are discussed in

Chapter 10 and some psychological approaches to a variety of growth patterns are discussed in Chapter 12.

## REFERENCES

1. American Heritage Dictionary of American Language, William Morris (ed). Boston: Houghton Mifflin Company, 1979.
2. Faigel HC: Developmental approach to adolescence. *Pediatr Clinic* **21**:358, 1974.
3. Marshall WA, Tanner JM: Variation in patterns of pubertal changes in girls. *Arch Dis Child* **44**:291, 1969.
4. Marshall WA, Tanner JM: Variation in patterns of pubertal changes in boys. *Arch Dis Child* **45**:13, 1970.
5. Tanner JM: Puberty, in *Fetus Into Man: Physical Growth from Conception to Maturity*. Cambridge, Harvard University Press, 1978, pp 60–70, 117–153.
6. Barnes HV: Physical growth and development during puberty. *Med Clin North Am* **59**:1305–1317, 1975.
7. Tanner JM, Whitehouse RH, Takaishi M: Standards from birth to maturity for height, weight, height velocity, and weight velocity for British children 1965, Parts I and II. *Arch Dis Child* **41**:454, 613, 1966.
8. Marshall WA: Growth and sexual maturity in normal puberty. *Clin Endocrinol Metab* **4**:3–25, 1975.
9. Ducharme JR, Collu R: Pubertal development: normal, precocious and delayed. *Clin Endocrinol Metab* **11**(Mar):57, 1982.
10. Lee PA: Normal ages of pubertal events among American males and females. *J Adoles Health Care* **1**:26, 1980.
11. Nydick M, Bustos J, Dale JH, et al: Gynecomastia in adolescent boys. *J Am Med Assoc* **178**:449, 1961.
12. Lee PA: The relationship of concentration of serum hormones to pubertal gynecomastia. *J Pediatr* **86**:212, 1975.
13. Beck W, Stubbe P: Endocrinological studies of the hypothalamo-pituitary-gonadal axis during Danazol treatment in pubertal boys with marked gynecomastia. *Horm Metabol Res* **14**:653, 1982.
14. LeRoith D, Sobel R, Glick SM: The effect of clomiphene citrate on pubertal gynecomastia. *Acta Endocrinol* **95**:177, 1980.
15. Zacharias L, Wurtman RJ, et al: Sexual maturation in contemporary american girls. *Am J Obstet Gynecol* **108**:833, 1970.
16. Finkelstein JW: The endocrinology of adolescence. *Ped Clin North Am* **27**(Feb):53, 1980.
17. Ojeda SR, Andrews WW, Advis JP, et al: Recent advances in the endocrinology of puberty. *Endocrine Rev* **1**:228, 1980.
18. Sizonenko PC: Endocrinology in pre-adolescents and adolescents, I. Hormonal changes during normal puberty. *Am J Dis Child* **132**:704, 1978.
19. Root AW: Hormonal changes in puberty, *Pediatr Ann* **9**:365, 1980.
20. Forest NG, Sizonenko PC, Cathiard AM, et al: Hypophyso-gonadal function in humans during the first year of life. *J Clin Invest* **53**:819, 1974.
21. Conte FA, Grumbach MM, Kaplan SL: A diphasic pattern of gonadotropin secretion in patients with the syndrome of gonadal dysgenesis. *J Clin Endocrinol Metab* **40**:670, 1975.
22. Gupta D: Changes in gonadal and adrenal steroid patterns during puberty. *Clin Endocrinol Metab* **4**:27–56, 1975.

23. Sizonenko PC, Paunier L: Hormonal changes in puberty: III. Correlation of plasma dehydroepiandrosterone, testosterone, FSH and LH with stages of puberty and bone age in normal boys and girls and in patients with Addison's disease or hypogonadism or with premature or late adrenarche. *J Clin Endocrinol Metab* **41:**894, 1975.

24. Parker L, Odell W: Control of adrenal androgen secretion by a new pituitary factor—cortical androgen stimulating hormone (CASH), Abstract. *Fed Proc* **25:**299, 1977.

25. Root AW: Endocrinology of puberty: I. Normal sexual maturation. *J Pediatr* **83:**1–19, 1973.

26. Boyar RM, Finkelstein JW, Roffwarg H, et al: Synchronization of augmented luteinizing hormone secretion with sleep during puberty. *N Engl J Med* **287:**582, 1972.

27. Judd HL, Parker DC, Yen SSC: Sleep-wake patterns of LH and testosterone release in pre-pubertal boys. *J Clin Endocrinol Metab* **44:**865, 1977.

28. Mortimer CH, McNeilly AS, Rees LH, et al: Radioimmunoassay and chromatographic similarity of circulating endogenous gonadotropin releasing hormone and hypothalamic extraction in man. *J Clin Endocrinol Metab* **43:**882, 1976.

29. Swerdloff RS: Physiological control of puberty. *Med Clin North Am* **62:**351–365, 1978.

30. Grumbach MM, Grave DH, Mayer FE: *Control of the Onset of Puberty.* New York, John Wiley & Sons, 1974.

31. Abraham GE, Odell WD, Swerdloff RS, et al: Simultaneous radioimmunoassay of plasma, FSH, LH, progesterone, 17-hydroxy-progesterone, and estrodiol-17β during the menstrual cycle. *J Clin Endocrinol Metab* **34:**312, 1972.

32. Wallach EE, Root AW, Garcia CR: Serum gonadotropin responses to estrogen and progesterone in recently castrated human females. *J Clin Endocrinol Metab* **31:**376, 1970.

33. Franchimont P: The regulation of follicle-stimulating hormone and luteinizing hormone secretion in humans, in Martini L, Ganong WF (eds). *Frontiers in Neuroendocrinology,* London, Oxford University Press, 1971, pp 331–358.

34. Swerdloff RS, Walsh PC, Jacobs HS, et al: Serum LH and FSH during sexual maturation in the male rat: The effect of castration and cyrptorchidism. *Endocrinology* **88:**120, 1971.

35. Motta M, Fraschini F, Martini L: "Short" feedback mechanisms in the control of anterior pituitary function, in Ganong WF, Martini L (eds), *Frontiers in Neuroendocrinology.* London, Oxford University Press, 1969, pp 211–253.

36. Hyppa M, Motta M, Martini L: "Ultra-short" feedback control of follicle-stimulating-hormone releasing factor secretion. *Neuroendocrinology* **7:**227, 1971.

37. Reiter EO, Root AW: Hormonal changes of adolescence. *Med Clin North Am* **59:**1289–1303, 1975.

38. Reiter EO, Grumbach MM: Neuroendocrine control mechanisms and the onset of puberty. *Ann Rev Physiol* **44:**595, 1982.

39. Kulin He, Grumbach MM, Kaplan SL: Changing sensitivity of the pituitary-gonadal hypothalamic feedback mechanism in man. *Science* **166:**1012, 1969.

40. Odell WD: The physiology of puberty: Disorders of the pubertal process, in DeGroot LJ (ed), *Endocrinology.* New York, Grune & Stratton, Volume 3, 1979, pp 1363–1379.

41. Odell WD, Swerdloff RS, Bain J, et al.: The effect of sexual maturation of testicular sensitivity to LH stimulation of testosterone secretion in the intact rat. *Endocrinology* **95:**1380, 1974.

42. Sizonenko PC, Cuendet A, Paunier L: FSH: Evidence for its mediating role on testosterone secretion in cryptorchidism. *J Clin Endocrinol Metab* **37:**68, 1973.

43. Frisch RE, McArthur JW: Menstrual cycles: Fatness as a determinant of minimum weight for height necessary for their maintenance or onset. *Science* **185:**149, 1974.

44. Frisch RE, Wyshak G, Vincent L: Delayed menarche and amenorrhea of ballet dancers. *New Engl J Med* **303:**17, 1980.

45. Dale E, Gerlach DH, Wilhite AL: Menstrual dysfunction in distance runners. *Obstet Gynec* **54:**47, 1979.

46. Kennedy GC, Mitra J: Hypothalamic control of energy balance and the reproductive cycle in the rat. *J Physiol* **166:**395, 1963.

47. Prader A, Illig R, Szeky J, et al: The effect of human growth hormone in hypopituitary dwarfism. *Arch Dis Child* **39:**535, 1964.

48. Tanner JM: Growth and endocrinology of the adolescent, in Gardner L (ed), *Endocrine and Genetic Diseases of Childhood*, ed 2. Philadelphia, WB Saunders Co, 1975, pp 14–64.

49. Minuto F, Barreca A, Ferrini S, et al: Growth hormone secretion in pubertal and adult subjects. *Acta Endocrinol* **99:**161, 1982.

50. Luna AM, Wilson PM, Wibbelsman CJ, et al: Somatomedins in adolescence: A cross-sectional study of the effect of puberty on plasma insulin-like growth factor I and II levels. *J Clin Endocrinol Metab* **57:**268, 1983.

51. Rosenfield RI, Furlanette R, Bock D: Relationship of somatomedin-C concentrations to pubertal changes. *J Pediatr* **103:**723, 1983.

52. Penfold JL, Smeaton TC, Gilliland JM, et al: Indices of serum androgens in normal puberty: Correlations of two indices with chronological age, bone age, and pubertal development in boys and girls. *Clin Endocrinol Metab* **15:**183, 1981.

53. Malvaux P, Beckers C, DeVisscher M: Dynamic studies on the inorganic iodine compartment and its exchanges during adolescence. *J Clin Endocrinol Metab* **25:**817, 1965.

54. Rallison ML, Dobyns BM, Keating FR, et al: Occurrence and natural history of chronic lymphocytic thyroiditis in childhood. *J Pediatr* **86:**675, 1975.

55. Frisch RE, Revelle R: Height and weight at menarche and a hypothesis of menarche, *Arch Dis Child* **46:**695, 1971.

56. Frisch RE: Nutrition, fatness, puberty, and fertility. *Comp Ther* **7:**15, 1982.

57. Scott EC, Johnston FE: Critical fat, menarche, and the maintenance of menstrual cycles: A critical review. *J Adoles Health Care* **2:**249, 1982.

58. Nutrition Committee, Canadian Pediatric Society: *Canad Med Assoc J* **129:**419, 1983.

59. Heald FP: Adolescent nutrition. *Med Clin North Am* **59:**1329, 1975.

60. Widdowson EM: A Study of individual children's diets. Medical Research Council Special Report Series No. 257, London, 1947, p 64.

61. Marino DD, King JC: Nutritional concerns during adolescence. *Ped Clins North Am* **27**(Feb):125, 1980.

62. World Health Organization Technical Report Series, Requirements of Ascorbic Acid, Vitamin D, Vitamin $B_{12}$, Folate, and Iron, No. 452. Geneva, FAO/WHO, 1970.

63. National Research Council: Recommended Dietary Allowances. Washington DC, National Academy of Science, 8th Edition, 1974.

64. Aksnes L, Aarskog D: Plasma concentrations of Vitamin D metabolites in puberty: Effect of sexual maturation and implications for growth. *J Clin Endocrinol Metab* **55:**94, 1982.

65. Steendijk R: Effect of puberty on rates of bone growth and mineralization. *Arch Dis Child* **55:**655, 1980.

66. The Ten State Nutrition Survey, 1968–1970, U.S. Department of Health, Education, and Welfare, DHEW Publication No. (HSM) 72-8133, pp V-82, 83.

67. Dreizen S, Spirakis CN, Stone RE: A comparison of skeletal growth and maturation in under-nourished and well-nourished girls before and after menarche. *J Pediatr* **70:**256, 1967.

68. Gross RT, Duke PM: The effect of early versus late physical maturation on adolescent behavior. *Ped Clin North Am* **27** (Feb):71, 1980.

69. Jones M, Bayley N, Macfarlane J, et al (eds): *The Course of Human Development*. Toronto, John Wiley & Sons, 1971.

70. Jones M, Mussen P: Self-conceptions, motivations and interpersonal attitudes of early- and late-maturing girls. *Child Dev* **29**:491, 1958.

# 6
# Standards
# for Normal Growth

To determine whether the growth of an individual or a group of individuals is normal, we require standards for growth to provide objective data to which the growth of an individual or group may be compared.

## STANDARDS FOR PHYSICAL MEASUREMENTS
Tanner suggests that growth data may (a) serve to identify individuals or groups of individuals within a community who require special care, (b) be used to identify an illness which influences growth or to define the response to treatment of children who are ill, or (c) be used as an index of the health and nutrition of a population or subpopulation (1). For these purposes, the standards of growth should be representative of the groups with whom they are to be compared. Only healthy children who do not have any known or suspected health problems should be used to develop such standards. It is critical that measurements be made accurately and the techniques of measurement standardized.

### Types of Measurements, Uses and Limitations
There are many types of measurements that can be made to describe the growth of children and adolescents. Measurements of height made on large numbers of children at different ages yield *cross-sectional data*. On a chart formed from this type of information, we may confidently compare a given height of a child at a given age with his colleagues of the same age and sex. But to test growth over a period of time, *longitudinal growth data* are required. These represent measurements of the same individuals over the entire course of their growth. If individuals are added to the series or dropped from the series during the data collection period, *mixed longitudinal and cross-sectional data* are obtained. The latter is the most practical form of expression of longitudinal growth patterns. The impor-

tance of longitudinal growth data becomes evident at puberty with its wide variation in time of onset of adolescent growth spurt and the variation in time and height of peak rate of growth. In cross-sectional studies, wide variations dampen the true appearance of the individual growth spurt; whereas longitudinal measurements tend to preserve and define the individual changes in growth.

Growth may be expressed as height or weight achieved by certain age (*achievement or distance data*), or a rate of height or weight change in a specific period of time (*velocity of growth*). Each form of measurement provides unique information. In Figure 6-1 are depicted the measurements of height made by a French nobleman on his son from early infancy to adulthood. They represent the earliest known complete individual longi-tudinal measurements available and demonstrate both height achievement at successive years and velocity of growth at 6-month intervals during the entire growth period of the son.

Most charts of growth currently in use by primary health care physicians display height and weight achievement measurements. Achievement charts are limited somewhat in describing the growth process through infancy, childhood, and adolescence. It is difficult to display the rapid growth of infancy and the slow growth of childhood on the same achievement chart. For this reason, we often use charts specifically designed for infancy. It is likewise difficult to display the rapid growth of adolescence on the same chart, especially with the blunting effect of the cross-sectional data. It is in these two regions of growth that velocity charts are particularly helpful in describing the changes in rate of growth which occur (Figure 6-1).

## Expression of Physical Data for Comparison

Measurements may be expressed in a variety of ways to describe the population measured and to allow a comparison of physical data. A common way to express normal populations is to find mean values and express the natural Gaussian curve in terms of percentiles. In such charts, mean values are represented by the 50th percentile and the range from 3rd to 97th percentile encompasses 94% of the measurements. Three percent of the normal measurements fall below the 3rd percentile and 3% above the 97th percentile (Figure 6-2). This range works well to describe the normal population but may be unsuitable to describe the child whose measurements fall either far below the 3rd percentile or far above the 97th percentile. For such measurements, additional information about the normal standard population may be required. For any population whose measurements follow a normal distribution, a mean value may be calculated and the range of measurements may be described as standard deviations from the mean. If one charts the mean heights with standard deviations at various ages, growth charts may be designed which are very similar to those using percentiles. Plus or minus 2 standard deviations includes about 95% of the normal range of measurements corresponding

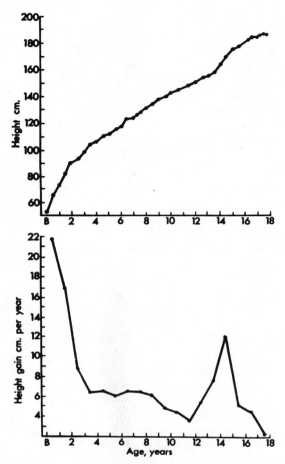

**Figure 6-1.** Growth in height. Progress of the son of Count Philibert de Montbeillard from birth to the age of 18 years. Upper graph, distance curve showing height reached at each age: lower graph, velocity curve, showing annual increments in height. (Reproduced by permission from Tanner JM: *Growth at Adolescence,* ed 2. Oxford, Blackwell Scientific Publications Ltd, 1962.)

almost identically to the 3rd and 97th percentiles. However, measurements below or above these measurements may also be described in terms of standard deviations from the mean, and more exact descriptions may be possible by using decimal fractions to describe the deviation of the measurements from the mean. For example, $-2.5$ SD means the measurements lies between 2 and 3 standard deviations below the mean (Figure 6-2). Note that this improves the precision of the description taken from the percentile chart from which we can only state that the measurement lies below the 3rd percentile.

# GROWTH STANDARDS

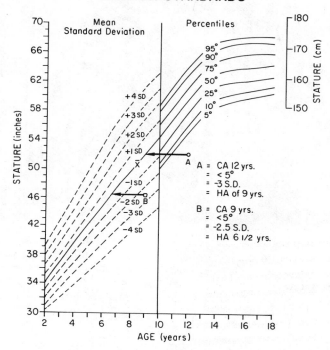

**Figure 6-2.**   Standard curves of height achievement. Comparison of measurements expressed as percentiles, mean ± S.D., and height-age (see text). Child A, with a chronologic-age (CA) of 12, is shown with a height below the 5° or −3 SD below the mean for 12 years or a height age (HA) of 9 years (horizontal intercepts 50th percentile @ 9 years). Similarly, child B, with a chronologic age of 9, may be said to have a height below the 5th percentile, −2.5 SD below the mean or HA of 6½ years.

Another way of relating a given measurement to those of the normal population of measurement is to describe the measurement in terms of average values by age. This is a concept popularized by the late Dr. Wilkins at Johns Hopkins University, and its utility lies in its simplicity. Given a height measurement of a child below the 3rd percentile, say minus 2.5 standard deviations at age 9, we say the measurement represents a height age of 6½. This means that an average child of age 6½ would have the same height measurement as the nine year old individual under consideration (Figure 6-2). This "height-age" is determined by comparing the actual height of the child with the age at which a horizontal line transects the 50th percentile or mean height line.

In general, charts constructed using percentile measurements of a population are best suited to describe normal populations and normal

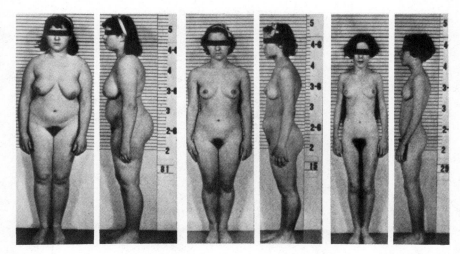

**Figure 6-3.** Somatotype as an expression of physique. Three 16-year-old girls are shown. The girl on the left displays typical characteristics of *endomorphy,* the girl in the center panel, *mesomorphy,* and the girl in the right panel, *ectomorphy* (see text). (Reproduced by permission from Lowrey GH: *Growth and Development in Children,* ed 7. Copyright © 1978 by Year Book Medical Publishers, Inc, Chicago.)

children. Either the mean with standard deviations or maturational age comparisons best describe the abnormally growing child. Achievement charts may be quite sufficient to describe the growth pattern of the average child, but the pattern of growth of the slow growing or rapidly growing child, and the early or late maturing child may be best described by velocity charts.

In addition to purely physical measurements such as height or weight, we may be interested also in measuring maturation, that is, the development of the child from an immature state to adulthood. This may be mapped in terms of growth and maturation of the bones or teeth which proceed through orderly steps of maturation. Maturation may also be mapped by stages of neurologic, mental, pubertal, social, or behavioral development (1). A means of assessing skeletal maturation is discussed below. Other measures of maturation will be included as they relate to physical growth or biological maturation.

## Measurement of Physique

It is sometimes useful to be able to describe the physique of a child with more than merely descriptive terms. To allow this, Sheldon introduced a somatotype numbering system (2). In this system, a child is rated from 1 to 7 for characteristics of endomorphy, mesomorphy and ectomorphy. In Figure 6-3, three girls are shown displaying typical features of *endomorphy*

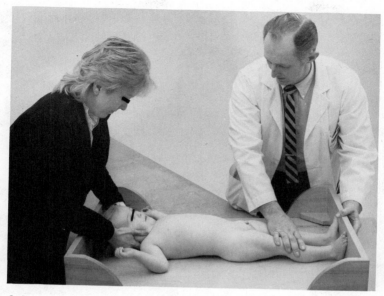

**Figure 6-4.** Technique for measurement of supine length using a board with right angle fixed head board and movable foot board with tape set into board for ease of accurate reading.

(711) such as obesity, round curves, softness; *mesomorphy* (171) muscular, angular, or athletic type; and *ectomorphy* (117) thin, asthenic, and usually tall. Although we have had little experience with the numbering system of Sheldon, we do often find physique description useful and would agree that photographs of children thought to have a growth disorder may be useful, not only for displaying physique, but for identifying syndromes associated with growth failure and for following the progress of growth.

## TECHNIQUES OF MEASUREMENT

It is important that physical measurements be made accurately and reproduceably. For this reason, techniques are described in detail to assure uniformity of measurements.

### Measurements of Length and Height

Supine *length* is usually preferred from birth to 2 years, and most growth charts are constructed to display normal standards of length during this period. The infant is measured in the supine position using a board with a right-angle fixed headboard and a movable foot board (Figure 6-4). The head is held against the headboard with the ear–eye plane vertical. The knees are held flat and the footboard moved up until the feet are against

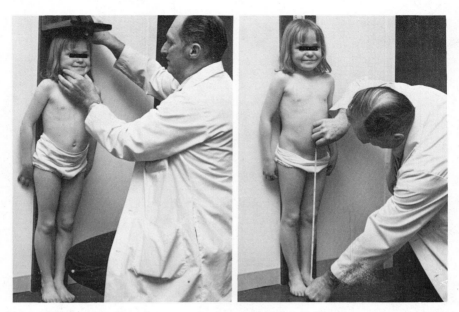

**Figure 6-5.** Technique for measurement of height and lower segment (pubis to floor). In the left panel, heels, buttocks, and shoulders are against the upright; eyes are looking straight ahead. A right angle device is lowered against the top of the head and height is read from the tape insert. In the right panel, a mark is made at the upper border of the pubic bone and distance from top of pubis to floor between feet is measured. This measurement should be performed in supine position if length comparisons are desired.

the footboard in a vertical position. The distance between the headboard and the footboard can be read off on an installed tape or between marks made at the head and foot. In the newborn infant, advantage may be taken of the reflex fencing position to obtain accurate length measurements. With the head turned to the side, the infant straightens one leg reflexly which is then used to perfect the measurement at the foot end. During chidhood, supine length averages 1 cm longer than standing height (1).

*Height* is measured in the standing position after 2 years, though length standards are available up to 36 months. Height should be obtained with the use of an apparatus that has a firm base, a tape affixed from the floor to at least 6 feet, and a right-angle board or other device above the head to give an accurate measurement. The child stands with back against the wall; heels, buttocks, shoulders, and back of head should all touch the wall (Figure 6-5). The head is erect with the ears and eyes in a horizontal plane. The child is told to stand at full height with heels flat on the base plate. The right-angle device is lowered until it touches the tip of the head and the measurement is read from the tape on the wall portion of the device (or measured from floor to the right-angle line at the top of the head). A weighted device (stadiometer developed by Whitehouse and Tanner) facilitates height measurement (3). The reproduceability of measurements with a free right-angle device is fairly good. Angle arms in weight machines are not generally accurate and should not be used in lieu of a right angle device. Note: There is a diurnal variation in height; a loss of about 0.7 cm occurs during the day because of compaction of the spinal column from the upright position (4).

*Sitting height* is measured with the subject's buttocks, shoulders, and head against the wall in a chair or on a box with a flat surface. The head of the child is held erect with ear–eye plane horizontal and a right-angle device is placed on the head, as with the measurement of height. The distance from buttocks to crown of head is recorded. Sitting height, when compared to total height, can give valuable information about relative length of limbs to trunk and can identify disproportionate growth (Appendix, Tables A-4 and A-6).

The ratio between *upper body segment* and *lower body segment* may also describe body proportions. The lower segment is measured with a firm tape from the upper edge of the symphysis pubis to the floor (Figure 6-5) or to the bottom of the heel in the supine position. The upper segment is obtained by subtracting the lower segment measurement from the total height or length. The measurements are expressed as a ratio of upper to lower segment (US/LS). This ratio expresses relative lengths of trunk and limbs which during growth undergo predictable changes. At birth, the legs represent about one-third the total body length, so the US/LS ratio is near 2/1 (1.7). By about 10 years of age, the legs have grown faster than the trunk and the ratio approaches 1.0. Standards for US/LS ratios by age allow interpretation of disproportionate growth (Appendix, Tables A-7 and A-8).

## Measurements of Weight and Skin Fold Thickness

Weight should be obtained on a reliable scale which is checked at intervals by "weights and standards". The infant may be weighed in a basket-type scale, the child on a standing scale. Weight may be recorded as pounds or kilograms and fractions thereof. The infant or child should be weighed either nude or lightly clothed, such as underpants or examination gowns. Weights do not distribute themselves in a normal curve but are skewed toward heavy weights. This skewed distribution invalidates the use of mean and standard deviations for expression of weight measurements in a population. Weights are more accurately defined in terms of percentiles.

To assess fat tissue deposition, we measure triceps and subscapular skinfold thickness. By convention, the left side of the body is used for these determinations. The triceps skinfold thickness represents limb fat

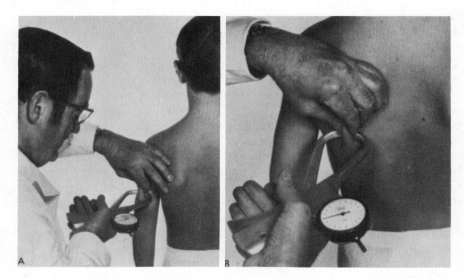

**Figure 6-6.** Technique for measuring skin fold thickness of triceps (A) and subscapular (B) regions (see text). (Reproduced by permission from Smith DW: *Growth and its Disorders*. Philadelphia, WB Saunders Co, 1977.)

deposition, and the subscapular skinfold thickness represents truncal deposits of fat. The technique for measurement is illustrated in Figure 6-6 and must be performed as exactly as possible (3). The triceps skinfold is measured halfway down the left upper arm with the left arm hanging relaxed at the subject's side. A point halfway between the shoulder (acromion) and elbow (olecranon) is marked on the dorsal surface of the arm. The skinfold is picked up just above the mark; calipers are applied to the skinfold just under the pinch point and relaxed to allow the spring-controlled constant pressure to be exerted, as illustrated in Figure 6-6. The caliper is designed to exert a constant pressure of 10 g/mm² at all openings.* The thickness of the double thickness of skin and subcutaneous tissue is read in millimeters to the nearest tenth millimeter from the caliper dial. The *subscapular skinfold* is picked up just below the angle of the left scapula at the fold in a vertial line as illustrated in Figure 6-6.

### Measurements of Skull and Face

*Circumference* of the skull (OFC) is measured with a nonstretchable tape in a plane over the occipital prominence above the ears and over the eyebrows. This measurement, usually recorded in centimeters, should

---

* Calipers for measuring skinfold thickness are obtainable from (1) R.E. Holtain, Holtain Ltd., Croswell, Crymmych, Penbrakshire, UK; or (2) Harvard Instruemnts, Inc., Boston, Mass.

represent maximal circumference of the skull in a horizontal plane. Although hair density will affect the circumference measurement, most infants in whom the accuracy of the measurements are most critical do not have heavy growth of hair and the effect of hair on the measurement is negligible. *Facial maturation* is subjective but occasionally useful as a measurement of delay in expected maturation. The maturation of the face is attributable primarily to the growth of the bridge of the nose and of the maxilla and mandible, especially with the coming of teeth. No standards exist and the accuracy of the assessment depends on the experience of the assessor and is one of "clinical impression".

## Miscellaneous Measurements

*Arm span* provides some information about body proportions. Arm span is measured from the center of the back to the tip of the longest finger with the arm held at shoulder height in the mid-plane of the body. Deviations of the arm forward or backward, or up or down will obviously affect the accuracy of the measurement. This measurement is doubled to obtain full span if the arms are of equal length or each is added separately if asymmetry is suspected. *Foot length* is measured with the foot in vertical position from the heel to the tip of the largest toe with the foot against a right-angle device. *Width of shoulder, hip, and head* can be measured with obstetric calipers. Shoulder width is measured between the acromial processes, hips at the intertrochanteric distance; the head is measured at biparietal width. Care should be taken to find the widest point overlying these bony processes.

## ASSESSMENT OF BIOLOGICAL MATURATION

The degree of biological maturation which has taken place in the growth process of an individual may be described in a number of different ways. Any tissue which undergoes specific, identifiable changes in the growth process and which has a specific end maturational state may be utilized to assess biological maturation.

## Indices of Maturation

In infancy, some indices of bone growth may be seen in the *size of fontanelles of the skull* and in the *form of the facial features*, especially of the nose and cheek bones. At birth, epiphyses are generally present in the distal femur and proximal tibia and progressive appearance of epiphyses can be charted throughout infancy. *Neurologic assessment* can be used not only to determine the state of maturity at birth (e.g., the Dubowitz criteria) but also to assess progress through infancy with the use of such instruments as the DDST, which assess developmental maturity.

In children, continued *maturation of the brain* can be assessed by behavioral or neurological stages of maturation. *Eruption of deciduous teeth* can

## INDICES OF MATURITY

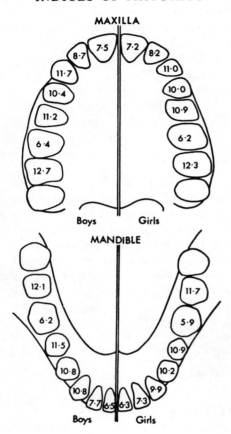

**Figure 6-7.** Mean times for eruption of *permanent* teeth. The first to appear is usually the first permanent molar in the lower jaw. The times of appearance of "wisdom" teeth are so variable that they have been omitted. (Reproduced by permission from Sinclair D: *Human Growth after Birth,* ed 3. London, Oxford Medical Publishers, 1978.)

give evidence of biologic maturity from ages 6 months to about 3 years, and the time of *eruption of permanent teeth* can allow an estimate of maturity from about 5 to 12 years (Figure 6-7). Over the entire period of growth, the changes occurring in the skeleton with appearance and *maturation of epiphyseal growth plates* probably provides the most reliable index of biologic maturity with the widest possible span, allowing identification of maturity at birth and extending to about age 17–18 before full maturity is achieved (5).

*Pubertal development* and *sexual maturation* provide recognizable indices of biologic maturation in adolescence. *Stages of pubertal development* are judged by visual inspection in comparison with photographic standards, and testicular size is visually compared with plastic models of known volume. (See Chapter 5.) In a study of the pubertal growth spurt, Hägg and Taranger found studies of puberty and skeletal development to be reliable maturation indicators but dental development less accurate (6).

## Skeletal Maturation

By far the most common means of assessment of biologic maturation is that of estimation of *skeletal maturation*. The reasons for this are several: (a) the changes which occur in bones of the maturing individual are roughly similar in all individuals, varying mainly in timing as an expression of delayed or accelerated maturation, (b) every center of ossification passes through a number of identifiable morphologic stages which may be identified as determiners of maturation; (c) all centers of bone maturation can be easily identified and recorded radiographically by means of x-rays of bones. Standards of maturity of bones and epiphyseal centers are usually based on maturation of a limited number of epiphyseal centers, those of the hand and wrist being most commonly chosen.

### Greulich and Pyle Atlas of Skeletal Maturation

The method of estimation of skeletal maturity used most widely in North America is that based on the atlas of hand and wrist by Greulich and Pyle (6). This atlas depicts by x-ray the average maturation of epiphyses of hand and wrist in male and female from newborn to full maturity. The standards are based on studies of middle-class children in Cleveland, Ohio from 1931 to 1942. Dr. T. W. Todd, who initiated the study, published standards from the early phases of the study in 1937 as *Todd's Atlas*. The Greulich and Pyle atlas, using standards derived from the complete study, was published in 1950 and revised and republished in 1959 (7).

In addition to approximately 60 photographic standards chosen to represent changes in osseous maturity at different ages from birth to approximately 19 years, the atlas contains tables of means and standard deviations for skeletal age for girls and boys, and maturity indicators of indivual bones and epiphyses of the hand describing the principle changes which occur in each bone from appearance at birth to full maturity (7). This information may be used by the radiologist to describe the level of maturation of the skeleton from an x-ray of the left hand and to describe the degree of delay or advancement of the skeletal maturation in standard deviations compared to the chronologic age.

The method of use of the Greulich–Pyle atlas is a simple matching procedure. The x-ray of the patient's hand and wrist is compared with the standard plates. There are 28 epiphyses and wrist bones plus two pisiforms in the hand and wrist, which may be used for the comparison with the subject's x-ray until one plate is found which best approximates the level of development of the patient. Skeletal development tends to occur in an orderly sequence, so it is usually possible to select a plate which approximately matches that of the subject. Skeletal age (bone age = BA) is recorded in years and months according to the nearest standard. According to the atlas, skeletal maturation is most accurately performed by comparing each of the bones of the hand and wrist and assigning to each a maturity age. Skeletal maturity is a modal expression of the sum of each of the bones of the hand and wrist.

There are often discrepancies between maturation of carpal bones and metacarpals or phalanges. To improve the reliability of the comparisons, Garn et al. have identified epiphyseal centers which have the highest statistical "communality", that is, tend to progress in a harmonious sequence together (8) (Figure 6-8). Because of their statistical communality, these centers are said to have maximum predictive value for skeletal maturation (8). When the subject's carpal development is at odds with the metacarpal or phalangeal development, we choose the skeletal maturity represented by the centers showing communality (Figure 6-8).

It is difficult to provide an atlas which accurately mirrors the average stage of maturity of children of different socioeconomic classes and of different races who mature at different rates. The Greulich–Pyle standards are advanced by 6 to 9 months over standards derived by Tanner and Whitehouse from a study of Scottish children (1). They may even be out-of-date for present-day American children who now mature at a different rate than children of the 1930s. The steady decline in age of menarche in North American girls reflects a need to re-evaluate our standards of biological maturation (skeletal maturation). In our hands the Greulich–Pyle standards, utilizing only the hand and wrist, do not represent the level of skeletal maturation sufficiently accurately in infancy (0–2 years). We prefer the Elgenmark method for this early age. The Elgenmark standards of skeletal maturation are based on the appearance of epiphyseal centers which normally occur in a specific sequence and in a relatively specific relation to each other. The estimate requires x-rays of one-half of the body to identify the total number of epiphyseal centers. The estimate of skeletal maturity (bone age) is expressed by the number of epiphyseal centers present. From tables prepared by Elgenmark, the level of skeletal maturity and a standard deviation of that estimate may be derived (9).

### Tanner–Whitehouse Maturity Scale

Tanner and Whitehouse describe a method of estimation of skeletal maturity based on a *"bone scoring method"* (*TW-2*) (1, 10). Each bone must progress through a certain number of identifiable stages to maturity involving changes in shape, conformity to neighboring bones, epiphyseal appearances, and eventual fusion. For each bone of the hand, Tanner and Whitehouse have identified 8 stages of maturity. To determine maturity levels, each bone in the hand radiograph is matched with the standard and its stage is rated from 1 to 8. Each stage has a score assigned so that the "sum of all the scores for all the bones represents the best overall estimate of skeletal maturity" (1). The score expressing maturity runs from 1 to 100, the latter representing full maturity of the skeleton. The maturity score may be converted to a "bone-age" by means of a table

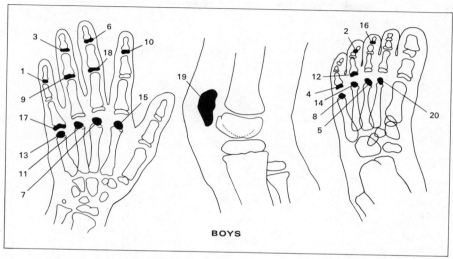

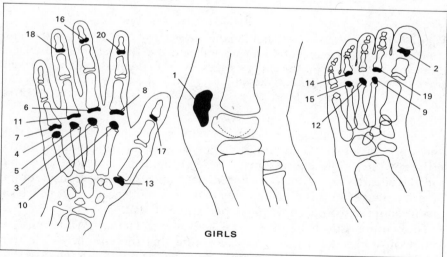

**Figure 6-8.** The twenty epiphyseal centers of the hand, knee, and foot which have the highest statistical "communality" and hence the greatest predictive value in assessment of skeletal maturation in boys and in girls. (Reproduced by permission from Garn SM, Rohman CG, Silverman FN: Radiographic standards for postnatal ossification and tooth calcification. *Med Radiogr Photogr* **43:**45, 1967.)

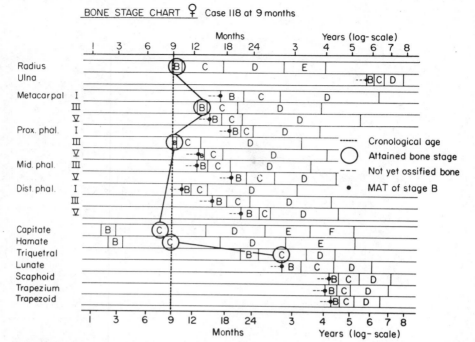

**Figure 6-9.** Bone stage chart showing the skeletal profile of a girl age 9 months demonstrating the method of Taranger et al. in expressing skeletal maturation as mean appearance time (MAT) of bone stages (see text). (Reproduced by permission from Taranger J, Bruning B, Claesson I, et al: Skeletal maturity-the MAT-method (mean appearance time of bone stages). *Acta Paediatr Scand* **258**(Suppl):109, 1976.)

relating chronologic age to maturity score for males and females. Boys and girls pass through identical stages of skeletal development but at different rates. The expression of skeletal maturity as a bone age takes the discrepancy in maturity between boys and girls into consideration. The "bone-age" in this case, represents the chronological age at which the given maturity score is at the 50th percentile (1, 10).

In a comparison between Greulich–Pyle and Tanner–Whitehouse assessment of skeletal maturity, Roche found that the Greulich–Pyle standards gave more advanced readings than did Tanner–Whitehouse standards (British children), suggesting that North American and Australian children mature earlier than do British children (11).

### Taranger–MAT System

Taranger et al. have suggested a method of assessment of skeletal maturity for infancy through childhood based on *mean appearance time* (MAT) of bone stages (12). They describe stages of maturity of each of 20 bones of the hand/wrist which are given alphabetical designations corresponding

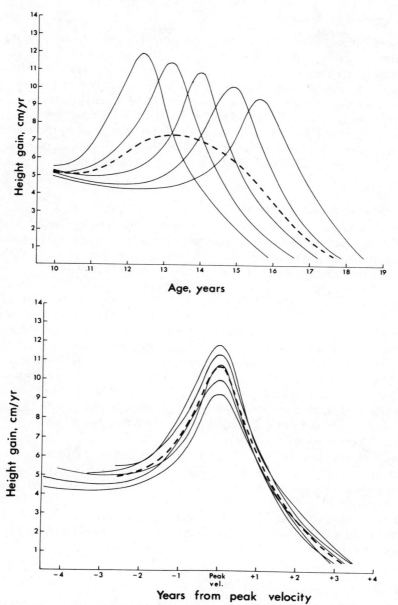

**Figure 6-10.** Velocity curves of the adolescent growth spurt showing the relation between mean velocities (dotted lines) and individual height velocity curves (solid lines). In the upper panel, the mean curve is constructed by averaging the values at each age, resulting in a blunted peak, not characteristic of the adolescent growth spurt. In the lower panel, the same subjects are plotted according to peak height velocity giving a mean curve more consistent with the true velocity curve of adolescence. (Reproduced by permission from Tanner JM, Whitehouse RH, Takaishi M: Standards from birth to maturity for height, weight, height velocity, and weight velocity for British children 1965, Parts I and II. *Arch Dis Child* **41**:454, 613, 1966.)

to stage of maturity. The stage of development of each bone is related to the chronologic age at which each stage is likely to appear (MAT) so that in assessing the state of development of each of the 20 bones and charting each on a *bone stage chart* (Figure 6-9), a graphic representation of bone stages is provided, similar to the "weighted bone scores" of the Tanner–Whitehouse method (12). The MAT method provides a graphic demonstration of variability of individual bones in conforming to the standard "mean appearance time". It allows "visual fit" judgments to be made of the overall maturity achieved by the bones of the hand of the subject (12) (Figure 6-9).

## Pubertal Maturational Indices

Growth rate, skeletal maturation, and sexual maturation should be considered together to allow a complete physiologic description of maturation during puberty. The growth spurt of adolescence, described in Chapter 5, can be most accurately displayed by means of growth velocity charts for height and weight. The adolescent growth spurt is not accurately displayed in growth standards based on averages at different ages because of the variability in time of onset of the growth spurt. The adolescent growth spurt is only depicted accurately if the peak height velocity is taken as reference point and the velocity curve constructed around the reference point (1) (Figure 6-10). Sexual development proceeds by stages from a prepubertal appearance to full adult sexual maturity. Stages for breast and pubic hair and time of menarche for girls and stages for pubic hair, genitalia, and testes for boys have been described in Chapter 5. Standards for stages of sexual development may be found in Figures 5-7, 5-8, and 5-11 and tabulated in Table 5-1.

Skeletal maturation bears a fairly close relationship to maturational events of puberty, corresponding most closely to time of menarche (13). Peak height velocity in females occurs shortly after breast tissue appears and in males about 2 years after the first sign of puberty (1). Menarche occurs about the time the distal phalangeal epiphyses fuse and the epiphyses in the ileal crest appear, corresponding to a skeletal maturation level of 13–13½ (6).

## GROWTH STANDARDS

For the assessment of growth progress of individual children in the office of the physician, longitudinal standards would be preferred. Growth standards for infants must be related to gestational age. Adolescent growth curves should be related to peak height velocity and must make allowances for early and late maturing adolescents. The standards should be from healthy, well-nourished, well-cared-for children. They should be accurately obtained and the study population should be sufficiently large that the appropriate variability around the mean will be meaningfully expressed.

Standards should reflect current growth patterns and, if possible, the genetic–racial patterns of the children to be examined.

Present standards do not satisfy all of these stipulations. Most data available on growth of children are obtained by cross-sectional studies. If we prefer longitudinal over cross-sectional data, we must choose from populations, not necessarily identical to our own in time or place, on whom such data are available. If we will restrict our standards to a circumscribed genetic–ethnic group, we may find few standards available. We are forced, therefore, to accept some compromise and to recognize the limitations in use of standards for the individual child or group of children whom we wish to study. Some standards are in metric and some in the English system of pounds and inches. To conveniently convert measurements from one system to the other, the following formulas may help:

$$cm \times 0.394 = inches$$

$$inches \times 2.54 = cm$$

$$kilograms \times 2.2 = pounds$$

$$pounds \times 0.454 = kilograms$$

### Newborn Standards

At the time of birth we are interested in measurements which will help us to evaluate the size of an infant in relation to its level of maturity, so measurements must be related to the gestational age of the infant. In Tables A-1 and A-2 of the Appendix we provide the data of Miller and Merrett, giving percentile distributions for length, OFC, and birth weight of newborn male and female infants by gestational age from 37 to 42 weeks. Comparisons of birth weight are made between first born and multiparous infants. The relationship between fetal measurements and gestational age are shown in Figures 2-7 and 2-8.

The maturity of the newborn may be assessed in a number of ways. Figure A-1 of the Appendix displays a newborn maturity rating system based on a scoring system of neuromuscular activity and physical maturity of the infant (14, 15). It is often helpful to classify infants by weight, length or OFC measurements as large (LGA), appropriate (AGA), or small (SGA) for gestational age. Figure A-2 of the Appendix displays charts for length, weight, and head circumference for preterm (gestational ages 26– 37 weeks), term (37–42 weeks), and postterm (after 42 weeks) infants to allow classification of newborns as LGA, AGA or SGA based on intrauterine growth (16, 17).

### Standards for Infancy and Early Childhood
### from Birth to 3 Years

During infancy and early childhood, growth standards must be able to display accurately the rapid changes in length, weight, and head circumference. From data compiled by the Fels Institute in Ohio, the National Center for Health Statistics (NCHS) has constructed growth charts for boys and girls from birth to 36 months with reference percentiles displaying length, weight, and head circumference for age (Appendix, Figures A-5 and A-6). Several laboratories which provide infant nutrition products have printed the charts and made them available for general use by physicians. The charts from the Fels Institute are mixed racial measurements and do not take into consideration the special growth characteristics of black or Chicano populations. Black children are smaller than white children at birth, but catch up and surpass white children during the first few years of life (18).

Head circumference measurements for boys and girls from birth to 3 years are included with the growth charts for children published by NCHS. For standards of head circumference from birth through adolescence, we may use tabulations of mean and SD by Tanner (Appendix, Tables A-4 and A-6) or the charts constructed by Nellhaus (19) (Appendix, Figures A-3 and A-4). The head circumference of boys at birth averages 0.5 cm greater than girls. By 3 years, boys' heads average 1.2 cm larger than girls, which can be seen either from tables (A-4 and A-6) or from the Nellhaus charts (Figures A-3, A-4).

## Standards for Childhood to Adolescence

Means and standard deviations by age from birth to 18 years for length or height, weight, height velocity, weight velocity, head circumference, and skinfold thickness are presented in Tables A-3 and A-4 of the Appendix for males and in Tables A-5 and A-6 for females.

### Height–Weight Measurements from Age 2 to 18

Growth charts for girls and boys, ages 2–18 years, have been constructed by the National Center for Health Statistics (NCHS) from current samples representative of girls and boys in the general U.S. population. The charts display stature and weight for age with reference percentiles (Appendix, Figures A-7 and A-8). The charts from NCHS provide achievement or distance information and are best designed to compare height and weight measurements of individuals with a group population. To assess rate of growth, velocity curves are necessary. Velocity curves for height and weight for boys and girls have been constructed by Tanner from data from Scottish children (5) (Table 6-1).

### Standards for Body Proportion and Pubertal Development

*The assessment of body proportion* can be made with either a measurement of sitting height (crown–rump length) or by expressing the ratio of upper segment to lower segment. Standards for sitting height by age may be found in Tables A-4 and A-6 in the Appendix. These data are from

British children expressed as mean and standard deviation in centimeters. In Tables A-7 and A-8 the change in body proportion as a ratio of upper segment to lower segment (US/LS) from birth to 18 years in males and females is displayed. For *standards for sexual development*, the reader is referred to the charts and discussion in Chapter 5, entitled "Growth and Maturation in Adolescence".

### Standards for Skin Fold Measurements

The standards chosen for skinfold thickness are from British children reported by Tanner and Whitehouse in 1975 (3). Charts have been prepared by Tanner for triceps and subscapular thickness in boys and girls from birth to 19 years (Table 6-1). Because the values of skinfold thickness with the caliper give a non-Gaussian frequency distribution, the measurements in millimeters are plotted in a logarithmic distribution in the charts. For calculation of mean and standard deviations, logarithmic transformations of the measurements are necessary. Means and standard deviations of skinfold thickness are tabulated in Tables A-4 and A-6 of the Appendix.

## HEIGHT OF PARENTS
## AND HEIGHT OF CHILDREN

The ultimate height that a child achieves is determined in large part by the heights of his parents (20). Simple observation suffices to affirm that tall parents generally produce tall children and short parents generally have short children. The height potential of children is statistically related to the mid-parent height (MPH), the average of mother's and father's heights. If both parents are of nearly the same height, the heights of the children tend to be very near the mean parental height. Whereas, if one parent is tall and one short, the range of heights of the children is quite wide (20).

Consideration of the effect that parental height might have on the height of the child becomes quite important when there is concern about abnormalities in growth. A child on the 3rd percentile may be perfectly normal if his parents are also short, but may have a clear growth abnormality if his parents are tall. The growth patterns of grown siblings, grandparents, uncles, and aunts may be of additional value in determining a child's growth potential, but the further one traces growth patterns from the immediate genetic pool of the child, the weaker the influence becomes (20).

### Standards of Height Allowing
### for Height of Parents

From data collected by the Fels Institute, Garn and Rohman have constructed tables of "parent specific standards" for height of boys and girls providing expected mean height in cm of boys and girls by age according to mid-parent stature (21). The tables provide standards for children ranging in age from birth to 19 years with parents whose mid-parent stature ranges from 161 to 178 cm. The effect on height from parents with mid-parent stature below or above these levels must be extrapolated. No data are available to test the validity of such extrapolations (Appendix, Tables A-9 and A-10). Tanner et al. have constructed similar charts which give percentile standards for boys' and girls' heights between ages 2 and 9 when parents' height is allowed for. The child's height is expressed as a percentile of the expected standard adjusted for the mid-parent height (20). This approach provides precise information concerning the degree to which the child conforms to an expected growth pattern adjusted for the height of parents.

### Calculation of Target Height
### Based on Mid-Parent Height

In addition to being able to determine how well the current growth of a child relates to expected patterns expressed by the mid-parent height, it is often useful to be able to judge how parental height will influence ultimate height of the child. Tanner suggests that a "target adult height" of a child may be displayed on a growth chart, allowing for mid-parent height by plotting an "adjusted mid-parent height" and percentile range on the growth chart of the child (20).

The adjusted mean expected height may be derived as follows:

1. For a boy:
    (a) Plot father's height* in cm at the adult end of the boy's growth chart (age 18 or 19).
    (b) *Add* 13 cm to mother's height† in cm and plot identically.
    (c) Find the mid-parent or average height between these plots: this represents the *mean target height* for the son adjusted for mid-parent height

$$[F + (M + 13] \div 2 = \text{Adjusted MPH}$$

    (d) add 8.5 cm above and below the mid-point target height to

---

* Heights of father or mother should be their height at 19–20 years of age or the highest adult height achieved. Height after 45–50 years begins to decrease, and if actual measurements are used, height corrections will be necessary by adding 1.5 cm to parental height at ages 45–55, and 3 cm at ages above 55.

† Mother's actual height must be adjusted for the average male–female difference in final height in order to plot mother's height on the appropriate percentile on the boy's chart. Mother's height + 13 cm will place mother at the correct percentile on the boy's chart. The reverse calculation must be done to adjust father's height to the appropriate percentile on the girl's charts.

approximate the target range from 3rd to 97th percentile for anticipated adult height for the son adjusted for mid-parent height

$$\text{Target height} = \text{MPH}_{adj} \pm 8.5$$

OR

(a′) Find the mid-parent height, that is, average of mother's and father's height in cm,* *add* 6.5 cm to get the "adjusted mid-parent height"

$$(\text{MPH} + 6.5) = \text{Adjusted MPH}$$

(b′) Plot the adjusted mid-parent height on the boy's chart at the end of the growth chart (age 18).

(c′) Add 8.5 cm above and below the adjusted mid-parent height to approximate the target range 3rd to 97th percentile for the anticipated adult height of the son adjusted for mid-parent height (20).

2. For a *girl*:

(a) Plot mother's height in cm at the adult end of the girl's growth chart, that is, at age 18.*

(b) *Subtract* 13 cm from father's height† in cm and plot identically.

(c) Find the mid-parent height or average between these plots, which represents the mean target height for the daughter adjusted for mid-parent height

$$[M + (F - 13)] \div 2 = \text{Adjusted MPH}$$

(d) Add 8.5 cm above and below the mid-point target height to approximate the target range of 3rd to 97th percentile for the anticipated adult height for a daughter adjusted for mid-parent height

$$\text{Target height} = \text{MPH}_{adj} \pm 8.5 \text{ cm}$$

OR

(a′) Find mid-parent height, that is, average of mother's and father's height in centimeters,* and *subtract* 6.5 cm to get an "adjusted" mid-parent height.

(b′) Plot the adjusted mid-parent height on the girls chart on the end of the growth chart, at age 18.

(c′) Add 8.5 cm above and below the adjusted mid-parent height to approximate the target range from 3rd to 97th percentile for the

## GENETIC GROWTH POTENTIAL

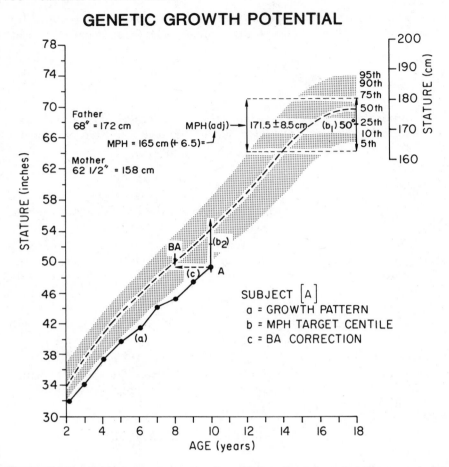

**Figure 6-11.** Achievement growth chart illustrating plot of mid-parent height adjusted according to Tanner (20) to describe the target growth centiles (b₁) or anticipated growth potential of the child adjusted for mid-parent height. Growth pattern of a child (A), age 10, with bone-age 8 years is shown with adjustments made for mid-parent height (b₁ & b₂) and for skeletal maturation (c) (see text).

anticipated adult height for a daughter adjusted for mid-parent height (20).

### Mid-Parent Height and Growth Assessment

Although the predicted target percentile does not specify standards of current growth, we have found it useful in familial stature aberrations to calculate the target range and determine whether the child of short (or tall) parents is indeed growing within a percentile appropriate for the mid-parent height. In families with history of delayed or accelerated growth patterns, additional adjustment of the expected growth potential may be indicated by skeletal maturation (as an indicator of biologic maturation). It is useful to adjust the height of the child to the appropriate percentile for height corresponding to the "bone age" rather than chronologic age to more accurately judge whether the child is fulfilling expected genetic potential. In Figure 6-11 we illustrate the concepts of adjusted mid-parent height, target or anticipated growth potential adjusted for mid-parent height, and adjustment of height percentile for skeletal age. Boy A, age 10, has a height of 125 cm or 49.5 inches and a bone age of 8 years. His height falls below the 3rd percentile for boys of age 10 and has consistently done so since age 2 [see growth pattern labeled (a)], but note that *velocity* of growth has been normal from age 2 to 10. The adjusted mid-parent height is 171.5 cm (25th percentile), and the target range (b$_1$) for adult height for sons in this family range from 180 to 163 cm. The son's current height, as position A, below the 3rd percentile is at the lowest point on the expected target range adjusted for mid-parent height (b$_2$). But if the growth potential is adjusted for a height of 125 cm at a bone age of 8 years (c), he now falls well within the range of expected height achievement adjusted for mid-parent height.

## PREDICTION OF MATURE HEIGHT

In a variety of circumstances, it may be useful not only to be able to assess current growth patterns or status, but to be able also to predict the continuation and culmination of the growth process. This is of particular concern to the tall girl who perceives problems of a social or psychologic nature if she grows to an "excessive" height. Potential adult height may be of importance to a short boy who perceives himself to be growing too slowly and unable to compete with his taller and more mature peers. In this case, not only is information concerning ultimate height desired, but timing of the events of the growth process, such as probable time of puberty and adolescent growth spurt, may be crucial as well. The child would like to know how much growth will occur and when. The ultimate growth of the spine may be of concern to the orthopedist in the treatment of scoliosis or the potential growth of legs when asymmetry suggests the need for equalizing growth in the short limb. The dentist interested in orthodentic measures, needs to know of variations in the expected appearance of permanent dentition.

An approximation of ultimate height may be derived from growth charts by simply identifying the percentile in which the child is growing and assuming that adult height will approximate the same percentile. Such assumptions fail to take into consideration the tempo of growth, that is, early or late maturing growth patterns.

## Bayer–Bayley–Pinneau Method

Tables of height prediction were first introduced by Bayley in 1946 and revised for use with the Greulich–Pyle atlas of skeletal maturation by Bayley and Pinneau in 1952 (22). This system of height prediction is based on the observation that there is a high correlation between skeletal maturation and proportion of adult height achieved. The tables are constructed for boys and girls of average, retarded, and accelerated rate of maturation. Tables for average rate of maturation include those subjects whose skeletal maturation is within 1 year of their chronologic age. For skeletal maturation retarded or accelerated by more than 1 year, separate tables are provided. In the tables, the height in inches is matched to the skeletal maturation to the nearest quarter year and the predicted mature height calculated from the percent of mature height achieved according to the skeletal maturation. Tables allow predicted height to be read directly from the intercept of skeletal age and height (Appendix, Tables A-11 and A-12).

The Bayley–Pinneau tables are constructed from measurements taken from 122 California children; 103 girls and 89 boys. Measurements were made every 6 months from 8 to 18 years, or until all epiphyses had closed (22). In general usage in this country for nearly three decades, the tables have been widely accepted as providing reasonably accurate height predictions for most average North American children. The applicability of the standards for height prediction in potentially tall children has been occasionally questioned. The tables tend to over-predict adult height in girls with skeletal ages of 14 years or more and to under-predict adult height in those who are retarded skeletally (23, 24). Height prediction in younger girls, ages 8 to 11, with retarded skeletal ages tend to be low and increase as the girls approach the age of menarche. Despite this drawback, height prediction tables of Bayley and Pinneau are of considerable help to clinicians anxious to obtain a reasonable estimate of adult height of an individual child. The charts of height prediction begin at about age 7 for boys and age 6 for girls. Bayley has suggested that use of mid-parent stature improves the accuracy of the prediction in earlier childhood (25), but no tables have been constructed to include earlier ages in the height prediction tables.

## Tanner–Whitehouse Method

Tanner et al. have devised a formula for calculation of adult height based on present height, chronologic age, and bone age. Additional corrections may be made for a mid-parent height by adding or subtracting one-third of the amount the mid-parent height deviates from the mean mid-parent height of the general population (168 cm) (26). The bone age used is determined by the Tanner–Whitehouse method or the RUS bone age. This system of bone age is based on the maturation of individual bones of the radius, the metacarpals, and the phalanges (26). Prediction is made through regression equations specific for each age as described by Tanner et al. (10, 26). Height, chronologic age, and bone age are multiplied by their respective coefficients, a constant is added, and adjustment made for mid-parent height. The height prediction, ±1 standard deviation, is then expressed as probable mature height.

## RWT System-Weighted Calculations

The Roche–Wainer–Thissen (RWT) method estimates the adult height of an individual from data recorded at a single examination. This method predicts the height at 18 years. Final adult status can be estimated by adding 8 mm in boys and 6 mm in girls (27). The data required are recumbent length,* nude weight, mid-parent stature, and skeletal age from hand-wrist x-ray (28). In determining the skeletal maturation, the Greulich–Pyle atlas is used to determine the maturity of each bone of the hand and wrist. In the RWT method of height prediction, each of the measurements—weight, length, mid-parent stature, and skeletal age—are "adjusted" by multiplying the value by a weighted constant (age and sex specific) which is assigned a positive or negative value (28). The algebraic sum of the positive and negative products yields the height prediction in cm (28).

## Limitations in Applications of Height Predictions

The use of any of the methods for height prediction provides a more sophisticated estimate of height prediction than use of age-related percentage of adult height achieved, or simple extrapolation from percentiles based on current growth measurements. All of the methods are reasonably accurate for children near the mean in tempo of growth, but all suffer various distortions of prediction at extremes of the growth pattern. Furthermore, the predictions are of questionable value in predicting final height achievements in pathologic states such as Turner syndrome, congenital adrenal hyperplasia, precocious puberty, and skeletal disorders that might affect the orderly maturation of the epiphyses. Nonetheless, height predictions can be very useful to the potentially tall, but otherwise nromal, girl and the small boy with delayed adolescence. Not only can ultimate height achievements be predicted, but the time of achievement can also be predicted with sufficient accuracy to provide the type of reassurance needed.

## COMPARISONS BETWEEN GROWTH MEASUREMENTS

It is often helpful to be able to compare one set of measurements of a child (e.g., height) with other measurements (e.g., weight or skeletal

---

* If only standing height is avialable, 1.25 cm is added to obtain estimate of recumbent length.

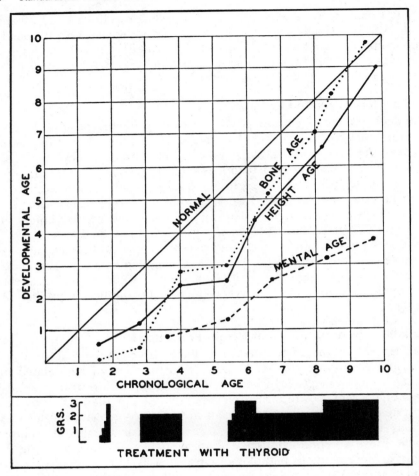

**Figure 6-12.** Chart expressing developmental age as a function of chronologic age to display simultaneously the developmental level of a variety of interrelated growth parameters. The figure displays growth and developmental relationships of a child with hypothyroidism. (Reproduced by permission from Wilkins L: *Diagnosis and Treatment of Endocrine Disorders in Childhood and Adolescence*, ed 3. Springfield, Charles C Thomas, 1965.)

maturation) and to be able to compare the growth pattern of one child with those of other children. We can describe the physique in tall, thin children and short, stocky children depending on interrelationships between measurements of length and weight. Similarly neurologic status, bone-age, IQ, and so on provide additional information that might be integrated into the pattern of growth and development. Some of these interrelationships are obvious from single measurements, but more infor-

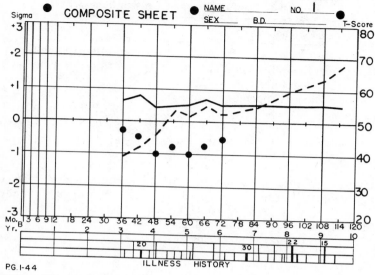

**Figure 6-13.**   Fels composite sheet demonstrating simultaneous recording of serial measurements of weight, height, and bone ossification expressed as deviations from the mean in terms of standard deviations (sigma). (Reproduced by permission from Sonntag LW, Reynolds EL: The Fels composite sheet: A practical method for analyzing growth progress. *J Pediatr* **26:**327, 1945.)

mation can usually be derived from serial measurements or trends. One can consider each growth parameter separately and note its relationship to patterns of norms for children of similar age or maturation, or one can compare height with other values of growth and maturation of the same child. Reassurance of harmonious growth is as important as identification of significant deviations from normal growth patterns calling attention to disease or some disorder affecting growth.

## Maturation Age Scale

Some years ago, Dr. Lawson Wilkins introduced a concept of comparing developmental age to chronologic age as a means of allowing comparison of a variety of measurable parameters of growth (29) (Figure 6-12). In the diagram, the maturational age is listed on one axis and the chronologic age on the other. "Developmental age" is the age at which any given measurement of growth would be at or near the 50th percentile. For example, the "height age" of a child is the age at which the child's measured height would represent the mean or average height. Similarly, the weight can be expressed as "weight age", the skeletal maturation as "bone age", neurologic status as "developmental-age", tooth eruption as "dental age", intellectual achievement as "IQ or mental age", and sexual maturation can also be expressed as "sexual age", at least during puberty.

### Table 6-1. Useful Charts of Growth Standards

| Designation | Availability |
| --- | --- |
| 1. *Newborn Maturity Rating* Neuromuscular and physical maturity scoring system for estimation of gestational age (Appendix, Figure 1). | Distributed by Mead Johnson Nutritional Division |
| 2. *Classification of Newborns* Charts of length, weight, and OFC by gestational age with LGA, AGA, and SGA determinations (Appendix, Figure 2). | Distributed by Mead Johnson Nutritional Division |
| 3. Chart of *head circumference* for boys and girls showing mean ± 2 standard deviations (2nd–98th percentile) by age from birth to age 18, from Nellhaus G, *Pediatrics* **41**:106, 1968 (Appendix, Figures 3 and 4). | Distributed by Mead Johnson Nutritional Division and Ross Laboratories |
| 4. Growth charts with reference percentiles for boys and girls from *birth* to *36 months* of age displaying *length, weight,* and *head circumference* for age and weight for length, constructed by the National Center for Health Statistics (NHCS) in collaboration with the Center for Disease Control (CDC) with data from the Fels Research Institute, Ohio (Appendix, Figures 5 and 6). | Distributed by Ross Laboratories and Mead Johnson Nutritional Division |
| 5. Growth charts with reference percentiles for boys and girls from *ages 2 to 18 years* of age displaying *stature* and *weight* for age and weight for stature, constructed by NCHS from data compiled from national samples representative of boys and girls in the general U.S. population (Appendix, Figures 7 and 8). | Distributed by Ross Laboratories and Mead Johnson Nutritional Division |
| 6. Charts of *height* and *weight velocity* with reference centiles (3rd–97th percentile) for boys and girls from ages 2 to maturity, showing percentiles for adolescent growth spurt when peak velocity occurs at an average age and for early and late limits of age, prepared by Tanner and Whitehouse, University of London, Institute of Child Health, from the Hospital for Sick Children, London, *Arch Dis Child* **51**:170, 1976. | Printed and distributed by Castlemead Publications, Swains Mill 4A Crane Mead, Ware, Hertsfordshire, England |

**Table 6-1. (Continued)**

| *Designation* | *Availability* |
|---|---|
| 7. | Charts of *subscapular* and *triceps skin thickness* (in millimeters for girls and boys) with reference percentiles (3rd–97th percentile) from birth to age 19, from Tanner and Whitehouse, *Arch Dis Child* **50:**142, 1975. | Printed and distributed by Castlemead Publications, Swains Mill, 4A Crane Mead, Ware, Hertsfordshire, England |
| 8. | *Denver Developmental Screening Test (DDST)* A developmental inventory for infancy and childhood showing visually mean and 95th confidence limits for each skill arranged into groups of gross motor skills, fine motor skills, personal–social, and language skills (Figure 3–7). | Developmental inventory sheets, testing kit, and instructions for administration available from University of Colorado Denver, CO (Dr. W. K. Frankenburg) |

In Figure 6-12, height, bone-age, and IQ are depicted for a boy with hypothyroidism who is short, with delayed bone maturation, and intellectual impairment. At a chronologic age of 6 years, the height age was that of an average 4-year-old, with similar delay in skeletal maturation, but the IQ showed severe retardation. At age 10, after several years treatment, the bone age approaches normal, but the IQ remains that of a 4-year-old. If all measurements of growth were average for the given chronologic age, they would all fall on the diagonal line of the graph. Accelerated maturation is depicted above the diagonal and delayed maturation below. In the diagram, comparisons among growth achievements can be recorded and considered simultaneously and trends toward, or deviations from, normal easily recognized.

## Comparisons by Deviation from Mean

The Fels Composite Sheet provides another means of displaying several kinds of growth data simultaneously over a period of time (30) (Figure 6-13). This system portrays measurements in relation to the mean for normal values for that measurement. A measurement may be compared to a mean value for a given age and the deviation of the measurement from the age specific mean calculated as standard deviation or decimal fraction thereof. This deviation is then plotted on the Fels Composite Sheet above or below the midline representing the mean. Any measurement for which tables of means and standard deviations of normal populations exist can be used in the comparative plot.

In Figure 6-13, deviation from the mean weight values are plotted with a solid line from age 3 to 10 years, height by a dashed line, ossification centers by dots. It can be readily appreciated that weight has remained fairly constant in relation to the mean, although a little over the mean; the osseous maturation seems to remain mildly retarded though again fairly steady. Height, however, moves from about 1 standard deviation below the mean to 2 standards above the mean; the child was short and stocky at 3 years but has become tall for his age and thin for his height at age 10 years.

It is evident that maximum information about growth patterns may be derived from accurate, serial measurements of as many facets of growth as is feasible, including serial trends of height, weight, osseous maturation, sexual development, dental age, etc. The more information that is available, the more readily the measurements can be compared effectively with norms and with other aspects of growth of the same child.

Table 6-1 lists the sources of useful charts of growth standards displayed in the Appendix.

## REFERENCES

1. Tanner JM: *Fetus Into Man: Physical Growth From Conception to Maturity.* Cambridge, Harvard University Press, 1978, pp 6–23, 78–86, 167–205.
2. Sheldon WH: *The Variety of Human Physique.* New York, Harper and Bros., 1940.
3. Tanner JM, Whitehouse RH: Clinical longitudinal standards for height, weight, height velocity, weight velocity, and stages of puberty. *Arch Dis Child* **51**:170, 1976.
4. Whitehouse RH, Tanner JM, Healy MJR: Diurnal variation in stature and sitting height in 12–24 year old boys. *Ann Hum Biol* **1**:103, 1974.
5. Sinclair D: *Human Growth After Birth.* London, Oxford University Press, 1978, pp 98–116.
6. Hägg U, Taranger J: Maturation indicators and the pubertal growth spurt. *Am J Orthod* **82**:299, 1982.
7. Greulich WW, Pyle SE: *Radiographic Atlas of Skeletal Development of the Hand and Wrist,* ed 2. Stanford, Stanford University Press, 1959.
8. Garn SM, Rohman CG, Silverman FN: Radiographic standards for postnatal ossification and tooth calcification. *Med Radiogr Photogr* **43**:45–66, 1967.
9. Elgenmark O: The normal development of the ossific centers during infancy and childhood: Clinical, roentgenologic, and statistical study. *Acta Paediatr Scand* [Suppl] **33**(1):1–79, 1946.
10. Tanner JM, Whitehouse RH, Marhsall WA, et al: *Assessment of Skeletal Maturity and Prediction of Adult Height.* London, Academic Press, 1975.
11. Roche AF, Davila GH, Eyman SL: A comparison between Greulich-Pyle and Tanner–Whitehouse assessments of skeletal maturity. *Radiology* **98**:273, 1971.
12. Taranger J, Bruning B, Claesson I, et al: Skeletal maturity—the MAT-method (mean appearance time of bone stages). *Acta Paediatr Scand* (Suppl **258**):109–120, 1976.
13. Marshall WA: Interrelationships of skeletal maturation, sexual development, and somatic growth in man. *Ann Hum Biol* **1**:29, 1974.
14. Ballard JL, Kazmaier K, Driver M.: A simplified score for assessment of fetal maturation of newly born infants. *J Pediatr* **95**:769, 1979.
15. Sweet AY: Classification of the low-birth-weight infant, in Klaus MG, Fararoff AA (eds.), *Care of the High-Risk Infant.* Philadelphia, WB Saunders Co, 1977, p 47.

16. Lubchenco LO, Hansman C, Boyd E: Intrauterine growth in length and head circumference as estimated from live births at gestational ages from 26–42 weeks. *Pediatrics* **37:**403, 1966.

17. Battaglia FC, Lubchenco LO: A practical classification of newborn infants by weight and gestational age. *J Pediatr* **71:**159, 1967.

18. Robson JRK, Larkin FA, Bursick JH, et al: Growth standards for infants and children: A cross-sectional study. *Pediatrics* **56:**1014, 1975.

19. Nellhaus G: Composite international and interracial Graphs. *Pediatrics* **41:**106, 1968.

20. Tanner JM, Goldstein H, Whitehouse RH: Standards for children's heights at ages 2–9 years allowing for height of parents. *Arch Dis Child* **45:**755, 1970.

21. Garn SM, Rohmann CC: Interaction of nutrition and genetics in the timing of growth and development. *Pediatr Clin North Am* **13:**353, 1966.

22. Bayley N, Pinneau SR: Tables for predicting adult height from skeletal age: Revised for use with the Greulich–Pyle hand standards. *J Pediatr* **40:**423, 1952.

23. Frasier SD, Smith FG Jr: Effect of estrogens on mature height in tall girls: A control study. *J Clin Endocrinol Metab* **28:**416, 1968.

24. Roche AF, Wettenhall HNB: The prediction of adult stature in tall girls. *Aust Paediatr J* **53:**13, 1969.

25. Bayley N: The accurate prediction of growth and adult height. *Mod Probl Paediatr* **7:**234, 1962.

26. Tanner JM, Whitehouse RH, Marshall WA, et al: Prediction of adult height, bone age, and occurrence of menarche at ages 4–16 with allowance for mid-parent height. *Arch Dis Child* **50:**14, 1975.

27. Roche AF, Davila GH: Late adolescent growth in stature. *Pediatrics* **50:**874, 1972.

28. Roche AF, Wainer H, Thissen D: The RWT method for the prediction of adult stature. *Pediatrics* **56:**1026, 1975.

29. Wilkins LW: Methods of endocrine study and diagnosis, clinical and developmental studies, in *Diagnosis and Treatment of Endocrine Disorders in Childhood and Adolescence* ed 3. Springfield, Charles C Thomas, 1965, pp 28–43.

30. Sontag LW, Reynolds EL: The Fels Composite sheet: A practical method for analyzing growth progress. *J Pediatr* **26:**327, 1945.

# 7

# Classification
# and Approach to
# Disorders of Growth

We define growth as aberrant if (a) height achievement is below the 3rd or above the 97th percentile, (b) the height velocity deviates more than 2 standard deviations above or below the mean height velocity for age, or (c) a pubertal growth spurt fails to occur within 2 standard deviations of the usual time for the pubertal growth spurt. It is acknowledged that a definition of abnormal growth at plus or minus two standard deviations will include about 5% of the normal population in the definition of abnormal, but it is deemed reasonable to consider the possibility of a growth disturbance at these limits so that treatable growth disturbances might be recognized before major deviations from normal occur.

For most of the growth disorders, weight changes occur in about the same proportion as height. Those conditions in which weight changes predominate—failure to thrive and obesity—will be taken up separately in Chapter 11. Measurements in head growth, body proportion, skinfold thickness, and so on can be referred to a mean and considered exceptional if they fall outside plus or minus two standard deviations from the mean. (Note: Weight forms a skewed curve and cannot be referred to arithmetic mean, but must be expressed in percentiles or logarithmic transformations.)

## FREQUENCY OF GROWTH DISORDERS

The frequency of growth problems in the general population at various ages is not known. We know that approximately 9% of all infants have low birth weights, but only about one-third of these are small for gestational age (1). We also know that about two-thirds of all infants shift channels of growth during the first 2 years of life (2). Our information beyond the

176

**Table 7-1. Growth Problems Seen in a Referral Endocrine Clinic**

| Disorder | Average Number/Year | Percentage of Visits |
|---|---|---|
| *Normal Growth Variants* | | |
| Familial short stature | 24 | 5.0% |
| Delayed growth pattern, constitutional | 35 | 7.2 |
| Familial tall stature/accelerated growth | 37 | 7.6 |
| Delayed adolescence | 33 | 7.8 |
| Subtotal | 129 | 27% |
| *Disorders of Growth* | | |
| Turner's syndrome | 27 | 5.5 |
| Precocious puberty | 22 | 4.5 |
| Hypothyroidism | 45 | 9.3 |
| Hypopituitarism | 25 | 5.2 |
| Intrauterine growth retardation, skeletal dysplasias, dysmorphic syndromes | 11 | 2.3 |
| Failure to thrive | 11 | 2.3 |
| Miscellaneous growth problems | 6 | 1.2 |
| Subtotal | 147 | 30% |
| Total seen for growth problems | 276/yr | 57% |

newborn period, however, is generally restricted to reports from clinics to which children have been referred for investigation of growth problems.

In Newcastle-upon-Tyne, all children born during 1960, who were at or below the 3rd percentile at 10 years of age, were studied by Lacey and Parkin (3). This study provides a glimpse into the panorama of growth disorders in children, although disorders of infancy that have a lethal potential or that may have been corrected would not be represented. Among the ninety-eight youngsters who were below the 3rd percentile, 82% were considered to be normal variants by Lacey and Parkin. They attributed the small size in these youngsters to small parents, slow maturation, or low birth weight, which was, in turn, related to small maternal size. In about one-third of the cases, the small size seemed related to poor social environment and Lacey and Parkin in a subsequent paper, discussed small size as a "disease of social environment" (4). The remaining 18% of the children who were below the 3rd percentile had a variety of genetic and systemic disorders, including Down's syndrome, mental deficiency, Hurler's syndrome, Still's disease, Fallot's tetralogy, chronic renal disease, and cystic fibrosis of the pancreas. Only one case of possible human growth hormone deficiency was discovered and no hypothyroidism. The relative rarity of endocrine disorders as a cause of short stature in this study is remarkable, although such a finding may not be uncharacteristic.

Growth problems are a common complaint in endocrine clinics. At the University of Utah, representing referral from a population of about two million, over half of the clinic visits are for growth problems (57%), and of these, about half (27%) are normal variants, such as familial short stature, excessive height or constitutional delayed or accelerated growth (Table 7-1). Of the remainder, Turner's syndrome, precocious puberty, thyroid disorders, and human growth hormone deficiency represent the major endocrine disorders.

## CLASSIFICATION OF GROWTH DISORDERS

Because of the wide variety of causes of growth disturbances, it is necessary to organize our approach to the infant or child with a growth disturbance so that we may recognize rapidly and readily those with normal variants of growth and those with problems amenable to therapy (5). We will draw attention to disturbances of growth which are *intrinsic* or which represent a *primary* defect within the growing cells, in contrast to those which occur because of *extrinsic* or *secondary* influences on growth. To facilitate the approach to growth disturbances we have chosen to organize growth disorders in age groups, considering separately those growth disturbances which are most likely to occur in infancy, childhood, and adolescence. These time periods correspond roughly to earlier descriptions of normal growth in infancy, childhood, and adolescence (Chapters 2 through 5).

Growth disturbances evident in *infancy* often have their onset during intrauterine life and may be traced back to intrinsic defects or genetic or chromosomal deficiencies or to absence or maldevelopment of an organ such as the thyroid. Small or large infants of small or large parents (normal variants), or infants born prematurely, are all infants with normal growth potential. Prematurity may present severe physiologic handicaps, but once overcome there is generally no permanent growth deficit. Extrinsic or environmental factors which affect growth of the fetus and infant include twinning, intrauterine growth retardation, congenital hypothyroidism, or diabetes in the mother. Basically, these infants have a normal growth potential, but this potential can only be realized if the extrinsic factors are prevented from interfering with growth at critical growth periods (Table 8-1).

Growth disturbances in *childhood* are frequently normal or familial aberrations in the tempo of growth, but systemic illnesses and endocrine deficiencies are also common during this period. Some of the postnatal onset growth disturbances may become evident in infancy and early childhood; hence, several may be included in both lists as causes of growth disturbances (Table 9-1).

*Adolescent* growth disturbances are closely related to the events of sexual maturation and are considered in relation to delayed or accelerated puberty, although systemic diseases and endocrine disorders unrelated to puberty also occur during this period of growth (Table 10-1).

We emphasize the recognition first of normal variants which do not necessarily require treatment. A great number of the growth disturbances of prenatal onset are not amenable to therapy. This is particularly true of primary or intrinsic defects such as chromosomal anomalies, genetic defects, and congenital malformations. In these circumstances, psychological acceptance may be the primary treatment provided. Guidelines for providing counseling concerning psychological problems associated with growth disturbances are discussed in Chapter 12.

## TAKING A HISTORY FOR GROWTH DISORDERS

The medical history of a child being seen for a growth disturbance is not greatly different from that required for any other childhood health problem, although certain kinds of information deserve emphasis.

The *family history* should include heights and weights of both natural parents and of natural siblings. Heights and weights of grandparents or other relatives will help to define the genetic pool from which the child comes. The tempo of parents' growth and time of puberty should be recorded. For girls, this is the time of mother's menarche but to determine father's growth pattern one may need to ask if he was slower or faster than friends in his pubertal growth spurt or if he grew much after finishing high school. A review of family health should include questions about growth problems, skeletal disorders, early or late puberty, and thyroid or other endocrine disorders.

The size of an infant is influenced strongly by the size of the mother, so height, prepregnant weight, and weight gained during pregnancy are helpful in determining the expected size of the newborn. *Gestational age* should be recorded as time from date of last normal menstrual period (menstrual age), or from 2 weeks after last normal menstrual period (true gestational age), and the birth weight and length should be plotted on a chart designed to show norms for gestational age (Appendix, Figure A-2). *Mother's health habits* during pregnancy should be recorded, including nutritional status, socioeconomic status, alcohol or drug ingestion, and smoking habits. Mother's *health during pregnancy* should be noted, including illnesses such as hypertension, toxemia, renal disease, anemia, and diabetes. Delivery complications should be described, including size and appearance of placenta.

A careful history should be taken of all measurements made during the child's life including birth weight, birth length, and OFC. *Serial length and weight measurements* should be sought and plotted on a longitudinal data growth chart to determine the *velocity* of growth. Anecdotal information on growth such as "failure to outgrow clothes" at expected times, though suggesting a trend in growth, are not a substitute for careful serial measurements. The more measurements available, the better a growth disturbance can be identified and characterized. It is especially important to identify at what period of a child's life a growth disturbance began.

It is important to determine any *general health problems* the child has experienced. Particular attention should be given to *nutrition*, teeth (time of appearance or shedding), prolonged illnesses, and drugs taken that might influence growth, such as corticosteroids, thyroid medications, and methylphenidate. Social or psychological problems should be sought, looking for a cause of the growth disturbance, as in deprivation syndrome, or an unfavorable response to small size or accelerated growth.

A *review of systems* is useful to identify disorders commonly associated with growth disturbances. Such a review might suggest anemia, hypothyroidism, diabetes insipidus, or other disorders masquerading as failure to grow. The time of onset of *puberty* in boys and girls should be recorded carefully. In a girl, the growth spurt begins soon after breast budding and growth is decelerating by the time of menarche. (See Chapter 5.) In boys, the time of onset of puberty is more difficult to determine since few boys note early testicular enlargement, and the change in size of penis may be somewhat gradual. The appearance of pubic hair will usually be remembered. Changes in voice and facial hair, though noticeable, occur late in puberty. The growth spurt begins later in the pubertal development of the boy, but for this reason, it is even more important to establish what timing one can from the pubertal events.

## PHYSICAL EVALUATION FOR GROWTH DISORDERS

The physical examination should describe current size, body proportions, and signs of illness or disease which might affect growth. Careful *measurements of length or height and weight* are needed. In infants and young children, head circumference (OFC) should also be obtained. If disproportionate growth is suspected, measurements of body proportions, such as sitting height or lower segment (pubis to floor measurements) as outlined in Chapter 6, should be performed.

In a young child, an estimate of *maturational level* may be suggested by facial features and by posture. In particular, the shape of the nose, the cheekbones, and the jaw undergo distinctive changes with maturation. In adolescent age youngsters, breast and pubic hair development in girls or testicular size, genital development, and pubic hair in boys may be evaluated according to the stages of Tanner. (See Chapter 5). The status of teeth and the timing of eruption or shedding of primary and deciduous teeth may be helpful in assessing maturational level during childhood and early adolescence (Tables 4-1 and 4-2).

Evidence of cardiac, renal, respiratory or digestive disturbances can be sought, as well as evidence of anemia and systemic signs of endocrine disorders. *Congenital anomalies* of hands, feet, face, head, and limbs should be noted, which might be helpful in identifying growth disturbances associated with specific congenital anomalies. The pterygium colli, cubitus valgus, ptosis, dysplastic nails, and low set ears of Turner's syndrome may allow recognition of the cause for growth disturbance and delayed sexual maturation characteristic of that syndrome. Of particular importance is an assessment of *nutritional status*, and with it, a careful examination of skin, hair, and nails. Skinfold thickness will display excess or scarcity of fat. (See Chapter 6.) Skin and hair consistency and other ectodermal lesions will often betray nutritional deficiencies.

Neurological or *developmental level* can usually be assessed by an abbreviated neurologic examination. In an infant, observation of strength, muscle tone, response to stimuli and reflexes, together with the use of a developmental checklist, such as the DDST (see Chapter 3), may provide adequate screening of the neurologic or developmental status. In an older child, simple tests of strength, coordination, gait, posture, and reflexes may suffice to identify neurologic aberrations associated with growth disturbances. Careful examination of the fundus of the eye, eye movements and visual fields are important. Intelligence rating of an older child may require more formal testing.

From the physical examination of the child suspected of growth disturbances, and particularly from serial measurements, it should be possible to determine whether the growth pattern is normal or sufficiently deviant to require further evaluation. The height or length should be adjusted for the parents' heights and for skeletal (biologic) age. If the height or length remains outside 2 standard deviations when corrected for mid-parent height and bone age, a pathologic cause for the growth disturbance should be sought. Rate or velocity of growth is more sensitive in showing recent trends in growth. Therefore, careful attention should be directed to aberrations in velocity of growth. Even though a child remains within normal standards for height and weight achievements, if the velocity of growth is more than 2 standard deviations from the mean for age (Appendix, Tables A-3 and A-5), a cause should be sought. If disproportionate growth or congenital anomalies are present, the cause should likewise be ascertained. When serial measurements are available so that velocity can be accurately displayed on appropriate charts and when measurements are adjusted for mid-parent height and maturational acceleration or delay, many supposed problems of growth vanish when they can be shown to be entirely normal for the circumstances (Figure 6-11).

## LABORATORY ASSISTANCE IN GROWTH DISORDERS

Because there are numerous causes for growth disturbances, ranging from congenital genetic syndromes to endocrine disorders, there can be no list of laboratory aids which will be useful in all circumstances. The choice of laboratory tests will be directed by the historical and physical evidence of the growth abnormality. It is customary, although not essential, to supplement the physical exam with a urinalysis, hemogram and chemistry screen, including electrolytes, calcium, phosphorus, alkaline phosphatase, and BUN or creatinine.

Determination of biologic level of maturation is helpful in determining whether the tempo of growth is consistent with the chronologic age or whether the child's growth should be compared with delayed or accelerated standards. *Skeletal maturation* (x-ray for bone age) is used most frequently to obtain this information. If disproportionate growth is discovered and a *skeletal dysplasia* is suspected, x-rays of skull, spine, pelvis, legs and arms will be needed to identify the degree and nature of the skeletal dysplasia and involvement of epiphysis, metaphysis, or diaphysis.

If congenital anomalies suggest a chromosomal abnormality, a *chromosomal karyotype* should be obtained, giving the cytogeneticist information about pregnancy, delivery, and congenital anomalies encountered. A syndrome can be sought from encyclopedias of congenital *anomalies*, such as *"Recognizable Patterns of Human Malformation"* by Smith (6) or *"Facial Anomalies"* by Gorlin et al. (7). Additional laboratory studies can be tailored to the specific genetic syndromes.

A *metabolic screen* will usually identify mucopolysaccharidosis, inborn errors of aminoacidemia or aminoaciduria, galactosemia, and sometimes congenital hypothyroidism. Specific tests for inborn errors of metabolism are found in Hsia's excellent book entitled *Inborn Errors of Metabolism* (8) or in more recent revisions (9). Among those inborn errors likely to be associated with growth failure are glycogen storage diseases, renal tubular acidosis, goitrous hypothyroidism, mucopolysaccharidosis, and a variety of aminoacidemias.

Specific testing will also be necessary if *endocrine disorders* are suspected as a cause of the growth disturbance. Disorders of the thyroid, pituitary, and adrenal are most likely to be involved in growth disturbances.

## Tests of Thyroid Function

The usual tests for identification of suspected hypothyroidism are plasma thyroxine ($T_4$) and thyroid stimulating hormone (TSH) measurements. In primary hypothyroidism $T_4$ is low and TSH is elevated. In milder cases of hypothyroidism, the $T_4$ may be in the normal range with mildly elevated TSH. $T_4$ measurements vary with each laboratory, but for children, normal values are usually in the 6–13 μg/dL range. At birth, levels of $T_4$ are higher (Table 7-2). Thyroxine levels of 6.5 μg/dL or less on newborn screening tests are considered low. (Some programs investigate an infant with initial $T_4$ below 7.0 or even 8.0 μg/dL.) TSH usually ranges from 2–8 μU/mL; levels above 15 μU/mL are usually considered abnormal in the neonate. However, each laboratory has a normal range, therefore it is necessary to compare levels in question with lab-established norms.

## Table 7-2. Normal Range for $T_4$, $T_3$, $T_3$ Resin Uptake, TBG, and TSH in Infancy and Childhood[a]

| Age | Total $T_4$ (μg/dL) Mean | Range | Total $T_3$ (ng/dL) Mean | Range | $T_3$ Resin Uptake (%) Mean | Range | TBG (mg/dL) Mean | Range | TSH (μU/mL) Mean | Range |
|---|---|---|---|---|---|---|---|---|---|---|
| Cord blood | 10.2 | 7.4–13.0 | 45 | 15–75 | 0.90 | 0.75–1.05 | 5.6 | — | 9.0 | 2.5–17.4 |
| 1–3 days | 17.2 | 11.8–22.6 | 124 | 32–216 | 1.15 | 0.90–1.40 | 5.0 | — | 8.0 | 2.5–13.3 |
| 1–2 weeks | 13.2 | 9.8–16.6 | 250 | — | 1.00 | 0.85–1.15 | — | — | — | — |
| 2–4 weeks | 11.0 | 7.0–15.0 | 160 | 160–240 | 0.95 | 0.80–1.15 | — | — | 4.0 | 0.6–10.0 |
| 1–4 months | 10.3 | 7.2–14.4 | 163 | 117–209 | 0.90 | 0.75–1.05 | — | — | <2.5 | <2.5 |
| 4–12 months | 11.0 | 7.8–16.5 | 176 | 110–280 | 0.98 | 0.88–1.12 | 4.4 | 3.1–5.6 | 2.1 | 0.6–6.3 |
| 1–5 years | 10.5 | 7.3–15.0 | 168 | 105–269 | 0.99 | 0.88–1.12 | 4.2 | 2.9–5.4 | 2.0 | 0.6–6.3 |
| 5–10 years | 9.3 | 6.4–13.3 | 150 | 94–241 | 1.00 | 0.88–1.12 | 3.8 | 2.5–5.0 | 2.08 | 0.6–6.3 |
| 10–15 years | 8.1 | 5.6–11.7 | 113 | 83–213 | 1.01 | 0.88–1.12 | 3.3 | 2.1–4.6 | 1.9 | 0.6–6.3 |
| Adult | 8.4 | 4.3–12.5 | 125 | 70–204 | 1.01 | 0.85–1.14 | 3.5 | 2.1–5.5 | 1.8 | 0.2–7.6 |

Reproduced by permission from LaFranchi, SA: Hypothyroidism, *Pediatr Clin North Am* **26**:33–51, February, 1979. (Data derived from Abuid JL, et al: *J Clin Endocrinol Metab* **39**:263, 1974; Chopra IJ, et al and Fisher DA, et al in Fisher DA, Burrows GN (eds): *Perinatal Thyroid Physiology and Disease*, New York, Raven Press, 1975; Fisher DA, et al: *J Clin Endocrinol Metab* **45**:191, 1977; O'Halloran MT, et al: *J Pediatr* **31**:916, 1972.)

[a] $T_4$, $T_3$, TSH, and TBG are measured by radioimmunoassay; $T_4$ measured by competitive protein binding is 15% lower. Range equals ± 2 SD from mean value.

183

$T_4$ levels are affected by the binding protein. Low total thyroxine-binding-globulin (TBG) will reduce the total $T_4$ to a "hypothyroid" level without affecting free thyroxine levels. Likewise, elevation of TBG will factitiously elevate the total $T_4$ into the "hyperthyroid" range without affecting free thyroxine appreciably. To screen for this possibility many labs perform a $T_3$ resin uptake, ($T_3$RU). The $T_3$RU varies inversely with the number of free binding sites on TBG. With a decrease in TBG and a low total $T_4$ there will be a rise in $T_3$RU; conversely a rise in TBG will result in a fall in $T_3$RU. Consideration of both $T_4$ and $T_3$RU will allow recognition of changes due to high or low levels of TBG.

To examine for a hyperthyroid state, plasma $T_4$, plasma $T_3$RIA (a measurement of circulating triiodothyronine) and thyroidal uptake of $^{131}I$ or $^{123}I$ at 2, 6 or 24 hours are most helpful. In hyperthyroidism, all three tests should be elevated, although in $T_3$ toxicosis, the $T_3$RIA is elevated out of proportion to the others. In questionable cases, the radioiodine uptake can be combined with treatment over a 7 day period with $T_3$ at a dosage of 75 µg/day (Werner suppression test). In normal individuals and in most subjects with lymphocytic thyroiditis, which can be confused with hyperthyroidism, there will be a suppression of thyroidal radioiodine uptake after $T_3$, but in hyperthyroidism, minimal suppression occurs. The use of radioiodine may be cumbersome and exposes the thyroid to some radiation from the radioisotope. The introduction of thyrotropin releasing hormone (TRH) enables us to test for thyrotoxicosis without radioiodine. TRH given i.v. results in elevation of TSH in normal individuals but no elevation is seen in hyperthyroid subjects (10, 11).

### Tests of Human Growth Hormone and Somatomedin

Since normal resting growth hormone levels range from 0–10 ng/mL, human growth hormone (hGH) release requires stimulation to separate subjects with normal growth hormone secretion from those with deficiency. Tests of hGH secretion have taken advantage of a number of physiologic and pharmacologic stimuli of growth hormone release including sleep, exercise, dopamine, arginine, glucagon, clonidine, and hypoglycemia (Table 7-3).

Although the rise of hGH 1 hour after beginning deep sleep was one of the first physiologic tests of growth hormone release described, its usage is very limited. The most commonly used *screening* test for hGH deficiency is the propranolol-augmented exercise test for growth hormone release (12, 13). Propranolol is administered orally in a dosage of 0.75 mg/kg up to a maximum of 40 mg. The subject rests 90 minutes and then exercises for 20 minutes by walking rapidly up and down stairs to induce fatigue but not exhaustion. Blood is drawn immediately after exercise and after a 20 minute rest for measurements of hGH by radioimmunoassay. A normal child will have a peak response of 7 ng/mL of hGH or more.

## Table 7-3.  Tests of Human Growth Hormone Release

| Test | Dosage | Time of GH Release |
|------|--------|--------------------|
| Exercise[a] | Growth hormone release related to strenuousness of exercise | 20–40 minutes after exercise is begun[c] |
| Sleep | hGH released during phase 3 and 4 of deep sleep | Peak 1 hour after beginning deep sleep[c] |
| Insulin-induced hypoglycemia | Regular insulin (CZI) 0.05–0.1 U/kg i.v. | 30–60 minutes after insulin administration[c] |
| Arginine-HCl (10%) | Infusion of 0.5 g/kg i.v. over 30 minutes (up to 30 g) | GH peak[c] often occurs after 30–60 minutes |
| Glucagon | 1.0 mg i.m. or s.c. | 120–150 minutes after administration[c] |
| L-dopa[a] | Oral dosage 125 mg/under 15 kg BW 250 mg/15–30 kg BW 500 mg/over 30 kg BW | 30–60 minutes after administration[c] |
| Clonidine[b] | 0.15 mg/m$^2$ oral | 30–120 minutes after administration[c] |

Reproduced by permission from Frasier SD: *Pediatric Endocrinology.* New York, Grune & Stratton Inc., 1980, pp 38–41.

[a] Propranolol (0.75 mg/kg) priming may be used before exercise or L-dopa to increase the response. Insulin-L-dopa or arginine-insulin tests may be performed sequentially.

[b] See reference 25.

[c] Peak hormone value of 7 ng/mL or more is considered normal (Frasier, cf above, suggests greater than or equal to 8 ng/mL as a normal response).

Among normal children there are some "nonresponders" to exercise-induced growth hormone secretion, but the use of propranolol to increase the sensitivity of the hypothalamus to exercise has improved the reliability to 90–100% of those tested (12). On occasion, propranolol may induce hypoglycemia, itself a stimulant for hGH release, but in this case, an unexpected side effect (14).

Diethylstilbestrol administered orally in a dose of 5 mg twice daily for 3 days also augments hGH release. A single morning serum sample on the fourth morning after 3 days of stilbestrol suffices as a screening test. Human growth hormone levels of 7 ng/mL or more are reported in 70% of normal subjects and levels below 4.0 ng/mL in subjects with hGH deficiency (15). Estrogen can improve sensitivity to exercise, L-dopa, or other provocative test substances. Glucagon, L-dopa, and clonidine have also been used as screening tests (described below under provocative tests).

The development of a sensitive, highly specific radioimmunoassay for *somatomedin C* (Sm C) has made use of Sm C levels feasible in the study of short stature both as a screening test for pituitary (hGH) deficiency and acromegaly (16), and as a definitive test in disorders of growth with normal hGH levels but low somatomedin activity or target tissue unresponsiveness (see Chapter 9). Patients with growth hormone deficiency generally have low Sm C levels, provided one takes into consideration the "developmental" age of the individual tested (16). Caution must be used in use of Sm C levels as a screening test for hGH deficiency in children under 6; below this age many normal children have low levels of Sm C, making it difficult to differentiate between normal and growth hormone-deficient children (16).

Since there always seem to be nonresponders to any of the screening tests for hGH release (17, 18), the diagnosis of hGH deficiency is reserved for those who fail to show a rise to a level of 7 ng/mL or more after two or more "*provocative*" tests. Although new tests are constantly being devised and tested, L-dopa, glucagon, clonidine, arginine infusion, and insulin-induced hypoglycemia are the provocative tests commonly used and accepted. The latter two are commonly performed together since both require no priming and both require i.v. administration of the provoking substance (19). For each of the definitive tests for hGH release, the subject must be fasting since glucose suppresses hGH release. Growth hormone releasing hormone (GRH) has recently been isolated and synthesized and is currently being tested as a stimulant for growth hormone release. This may eventually replace the pharmacologic stimulating substances currently being used.

*L-dopa* has been used extensively as a provocative test for release of growth hormone because it does not require intravenous administration nor monitoring of blood sugars; it is associated with few undesirable side effects (20) except for nausea. Testing is performed after an overnight fast. Levodopa is administered in a dose of 125 mg to subjects weighing less than 15 kg, 250 mg to those between 15–30 kg, and 500 mg to those weighing more than 30 kg (Table 7-3). [Porter et al. suggest a dosage of 500 mg/1.73 $m^2$ (21).] Blood samples are drawn for hGH determination at 30, 60, and 90 minutes after ingestion of levodopa. Used alone, without any previous "sensitization," Fass et al. found a 20–30% false positive rate with levodopa, about the same false positive rate as is seen with sleep-induced growth hormone release. However, when propranolol was added to the levodopa in a dosage of 0.75 mg/kg up to 40 mg, the rate of false positives (i.e., normal children who failed to achieve normal response) dropped to 5% (22). Propranolol must be used with caution because of its tendency to promote hypoglycemia (14). Sensitivity can also be increased by pretreatment with L-dopa. For pretreatment, levodopa is administered orally at one-half the test dose three times daily for 2 days preceding the test (21). A normal subject should reach hGH level of 7 ng/mL or more at 60 or 90 minutes after the administration of levodopa.

*Glucagon* also provokes release of human growth hormone. Glucagon, 1 mg is administered i.v. or i.m. and blood samples for hGH are obtained at 0, $2\frac{1}{2}$, and 3 hours after administration of glucagon. A rise to a peak level of 7 ng/mL or more is considered a normal response. Nausea after administration of glucagon has been a fairly regular occurrence and can cause some discomfort, but it is transient and does not affect the validity of the test.

Recent reports of the use of oral *clonidine* suggest that it may be as reliable as insulin-induced hypoglycemia in stimulating release of human growth hormone, requires no pretest preparation or "sensitization", and is virtually free of any side effects except drowsiness (24-26). If experience bears out the claims made in early reports, clonidine may replace some of the more cumbersome or complicated testing procedures. After an overnight fast and 15 minutes of rest, a single oral dose of clonidine, 0.15 mg/m$^2$ body surface area is given. Blood samples for hGH are drawn at 0, (30), 60, 90, and (120) minutes. Adequate growth hormone release is reported in 94% of subjects (24-26). For a screening test, 25μg of clonidine may be administered orally with blood samples for hGH obtained at 0 and 90 minutes (26).

*Arginine* is infused in a dosage of 0.5 g/kg over 30 minutes. (Arginine is available as a 5 or 10% solution of arginine in sodium chloride commercially.) Blood samples for hGH are obtained at 0 (i.e., at the conclusion of the infusion), and at 30, 60 and 90 minutes (27). The same standards for growth hormone levels apply as above.

*Hypoglycemia*-induced growth hormone release has generally been accepted as the standard to which most of the other tests have been compared. Hypoglycemia is induced with intravenous insulin 0.05−0.1 unit/kg body weight. (Note: This test should not be used in subjects with known symptomatic hypoglycemia.) Blood glucose is sampled at 0, 20, 30, 40, and 60 minutes to define the nadir of blood sugar which provokes hGH release. Blood is sampled for hGH at 0, 30, 60, 90, and 120 minutes after administration of i.v. insulin. Normal subjects achieve peak hGH levels of at least 7 ng/mL. Growth hormone deficient subjects are usually under 4 ng/mL on all specimens (17). Levels in between may represent the limits of accuracy of the method of measurement or may reflect subjects with partial hGH deficiency. In such circumstances, it is desirable to prime the subject with estrogen and repeat the study. In *adolescent aged* children with delayed puberty, pretreatment of girls with estrogen and of boys with testosterone must be performed before provocative tests can reliably be performed; many such youngsters fail to release hGH until primed with gonadal steroids (28).

*Somatomedin* activity is constant throughout the day because of the long biological half-life of Sm C complexed with its carrier protein. Somatomedin (Sm C) can be measured by a specific and sensitive radioimmunoassay, as well as a number of other methods; no stimulation is needed. Sm C can be measured simultaneously with hGH during any of the provocative tests for hGH release. The sample required is a fresh frozen plasma sample which must be delivered to the laboratory frozen. Normal ranges by sex and by age are reported by each reference laboratory. Levels are low through childhood ranging from 25-250 ng/mL (0.1–1.0 U/mL). Usual adult levels (~250 ng/mL or ~1.0 U/mL are reached by about 10–12 years of age (earlier in girls) but there is a temporary rise above these levels during puberty. Levels of 250–800 ng/mL (1.0–3.2 U/mL) are seen in girls during puberty with peak at about 13 years, while levels of 150–750 ng/mL (0.6–3.0 U/mL) are seen in pubertal boys with a peak at about age 15.

### Tests of Pituitary Function

In children with growth failure in whom hypopituitarism is suspected, complete testing of all pituitary hormones is now possible and feasible. *Growth hormone* measurement requires stimulation tests, as discussed above. *Thyroid stimulating hormone* (TSH) can be measured in plasma by radioimmunoassay. The range of normal is usually reported as 2 to 8 µU/mL. Levels are elevated in primary hypothyroidism but hypopituitary levels overlap with the lower ranges of normal. Thyrotropin releasing hormone (TRH) can be administered to provoke maximal secretion of TSH. TRH is administered i.v. over 30 seconds in a dose of 7 µg/kg (up to 400 µg) and blood is sampled for TSH at 0, 15, 30, and 60 minutes through a heparinized indwelling needle. An increment of 10–30 µU/mL above the baseline level of TSH is usually seen in normal children and no rise is seen in hypopituitary subjects (10, 11). Prolactin levels also rise in response to TRH; the maximal response occurs at 15–30 minutes with a three- to five-fold increase in prolactin level in children (31). *Adrenocorticotropic hormone* (ACTH) can also be measured by radioimmunoassay, but the test is difficult because of lability in plasma and other assay problems. ACTH secretion can be provoked by hypoglycemia induced by insulin. Peak response usually occurs about 45 minutes after the insulin is given. A cortisol rise mediated via ACTH may be detected 60–90 minutes after the insulin is administered. In an individual with normal pituitary–adrenal function, the serum cortisol should exceed 30 µg/dl. Metyrapone can also be used to test for ACTH-adrenal response (32). Metyrapone, which blocks 11-hydroxylation, is administered in a single dose of 30 mg/kg with milk at midnight. This blocks production of cortisol, which by negative feedback stimulates release of ACTH. Next morning at 8:00 a.m. a blood sample is obtained (heparinized so that plasma may be drawn off) for measurement of ACTH and 11-deoxycortisol. In normal individuals both ACTH and

11-deoxycortisol will rise. The ACTH level should rise above 100 pg/mL and the 11-deoxycortisol above 7 ug/dl. In hypopituitary subjects neither ACTH nor 11-deoxycortisol will demonstrate the characteristic rise (32). *Gonadotropins* (FSH and LH) can be measured in blood or urine of adolescents (See Chapter V). Before puberty, levels obtained from a subject may be compared to the usual range for age (33-36). After mid-puberty, clomiphene and GnRH may be used to stimulate the release of FSH and LH (37). When clomiphene is administered to prepubertal children, suppression of gonadotropins is observed. By midpuberty, a gonadotropin rise is seen with a dosage of 50–100 mg/day for 5 days. To determine gonadotropin release in subjects suspected of pituitary deficiency, we prefer stimulation with GnRH. The subject is given 2.5 µg/kg of GnRH (LH-RH) as an intravenous bolus and samples for FSH and LH measurements are drawn at 0, 30, 60, and 90 minutes. Incremental rises in LH and FSH are correlated with skeletal maturation (bone-age) rather than chronologic-age (39).

We commonly combine TRH, insulin, and GnRH intravenously to allow simultaneous measurement of multiple pituitary hormones. The recently successful synthesis of GRH (growth hormone releasing hormone) and CRH (corticotropin releasing hormone) makes possible a quadruple hypothalamic hormone stimulation test for pituitary hormone response. TRH, GnRH, GRH, and CRH can all be given simultaneously with measurement of TSH, Prolactin, LH, FSH, hGH and ACTH.

## ASSESSMENT OF SHORT STATURE

In the assessment of a child suspected of a growth aberration, the first consideration is to look for evidence of normal variation (40). In the child studied for short stature we pay particular attention to velocity of growth. If the child has a normal growth velocity for age, neonatal history, family history, physical exam, and bone-age x-ray should lead to differentation of familial short stature, constitutional delayed growth of intrauterine growth retardation (Table 7-4).

If growth velocity is subnormal for age, systemic illnesses and endocrine disorders that can slow growth must be considered. Nonendocrine disorders may be evident from physical exam or appropriate lab testing. (Table 7-4). Thyroid function tests and delayed bone age will direct attention to hypothyroidism with characteristic patterns for primary versus secondary deficiency. Karyotype and gonadotropins should be performed in a euthyroid short phenotypic female to discover Turner's syndrome. Growth hormone deficiency or psychosocial dwarfism can be defined with growth hormone tests; Laron dwarfism and biologically inactive growth hormone from measurement of somatomedin and the response of somatomedin (and rate of growth) to growth hormone administration (41). (See Table 7-4).

## Table 7-4. Differential Diagnosis of Short Stature

A. NORMAL GROWTH VELOCITY FOR AGE
   *(nonendocrine normal variants)*
   Bone-age x-rays
       Family history of short stature in childhood, delayed adolescence and normal adult stature. Normal physical examination and delayed bone-age.
       **Constitutional delay in growth and adolescence.**
       Family history of short adult height and normal timing of puberty. Normal physical exam and normal bone-age.
       **Genetic (familial) short stature.**
       Low birth weight for gestational age. Family history of normal height. Normal or characteristic physical findings and variable bone-age.
       **Intrauterine growth retardation.**

B. SUBNORMAL GROWTH VELOCITY FOR AGE
   *(chronic nonendocrine disease)*
   CBC, UA, Chemistry Panel.
   Other studies as indicated
       Symptoms and signs of renal, GI, cardiac, neurologic, etc., involvement with appropriate lab abnormalities.
       **Systemic disease affecting growth rate.**
   *(endocrine disorders)*
   Thyroid function tests: Serum $T_4$/TSH/thyroid antibodies.
   Bone-age x-rays
       Symptoms and signs of hypothyroidism, delayed bone-age, low serum thyroxine ($T_4$), high serum TSH, and elevated serum antithyroid antibodies.
       **Primary hypothyroidism (thyroiditis).**
       Symptoms and signs of hypothyroidism, delayed bone-age, low $T_4$ and low serum TSH.
       **Hypothalamic or pituitary hypothyroidism.**
   *(euthyroid, phenotypic female)*
   Karyotype.
   Serum gonadotropins (FSH, LH).
   Bone-age x-ray
       Low birth weight (IUGR), physical stigmata of Turner's syndrome, elevated serum gonadotropins, abnormal X chromosome, delayed bone-age.
       **Turner's syndrome (or variant).**
   *(euthyroid, normal karyotype)*
   Growth hormone screen with exercise, L-dopa, or clonidine.
   Bone-age x-ray
   Definitive growth hormone tests if screen not normal
       Short stature, subnormal growth velocity for age, delayed bone-age, failure of growth hormone to respond to screen and definitive tests.
       **Growth hormone deficiency.**
       **Psychosocial dwarfism (transient growth hormone deficiency).**
   *(normal growth hormone response in subject with clinical picture of growth hormone deficiency)*

**Table 7-4. (Continued)**

Somatomedin determination.
Somatomedin generation test (response to growth hormone)
   Low somatomedin-C, no response to growth hormone.
   **Laron dwarfism**.
   Low somatomedin-C, short stature, subnormal velocity of growth, delayed bone-age, normal somatomedin and/or growth rate after growth hormone administration.
   **Biologically inactive growth hormone**.

Reproduced by permission from Frasier SD: *Pediatric Endocrinology*. New York, Grune & Stratton Inc, 1980, pp 55–118.

## REFERENCES

1. Miller HC, Merritt TA: *Fetal Growth in Humans*. Chicago, Year Book Med Publ Inc, 1979.
2. Smith DW, Truog W, Rogers JB, et al: Shifting linear growth during infancy: Illustration of genetic factors in growth from fetal life through infancy. *J Pediatr* **89**:225, 1976.
3. Lacey KA, Parkin JM: Causes of short stature: A community study of children in Newcastle-upon-Tyne. *Lancet* **1**:42, 1974.
4. Lacey KA, Parkin JM: The normal short child. *Arch Dis Child* **49**:417, 1974.
5. Smith DW: *Growth and Its Disorders*. Philadelphia, WB Saunders Co, 1977, pp 62–69, 120–121.
6. Smith DW: *Recognizable Patterns of Human Malformation*. Philadelphia, WB Saunders Co, 1976.
7. Goodman RM, Gorlin RJ: in *Atlas of the Face in Genetic Disorders*, ed 2. St. Louis, Mosby, 1977.
8. Hsia DYY: *Inborn Errors of Metabolism*, ed 2. Chicago, Year Book Med Publ Inc, 1966.
9. Buist NRM: Metabolic screening of the newborn infant. *Clin Endocrinol Metab* **5**:265, 1976.
10. Ormston BJ, Garry R, Cryer RJ, et al: Thyrotropin releasing hormone as a thyroid function test. *Lancet* **2**:10, 1971.
11. Foley TP Jr, Owens J, Hayford JT, et al: Serum thyrotropic responses to synthetic thyrotropin releasing hormone in normal children and hypopituitary patients: A new test to distinguish primary releasing hormone deficiency from primary pituitary hormone deficiency. *J Clin Invest* **51**:431, 1972.
12. Maclaren NK, Taylor GE, Raiti SM: Propranolol-augmented, exercised-induced human growth hormone release. *Pediatrics* **56**:804, 1975.
13. Shanis BS, Moshang T Jr: Propranolol and exercise as a screening test for growth hormone deficiency. *Pediatrics* **57**:712, 1976.
14. Hesse B, Pedersen JT: Hypoglycemia after propranolol in children. *Acta Med Scand* **193**:551, 1973.
15. Bacon GE, Lowrey GH, Knoller M: Comparison of arginine infusion and diethylstilbestrol as a means of provoking growth hormone secretion. *J Pediatr* **75**:385, 1969.
16. Clemmons DR, Van Wyk JJ: Factors controlling blood concentration of somatomedin C. *Clin Endocrinol Metab* **13**(Mar):113, 1984.
17. Frasier SD: A review of growth hormone stimulation tests in children. *Pediatrics* **53**:929, 1974.

18. Lin T, Tucci JR: Provocative tests of growth hormone release: A comparison of results with various stimuli. *Ann Intern Med* **80**:464, 1974.

19. Penny R, Blizzard RM, Davis WT: Sequential arginine and insulin tolerance tests on the same day. *J Clin Endocrinol Metab* **29**:1499, 1969.

20. Weldon VU, Bupta SK, Haymond MW, et al: The use of L-dopa in the diagnosis of hyposomatotropism in children. *J Clin Endocrinol Metab* **36**:42, 1973.

21. Porter BA, Rosenfield RC, Lawrence AM: The levodopa test of growth hormone secretion in children. *Am J Dis Child* **126**:589, 1973.

22. Fass B, Lippe BM, Kaplan SA: Relative usefulness of three growth hormone stimulation screening tests. *Am J Dis Child* **133**:931, 1979.

23. Mitchell ML, Suvunrungsi P, Sawin CT: Effect of propranolol on the response of serum growth hormone to glucagon. *J Clin Endocrinol Metab* **32**:470, 1971.

24. Gil-Ad I, Topper E, Laron Z: Oral clonidine as a growth hormone stimulation test. *Lancet* **2**:297, 1979.

25. Lanes R, Hurtado E: Oral clonidine—An effective growth hormone releasing agent in prepubertal subjects. *J Pediatr* **100**:710, 1982.

26. Laron Z, Gil-Ad I, Topper E, et al: Low oral dose of clonidine: An effective screening test for growth hormone deficiency. *Acta Paediatr Scand* **71**:847, 1982.

27. Root AW, Saenz-Rodriguez C, Bongiovanni AM, et al: The effect of arginine infusion on plasma growth hormone and insulin in children. *J Pediatr* **74**:187, 1969.

28. Martin LG, Grossman MS, Conner TB: Effect of androgens on growth hormone secretion and growth in boys with short stature. *Acta Endocrinol* **91**:201, 1979.

29. Hintz RL: Plasma forms of somatomedin and the binding protein phenomenon. *Clin Endocrinol Metab* **13**(Mar):31, 1984.

30. Hall K, Sara VR: Somatomedin levels in childhood, adolescence, and adult life. *Clin Endocrinol Metab* **13**(Mar):91, 1984.

31. Kleinberg DL, Noel GL, Frantz AG: Galactorrhea: A study of 235 cases including 48 with pituitary tumors. *New Engl J Med* **295**:659, 1977.

32. Limal JM, Basmaciogullari A, Rappaport R: Evaluation of single oral dose metyrapone tests in children with hypopituitarism. *Acta Pediatr Scand* **65**:177, 1976.

33. Raiti S, Johansen A, Light C, et al: Measurement of immunologically reactive follicle-stimulating hormone in serum of normal male children and adults. *Metabolism* **18**:234, 1969.

34. Johansen AJ, Guida H, Light C, et al: Serum luteinizing hormone by radioimmunoassay in normal children. *J Pediatr* **74**:416, 1969.

35. Raiti SM, Light C, Blizzard, RM: Urinary follicle-stimulating hormone excretion in boys and adult males as measured by radioimmunoassay. *J Clin Endocrinol Metab* **29**:884, 1969.

36. Baghdassarian A, Guida H, Johansen A, et al.: Urinary excretion of radioimmunoassay-able luteinizing hormone (LH) in normal male children and adults according to age and stage of sexual development. *J Clin Endocrinol Metab* **31**:428, 1970.

37. Raiti S: Endocrine causes of short stature. *Postgrad Med J* **62**:81, 1977.

38. Kulin HE, Grumbach MM, Kaplan SL: Gonadal–hypothalamic interaction in prepubertal and pubertal man: Effect of clomiphene citrate on urinary follicle-stimulating hormone and luteinizing hormone and plasma testosterone. *Pediatr Res* **6**:162, 1972.

39. Alsever RN, Gotlin RW: Increments from baseline in serum concentrations of FSH and LH after intravenous bolus administration of LH-RH (Table 2-4), *Handbook of Endocrine Tests*. Chicago, Year Book Medical Publishers, 1978, p 19.

40. Zachmann M: Diagnosis of treatable types of short and tall stature. *Postgrad Med J* **54**(2):121, 1978.

41. Frasier SD: *Pediatric Endocrinology*. New York, Grune & Stratton Inc, 1980, pp 55–118.

# 8
# Growth Disorders in Infancy

Growth disturbances discussed in this chapter are those of prenatal onset, or those usually recognized in the neonatal period or early infancy. The divisions drawn between infancy and childhood are arbitrary and imperfect and there will be overlap, however, the large number of growth disorders occurring in the newborn period necessitates narrowing discussion in this chapter to those recognizable in infancy.

## CLASSIFICATION OF GROWTH DISORDERS IN INFANCY

In Table 8-1 we have classified the growth disorders of infancy into three general groupings: (a) normal variants, (b) growth deficiency disorders, and (c) growth excess disorders.

### Normal Variants

Normal variants are by definition not "disorders" at all, but merely represent natural extremes of infant growth which must be distinguished from pathological disturbances of growth in infancy. In terms of numbers among those considered to have growth disturbances in infancy, normal variants are the most common, especially if one encompasses within the definition those born prematurely but of appropriate size for gestational age.

### Growth Deficiency Disorders

Growth deficiency disorders are divided into (a) intrinsic or primary disorders and (b) extrinsic or secondary disorders. Among the former are infants with chromosomal anomalies, skeletal dysplasias, and congenital malformation syndromes associated with disturbances in size of the infant. These disorders have their onset prenatally and are considered to represent primary defects in the regulators of growth or in the growing tissues

## Table 8-1. Classification of Growth Disorders of Infancy

1.  Normal Growth Variants in Infancy
    A.  Small for Gestational Age Infants
        (a)  Familial Short Stature
        (b)  Parity, Race, Sex, Maternal Size
    B.  Large for Gestational Age Infants
        (a)  Familial Tall Stature
        (b)  Parity, Race, Sex, Maternal Size
    C.  Prematurely Born Infants
2.  Growth Deficiency Disorders in the Neonate
    A.  Intrinsic Growth Deficiency
        (1)  Chromosomal Imbalance Syndromes
            (a)  Chromosomal Excess Syndromes
                (i)  Down's Syndrome
                (ii)  Other Chromosomal Trisomies
                (iii)  Multi-X Syndromes
            (b)  Chromosomal Deletion Syndromes
                (i)  Turner's Syndrome
                (ii)  q-/p- Deletion Syndrome
                (iii)  Cri-du-chat Syndrome
        (2)  Skeletal Dysplasias (Genetic)
            (a)  Osteochondordysplasias
                (i)  Nonlethal Chondrodysplasias
                    a.  Achondroplasia
                    b.  Chondroectodermal Dysplasia
                    c.  Other Chondrodysplasias (see Table 8-5)
                (ii)  Lethal Chondrodysplasias
                    a.  Achondrogenesis
                    b.  Thanatophoric Dwarfism
                    c.  Other Lethal Chondrodystrophies (see Table 8-6)
            (b)  Abnormalities of Bone Density
                (i)  Hypophosphatasia
                (ii)  Osteogenesis Imperfecta Congenita
                (iii)  Osteopetrosis
        (3)  Inborn Errors of Metabolism
            (a)  Gangliosidosis Type 1 (Generalized gangliosidosis)
            (b)  Mucolipidosis II (I-Cell disease)
        (4)  Dysmorphic Syndromes with Short Stature
            (a)  Congenital Hypoplasia with Dysmorphic Features
                (i)  Silver–Russell Syndromes
                (ii)  Other Hypoplasia Syndromes (see Table 8-8)
            (b)  Dysmorphic Syndromes with Short Stature
                (i)  Progeria
                (ii)  Other Dysmorphic Syndromes (see Table 8-9)
    B.  Extrinsic Growth Deficiency
        (1)  Multiple Pregnancy, Twinning
            (a)  Intrauterine Crowding

**Table 8-1. (Continued)**

    (2)   Fetal Growth Retardation (IUGR)
- (a)   Fetal Factors
  - (i)   Chromosomal Aberrations
  - (ii)   Skeletal Dysplasias
  - (iii)   Congenital Malformation Syndromes
  - (iv)   Inborn Errors or Metabolism
- (b)   Maternal Medical Complications
  - (i)   Intrauterine Infections
  - (ii)   Maternal Hypertension and Other Diseases
  - (iii)   Abnormalities of Uterus/Placenta
- (c)   Maternal Behavior or Condition in Pregnancy
  - (i)   Socioeconomic Status
  - (ii)   Nutritional Condition
  - (iii)   Maternal Age
  - (iv)   Medications, Drugs
- (d)   Environmental Factors
  - (i)   Altitude
  - (ii)   Radiation
  - (iii)   Toxic Substances in Environment

    (3)   Congenital Endocrine and Metabolic Disorders
- (a)   Congenital Hypothyroidism
- (b)   Congenital Hypopituitarism
- (c)   Inborn Errors of Metabolism
  - (i)   Congenital Adrenal Hyperplasia
  - (ii)   Galactosemia
  - (iii)   Glycogen Storage Diseases
  - (iv)   Laron Dwarfism

3.  Growth Excess Disorders of Infancy
- A.  Intrinsic Factors
  - (1)   LGA Infants with Congenital Anomalies
    - (a)   Beckwith–Wiedeman Syndrome
    - (b)   Cerebral Gigantism
    - (c)   Weaver's or Marshall's Syndrome
  - (2)   LGA Infants with Chromosomal Abnormalities
    - (a)   XYY Syndrome
    - (b)   Trisomy 8 Syndrome
- B.  Extrinsic Factors
  - (1)   Infant of Diabetic Mother
  - (2)   Hyperthyroidism
  - (3)   Nesidioblastosis

themselves. The extrinsic disorders, which are generally more open to manipulation, include multiple pregnancies, intrauterine growth retardation, congenital endocrine deficiencies, and inborn errors of metabolism.

Although the variety of primary growth disorders in infancy is great, they are individually and collectively rare with a few exceptions. Down's syndrome, Turner's syndrome, achondroplasia, osteogenesis imperfecta, and perhaps Silver–Russel syndrome are of frequent enough occurrence that they may be recognized by most students of infant growth failure. Recognition of many of the other primary growth disorders of infancy is beyond the ken of the average student of growth. The extrinsic or secondary growth deficiencies of infancy are more common. Twinning occurs in a little over 1% of pregnancies and intrauterine growth retardation (small-for-dates infants) in close to 3% of live born infants (1,2). Congenital hypothyroidism is less common, occurring in approximately 1 in 4000 live births (3).

### Growth Excess Disorders

Growth deficiency disorders in infancy are far more common than growth excess disorders, both in varieties and in numbers affected. Though large-for-dates (LGA) infants are by definition nearly as common as small-for-dates (SGA) infants, they are almost all normal variants. There are a few rare intrinsic or primary disorders associated with LGA infants, but infants of diabetic mothers (IDM) constitute the single most common growth excess disturbance in infancy. The pathologic physiology of this disorder has been extensively studied and appropriate intervention therapy to improve the outcome is continuing to evolve (4).

### NORMAL GROWTH VARIANTS IN INFANCY

Each infant's growth is unique and is affected by genetic endowment, size of mother, race, sex, and parity. It is no surprise, therefore, that normal variation in size at birth is quite considerable. The mean weight at birth may vary among ethnic groups from 2.40 kg to 3.88 kg, a difference of 1.48 kg, and the normal range of birth-weight at term within a population may extend from 2500 g to 4275 g (5).

### Definition of Normal Variants

Since our definitions of large-for-dates (LGA) and small-for-dates (SGA) are based on statistical criteria according to weight for gestational-age at birth, some infants so designated will be perfectly normal. Some of the factors known to affect the size of the infant at birth are known so that corrections of birth-weight or length can be made to refine the definition of the infant who is smaller or larger than expected.

The natural disparity between male and female infants can be taken into consideration by using separate standards (Appendix Tables A-1, A-

2) or by applying standard corrections which vary according to gestational-age. Similar corrections can be applied for parity and race (Figure 2-8). First born infants are smaller than subsequent infants because of uterine constraint (Tables A-1, A-2). Black infants are smaller at birth than white infants. Race specific charts may need to be used for ethnic groups or races other than North American white and black infants (6). Corrections for tall and short mothers have been devised by Thomson (7). Using whatever corrections in birth weight seem appropriate, we can determine if the infant is likely to represent a normal variant related to sex, race, parity, or maternal size.

## Growth Patterns in SGA and LGA Infants

Some SGA infants are long and thin, others of appropriate weight for length, and still others short and thin. Some LGA infants are obese, while others are perfectly proportioned. The growth pattern during infancy depends to some extent on the relationship of weight to length. SGA infants who are thin, but of normal length for gestational-age, have a normal growth potential and gain weight rapidly after birth (8). By contrast, SGA infants who are both short and thin have limited growth potential or "latitude" (9). Large-for-date infants appear to have considerable growth "latitude" and tend to "lag-down" in growth after birth. "The large infant can afford to grow at a rate that suits his own unique developmental pattern" (9). Most LGA infants are either variants of normal or infants of diabetic mothers.

Infants of small or large parents may be small or large at birth, but with corrections for parity, sex, race, and maternal size, the infant size should fall within an appropriate range for parental size. Subsequent growth may be expected to follow the pattern suggested by genetic endowment from the parents. Many infants exhibit a natural catch-up or lag-down growth pattern during the first year to year and a half of growth, approaching the target patterns suggested by the genetic patterns of their parents.

## Premature Infants

Finally, we must identify those infants termed small who are in reality appropriate for gestational age but who are born prematurely. This can be ascertained by the use of figures or tables giving appropriate weights or crown/foot length for infants of different gestational-ages (Table 2-2, Figure 2-8, or Figure A-2 in Appendix). Infants who are born prematurely but are of appropriate size for their gestational age do not generally have a primary growth disorder but may have early growth disturbance because of physiologic immaturity interfering with appropriate nutritional intake; that is, respiratory distress syndrome, hyperbilirubinemia, poor suck reflex, and so on. Once these physiologic handicaps are overcome, prematurely born infants generally exhibit "catch-up" growth, in an attempt to return to the growth pattern normal for their stage of development which was interrupted by the premature birth. This growth will be influenced, of course, by any congenital anomalies or residual damage sustained during the neonatal period because of immaturity (10).

## GROWTH DEFICIENCY DISORDERS

The growth deficiency disorders include both intrinsic and extrinsic factors which interfere with growth either in utero or in the immediate postnatal period.

### Intrinsic Growth Deficiency Disorders

Intrinsic growth disorders imply a basic or primary problem in growth of tissues, especially skeletal, in utero. Malproportionate growth is a characteristic feature of skeletal dysplasias while, as Smith points out, "linear growth deficiency is a feature in the majority of dysmorphic syndromes which have a prenatal onset" (11). Some of the primary (intrinsic) disorders of growth are attributable to deletions or duplications of chromosomal material; others appear to be transmitted as genetic traits, while many are sporadic in appearance and of uncertain etiology. We shall consider the disorders in groups with similarities of etiology or of characteristics, acknowledging that many growth problems of infancy defy categorization by our present understanding.

#### *Chromosomal Imbalance Syndromes*

Both chromosomal duplication and chromosomal deletion can produce syndromes with characteristic patterns of malformation and growth deficiency. Most of these syndromes are associated with mental deficiency, but otherwise display rather diverse patterns of malformation.

#### *Chromosomal Excess Syndromes*

Table 8-2 lists the syndromes with chromosomal aneuploidy which are associated with primary growth deficiency (12). *Down's syndrome* (Trisomy 21) is both the best known and the most common of the chromosomal duplication syndromes. Lacey and Parkin found Down syndrome to be the most common cause of prenatal growth deficiency in a study of 10 year olds in Newcastle-upon-Tyne (13). The disorder has an incidence of 1 in 660 newborns, making it the most common pattern of malformation (12). Growth deficiency may be present at birth or begin in the neonatal period and is of variable degree.

Down's syndrome can usually be recognized at birth by a characteristic facial appearance (Figure 8-1). The infant has inner epicanthal folds, upward lateral slant of the palpebral fissures, flat facies, speckling of the iris, small nose with low nasal bridge, and small ears. Infants with Down's syndrome are usually hypotonic and have a tendency to hold the mouth

**Table 8-2. Chromosomal Excess Syndromes Associated with Growth Deficiency**

| Syndrome | Characteristic Malformations | Growth | Prognosis |
|---|---|---|---|
| Down's syndrome Trisomy 21 | Hypotonia, hyperflexibility, brachycephaly, flat face, slanting palpebral fissures, small nose, inner epicanthal folds, clinodactyly 5th finger, congenital heart disease, pelvic dysplasia | Small at birth, hypoplastic teeth, slow growth, delayed adolescence | Mental deficiency, male infertile, infant mortality of 44% from CHD, frequent infections, hypothyroidism |
| Trisomy 18 syndrome | Small mouth, short palpebral fissures, clenched hand with overlapping fingers, low arch dermal finger pattern, short sternum, CHD | Congenital hypoplasia, small at birth (mean 2340 g), polyhydramnios, small placenta | Failure to thrive, feeble, poor suck, hypertonic muscles, mental deficiency, 90% mortality by 1 year of age |
| Trisomy 13 syndrome | Holoprosencephaly (defects of eye, nose, lip and forebrain) scalp skin defect, CHD (80%), VSD, PDA, ASD, polydactyly, hyperconvex nails | Congenital hypoplasia (mean 2480 g) | Mental deficiency, 80% + mortality by 1 year |
| Trisomy 8 syndrome | Thick lips, deep-set eyes, camptodactyly, prominent ears | Mild to moderate growth deficiency | Mild to severe mental deficiency |
| XXXXY syndrome | Hypotonia, wide-set eyes with slanted palpebral fissures, inner epicanthal folds, limited elbow pronation, abnormal dermal ridge pattern cryptorchidism with hypogenitalism | Low birth weight, short stature, delayed bone age | Mental deficiency, infertility |
| Penta-X syndrome (XXXXX) | Slanted palpebral fissures, PDA, clinodactyly | Postnatal growth deficiency | Mental deficiency |

Adapted by permission from Smith DW: *Recognizable Patterns of Human Malformations*, ed 3. WB Saunders Co, Philadelphia, 1982.

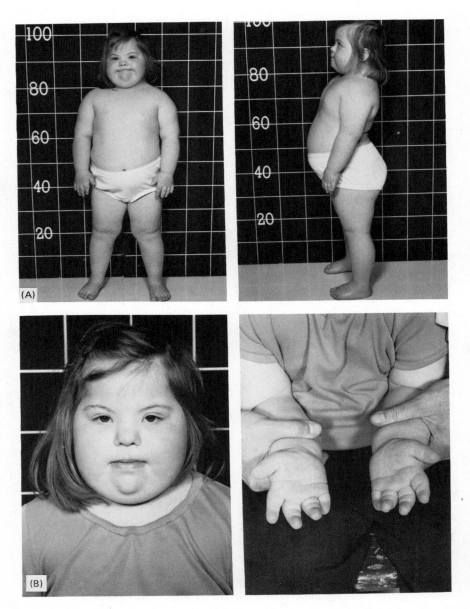

**Figure 8-1.** Child with Down's syndrome (age 10 years) showing short stature (<5°), typical facial features (inner epicanthal folds, upward slanting of palpebral fissures, flat face, small nose with low nasal bridge, and open mouth), and hands with short fingers.

open allowing the tongue to protrude (but the tongue is not enlarged as in cretinism). The hands have short metacarpals and phalanges, a simian crease and clinodactyly of the fifth finger. There is a wide gap and a plantar crease between the first and second toes. Characteristic dermal patterns can be see on the hands and feet. The skin is dry and hyperkeratotic, though not necessarily in the newborn period. The hair is fine, soft, and often sparse (14).

Growth is slow in early childhood with delay in skeletal maturation. Cardiac anomaly is present in 40% of infants with Down's syndrome, most commonly atrioventricular communis. Many of the infants with cardiac anomalies die in infancy. Increased susceptibility to lower respiratory problems may pose an additional threat, but after infancy, the mortality rate is not much greater than normal. Chronic persistent low grade infections, however, are frequent. Mental deficiency is invariable with IQ's in the range of 25–50. Hypotonia tends to lessen with age, however, mental deficiency becomes comparatively worse (12, 15).

Down's syndrome is the expression of a Trisomy 21; full Trisomy 21 in 94% and mosaicism or translocations in the remainder. Trisomy 21 is more likely to occur at older maternal age. The general recurrence rate is about 1%, but the recurrence rate for translocation carriers is much higher (12). All of the chromosomal excess syndromes are associated with mental deficiency, quite profound in all but 8 Trisomy (mosaic). Fetal growth retardation occurs in 18 Trisomy, 13 Trisomy and the XXXXY syndrome; birth-weight is low and subsequent growth is deficient as well. Infants with 18 Trisomy exhibit severe failure to thrive, associated with feebleness and poor suck, and over 90% die within the first year. Infants with 13 Trisomy have congenital heart disease (80%) and superficial facial/cranial deficits which often lead to death (over 80%) within the first year. Intrauterine growth is less compromised in Trisomy 8 and penta-X syndrome, but postnatal growth is usually affected and mental deficiency still clouds the prognosis. Each of the syndromes may be suspected from the characteristic malformation patterns and verified by karyotype patterns (12).

### Chromosomal Deletion Syndromes

Deletion or loss of chromosomal material results in patterns of malformation, all of which are characterized by growth deficiency. Table 8-3 lists the syndromes characterized by deletion of genetic material and growth failure (12).

*Turner's syndrome* (XO) is the most common chromosomal deletion syndrome associated with short stature. Deletion of the sex chromosome is accompanied by lack of gonadal tissue with a female phenotype, small stature, and characteristic somatic anomalies. A single X chromosome (45 XO) is found in about 1 in 5000 live births, a result of faulty chromosome distribution (nondisjunction) (12). It is generally a sporadic event, but

**Table 8-3. Chromosomal Deletion Syndromes Associated With Growth Deficiency**

| Syndrome | Characteristic Malformations | Growth | Prognosis |
|---|---|---|---|
| Turner's syndrome (XO, XO/XX) (XXp-, XXqi) (XO/XY) | Congenital lymphedema, cutis laxa (webbed neck), shield shaped chest with wide nipples, cubitus valgus, low posterior hairline, dysplastic nails, pigmented nevi, renal and cardiac anomalies | Low birth weight, short stature, slow growth, no adolescent growth spurt | Short adult height, sexual infantilism, infertility |
| Cri-du-chat syndrome, 5p-deletion | Cat-like cry, microcephaly, hypertelorism, down slanting palpebral fissures, epicanthal folds, simian creases, CHD | Low birth weight (under 2500 g), slow growth | Severe mental deficiency (IQ 20–30), hypotonia |
| 4p-syndrome, 4p-deletion | Hypertelorism, broad, beaked nose, microcephaly, low-set ears, cleft lip/palate, "fish" mouth, hypospadius, cryptorchidism | Severe growth deficiency, low birth weight | Severe mental deficiency, seizures, frequent respiratory infections, death in childhood |

| 13q-syndrome, 13q-deletion | Microcephaly, trigonocephaly holoprosencephaly, low-set, slanting ears, retinoblastoma, prom. nasal bridge, small or absent thumbs, clinodactyly, hypospadius, cryptorchidism | Prenatal growth deficiency | Severe mental deficiency |
| --- | --- | --- | --- |
| 18p-syndrome, 18p-deletion | Microcephaly (mild), ptosis of eyelids or epicanthal folds, hypertelorism, round face, wide mouth (cupid bow), large protruding ears, pectus excavation | Mild to moderate growth deficiency | Mental deficiency, life expectancy normal |
| 18q-syndrome, 18q-deletion | Nystagmus, midfacial hypoplasia, microcephaly, prom. anti-helix or anti-tragus, narrow ear canal, whorl digital pattern, cryptorchidism, hypoplastic labia | Small stature | Mental deficiency, poor coordination hypotonia, visual and hearing problems |
| 21q-syndrome, 21q-deletion | Down slanting palpebral fissure, large, malformed ears, micrograthia, redundant eyelids | Low birth weight (under 2500 g), moderate to severe growth deficiency | Severe mental deficiency, hypotonia |

Adapted by permission from Smith DW: *Recognizable Patterns of Human Malformations*, ed 3. WB Saunders Co, Philadelphia, 1982.

multiple recurrences in siblings have occurred (16). Characteristic anomalies are also seen in varying degree in individuals with partial X chromosome deletions (XXp-XXqi) and in individuals with mosaic patterns. Mosaicism appears to be as common as the full chromosomal deletion pattern. Short stature and somatic anomalies are most consistently associated with loss of the short arm of the X chromosome (17). Individuals with XY/XO mosaicism exhibit varying degrees of gonadal and genital maldevelopment. Gonadoblastoma may develop in the dysgenetic gonad. Individuals with single X chromosome (XO) have normal external and internal female sex organs, but the gonads are underdeveloped and are usually replaced by a "streak" of very primitive gonadal tissue.

Small size is often evident at birth, the mean birth weight being 2900 g (12). In addition, puffiness of the hands and feet (lymphedema) and redundancy of the skin at the back of the neck (cutis laxa) may be present at birth, directing attention to the presence of the chromosomal anomaly (Figure 8-2). The appearance in infancy was first described by Ullrich in 1930 (18) in a group of infants, some of whom later displayed typical features of Turner's syndrome. At the time of his original report, Ullrich attributed the lymphedema to migrating CSF fluid, similar to that seen in mice by Bonnevie, and suggested the name "status Bonnevie–Ullrich" for affected infants (19). Though the suggested pathogenesis was inaccurate (hypoplasia of lymph channels appears more likely) (20), Ullrich did describe quite faithfully the typical appearance of an infant with Turner's syndrome and, in European literature, the syndrome is aptly named the Ullrich-Turner syndrome.

In infancy, the diagnosis of Turner's syndrome is made by recognition of cutis laxa and lymphedema and by making a thorough search for associated somatic anomalies in an infant small-for-date; the chromosomal deletion pattern is confirmed by karyotype. The consistent features of the syndrome are short stature and gonadal dysgenesis, neither of which may be evident in the newborn period. It is imperative, therefore, to bear in mind the possibility of Turner's syndrome when considering the cause of short stature and/or sexual infantilism in a girl at any age.

The congenital lymphedema usually improves during infancy, although some puffiness of hands and fingers or of feet and toes may persist into childhood. The loose folds of skin at the nape of the neck usually persist as webbing of the neck (pterygium colli). Linear growth is below normal from early infancy, usually proceeding at about one-half to three-fourths normal velocity. Frequent ear infections may be seen in infancy and childhood. Coarctation of the aorta may require repair in infancy if heart failure threatens. Otherwise, the infant with XO Turner's syndrome leads a healthy life and though small, thrives (12, 17, 21). The effects of the syndrome on growth and development in childhood and at puberty will be described in Chapters 9 and 10 respectively.

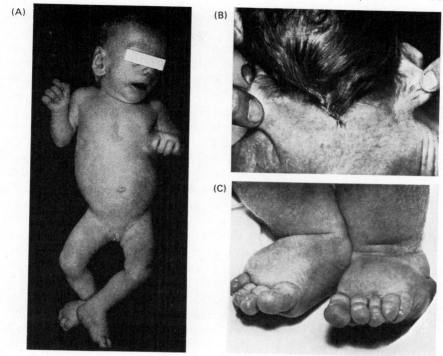

**Figure 8-2.**  Infant with Turner's syndrome showing cutis laxa (B) and puffy hands and feet (A, C) typical of status Bonnevie–Ullrich. (8-2 A Reproduced by permission from Haddad HM, Wilkins L: Congenital anomalies associated with gonadal aplasia—review of 55 cases, *Pediatrics* **23**: 885, 1959, copyright American Academy of Pediatrics 1959; 8-2 B and C reproduced from Boehnke H, Lenz W: Ullrich–Turner Syndrom bei zwei Schwestern. *Z Kinderheilkd* **84:**197, 1961.)

Except for Turner's syndrome, the chromosomal deletion syndromes associated with growth deficiency are characterized by moderate to severe mental deficiency, changes in muscle tone, seizures, and in one case, hearing and visual problems. Some are incompatible with long life but, in general, are not as life-threatening as the chromosomal excess syndromes. Congenital hypoplasia (low-birth-weight) is characteristic of most of the syndromes; slow postnatal growth is seen in the remainder. Each is recognizable from characteristic patterns of malformations and can be identified by karyotype (12).

### Skeletal Dysplasias

The skeletal dysplasias are a group of disorders in which there is a primary or intrinsic disturbance of bone formation. Any disorder which primarily affects the skeleton will also affect growth of the infant or child. The dysplasias affect size and shape of limbs, trunk or skull, frequently resulting in disproportionate growth (22). A primary disorder of the trunk, as in spondyloepiphyseal dysplasia, produces a short individual with normal limbs but short trunk. An individual with achondroplasia, on the other hand, has normal trunk length, but is short because of dysplasia of the limbs.

Names assigned to skeletal dysplasias often describe the part of the skeleton affected. A dysplasia with primary involvement of the epiphyses of long bones is called an *epiphyseal* dysplasia; primary involvement of the metaphysis, a *metaphyseal* dysplasia, and of the diaphysis, a *diaphyseal* dysplasia. Involvement of the spine is described by the prefix *"spondylo"* as in spondyloephiphyseal or spondylometaphyseal dysplasias. Proximal shortening of the limb, as in achondroplasia, is termed *rhizomelic* shortening, middle segment shortening as in ulnofibular dysplasia, *mesomelic* and distal shortening, as in acrodysostoses, *acromelic* shortening. A twisting of the limbs is termed *diastrophic* dysplasia, a changing dysplasia is termed *metatropic* and a dysplasia ending in early death, *thanatophoric* (death-seeking) (23).

Many dysplasias share radiographic features but are different histologically, have a different pathogenesis, or have characteristic clinical features. Many of them resemble each other clinically but differ in pathogenesis or radiographic features. Most of the skeletal dysplasias appear to be the product of genetic mutations and in most a specific inheritance pattern has been suggested.

With so much diversity in pathogenesis, radiographic features, and clinical presentation, it has been difficult to agree on a unifying classification of the skeletal dysplasias. An international nomenclature for constitutional diseases of the bone, proposed in 1970 with revision in 1977, divides the skeletal dysplasias into two major groups—the *osteochondrodysplasias*, that is, abnormalities of cartilage or bone growth development, and the *dysostoses* or malformation of individual bones (23). Most of the disorders in which infant growth is affected fall into the osteochondrodystrophies, which are further divided into three groups: (a) the chondrodystrophies (achondroplasia), (b) the exostoses, and (c) the abnormalities of bone density, (osteogenesis imperfecta) (24). Rimoin has recently suggested a new pathophysiologic classification of the skeletal dysplasias which emphasizes the site and mechanism of the defect, bypassing the common descriptive names in an attempt to unify those skeletal dysplasias which appear to have a common pathogenesis (25). For our purposes, the skeletal dysplasias will be considered in groups suggested by the international classification. We have made an attempt to emphasize those most likely to affect growth of the fetus or infant in this chapter and will discuss some additional dysplasias which usually present in late infancy or childhood, in a subsequent chapter.

Skeletal dysplasias should be suspected in any infant with disproportionate growth—either short trunk or short limbs. Additional dysmorphic
features characteristic of specific skeletal dysplasias may be helpful in
identifying the specific dysplasia. Clinical and radiographic features,
together with genetic patterns in the family, will be of help in the diagnosis
of skeletal dysplasias. Accurate measurement of head, trunk, and limbs is
essential.

### Chondrodystrophies

Clinical and radiographic features of the nonlethal chondrodystrophies
most likely to present in the neonatal period are displayed in Table 8-4.

*Achondroplasia,* inherited as an autosomal dominant trait, is the most
common and best known of the chondrodystrophies with a frequency of
about 25 per million births. Approximately 80% are sporadic and represent
new mutations (26). The basic defect in achondroplasia is slow or irregular
ossification of cartilage at the growth plate of endochondral bones. Infants
with achondroplasia characteristically have a large head, normal-sized
trunk, and short extremities. The limb shortness is chiefly rhizomelic,
affecting mainly humerous and femur (Figure 8-3). The fingers are short
and when extended, a wedge-shaped gap between the third and fourth
fingers gives the hand a trident shape. The child with achondroplasia
stands with a pelvic tilt, producing a noticeable lumbar lordosis. The gait
is waddling and the lower extremities are bowed. Spinal deformity may
lead to cord compression and neurologic signs. The endochondral base
of the cranium is small, but the bones of the vault, which are membranous
bone, continue to grow, resulting in a macrocranial appearance with
prominent forehead. Deficiency of endochondral growth of some facial
bones results in a "scooped-out" or saddle appearance to the nose and
hypoplasia of the maxilla, while there is overgrowth of the mandible. With
the large head is often found some degree of hydrocephalus, the cause
for which is still conjectural (27).

Diagnosis is generally made by the characteristic radiologic features
(Table 8-4). Tubular endochondral bones are short and thick with flaring
metaphyses and irregular epiphyses. Achondroplasia resembles other
short-limbed chondrodystrophies, but the large head and the characteristic
radiographic changes allow a specific diagnosis.

The final average height of adults with achondroplasia is 129 cm in the
female and 143 cm in the male (28). Sitting height is normal. All of the
shortening is in the limbs. Skeletal age is normal at birth, becomes delayed
during early childhood, but catches up at the time of the adolescent
growth spurt with early closure of epiphyses. Mentality is normal, though
some psychological adjustments must be made for the disadvantages of
dwarfism. Infants with achondroplasia are healthy and develop normally.
Although there is no treatment of the chondrodystrophy, early orthopedic
correction of deformities may improve function and appearance (28).

**Table 8-4A. Newborn Skeletal Dysplasias (Chondrodystrophies): Clinical Features**

| Dysplasia (Inheritance) | Head and Neck | Chest and Trunk | Limbs | Skull |
|---|---|---|---|---|
| Achondroplasia (AD) | Large head, bulging forehead, low nasal bridge, prominent mandible | Slight rib flaring, normal length, lordosis | Rhizomelic shortening; bowed legs, folds of skin, short, broad hands and feet | Large calvarium, short base, small foramen magnum |
| Asphyxiating thoracic dysplasia (Jeune) (AR) | | Long, narrow; prominent rosary; respiratory distress | Variable shortening; short broad hands and feet; ± polydactyly | |
| Chondroectodermal dysplasia (Ellis–van Creveld) (AR) | Midline puckering of upper lip; ± natal teeth, peg-shaped | Long narrow chest ± congenital heart disease, ASD, single atrium | Polydactyly of hands, ± of feet; acromesomelic shortening; nail dysplasia; genu valgum | |
| Diastrophic dysplasia (AR) | Acute swelling of pinnae of ears | | Short with club feet; hitch-hiker thumbs; joint contractures | |
| Cartilage–hair hypoplasia (McKusick) (AR) | Fine sparse hair and eyebrows | | Short; lax ligaments; short pudgy hands | Hair sparse and fine |
| Metatropic dysplasia (AR) | | Tail-like sacral appendage | Prominent joints | |
| Spondyloepiphyseal dysplasia congenita (Spranger–Wiedmann) (AD) | Round flat face, short neck; prominent eyes, ± cleft palate | Short barrel chest, ± pectus carinatum | Mild rhizomelic shortening; normal hands ± club feet | |

**Table 8-4B. Newborn Skeletal Dysplasias (Chondrodystrophies): Radiological Features**

| Dysplasia (Inheritance) | Ribs | Vertebrae | Pelvic Bones | Limb Bones |
|---|---|---|---|---|
| Achondroplasia (AD) | Short, cupped anteriorly | Narrowing of lumbosacral interpedicular distance | Round ilia, small sacrosciatic notches | Short, thick; oval radiolucency in proximal femur and humerus |
| Asphyxiating thoracic dysplasia (Jeune) (AR) | Very short, cupped anteriorly | | Square, short; flat acetabula; spurs at ends of acetabula | Premature ossification, capital femoral epiphyses; broad proximal metaphyses |
| Chondroectodermal dysplasia (Ellis–van Creveld) (AR) | Short ± | | Squared ilia with hook-like spurs at acetabula | Acromesomelic shortening, thick metaphyseal flaring |
| Diastrophic dysplasia (AR) | | ± Scoliosis and lumbar interpedicular narrowing | | Short with broad metaphyses; delayed epiphyseal ossification |
| Cartilage–hair hypoplasia (McKusick) (AR) | Splayed and cupped anteriorly | | | Slight bowing of femora ± expanded metaphyses |
| Metatrophic dysplasia (AR) | Short, flared cupped anteriorly | Tongue-like flattening; wide intervertebral spaces | Hypoplastic crescent-shaped ilia; low set anterior iliac spines | Short, broad club-like |
| Spondyloepiphyseal dysplasia congenita (Spranger–Wiedmann) (AD) | | Flattened; dorsal wedging (pear-shaped) | Absent ossification of pubic bones | Absent epiphyses of hips, knees; absent ossification of tarsal centers |

Reproduced by permission from Sillence DO, Rimoin DL, Lachman R: *Pediatr Clin North Am* **25**:453, August, 1978.
Abbreviations: AD = autosomal dominant, AR = autosomal recessive, NK = not known.

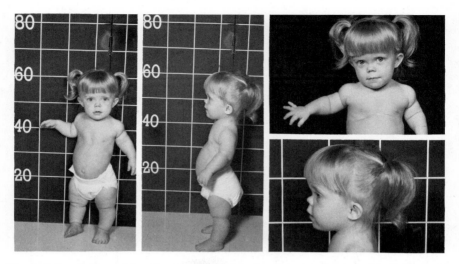

**Figure 8-3.** Infant with achondroplasia showing shortened extremities (rhizomelic shortening), skin folds over upper arms and legs, trunk of normal length with noticeable lumbar lordosis, apparent macrocranium and underdeveloped nasal bridge, and stubby hands with wedging of fingers. (Courtesy of John Carey, M.D.)

*Asphyxiating thoracic dysplasia* (Jeune syndrome) is characterized by a small thoracic cavity, respiratory distress, and respiratory insufficiency. Infants that survive the neonatal period, have frequent respiratory infections in childhood. There is variable shortening of the extremities and often polydactyly (29).

*Chondroectodermal dysplasia* (Ellis–van Creveld syndrome) is an autosomal recessive disorder found in a particularly high incidence among the Old Order Amish in Pennsylvania (30). Limbs are shortened distally (acromesomelic) and polydactyly is common. The hair, teeth (often present at birth), and the nails are dystrophic. A midline puckering of the upper lip is termed "partial cleft lip" by affected families. Congenital heart disease is present in nearly one-half of affected children.

*Diastrophic dysplasia* is identifiable at birth from the short limbs (micromelic), twisting of the hands and feet, and swelling and deformity of the ears. The diastrophic features of the dysplasia progress during life and some children never walk or stand. Laxity of ligaments and musculature frequently leads to joint subluxation and eventual joint destruction.

*Hypochondroplasia* is a chondrodystrophy with "generalized bony changes resembling those of classic achondroplasia but less marked in degree" (31). The limb shortening of hypochondroplasia is rhizo-mesomelic. The head is normal; long bones are short and thickened. Mental retardation may be present in over one-third, in contrast to achondroplasia, but the spinal cord compression problems common in achondroplasia are not seen in hypochondroplasia (32).

*Metaphyseal chondrodysplasia* (Cartilage—Hair Hypoplasia) is a rare chondrodysplasia characterized by disproportionate shortening of the lower extremities and fine, sparse, light-colored hair (33). A deficiency in cell-mediated immunity, lymphopenia and neutropenia leads to increased susceptibility to a number of infections. Sinus and pulmonary infections are common and varicella infections may be life-threatening (30).

*Metatrophic dysplasia* is characterized by "changing" body proportions with growth. At birth, the infant resembles achondroplasia, with short extremities, long trunk, and narrow thorax. With time, severe kyphoscoliosis develops with such deformity of the trunk that they resemble the short-trunk dysplasias. Neonatal death may occur from respiratory insufficiency or pulmonary aspiration.

*Spondyloepiphyseal dysplasia congenita* presents at birth with short trunk and relatively long extremities; the neck is short and it appears to rest directly on the shoulders. The chest is short and barrel-shaped and the thoracic kyphosis and lumbar lordosis are exaggerated. The eyes are prominent, usually myopic, and retinal detachment may occur.

### Lethal Chondrodystrophies Recognizable at Birth

The chondrodystrophies presented in Table 8-5 are incompatible with life, and their identification is important primarily for genetic reasons and not becaues they have any profound influence on growth. These include *achondrogenesis* in which there is almost complete lack of ossification of bones (28), the *camptomelic* or "bent extremity" syndrome (34), and *thanatophoric* dwarfism (35), which takes its name from a Greek term meaning "constantly bearing death".

### Abnormalitites of Bone Density

Of the osteochondrodysplasias affecting bone density, only two have forms which may be manifest in the neonatal period (Table 8-6).

In the severe form of *hypophosphatasia*, there is almost complete lack of mineralization of the skeleton and the baby is either born dead or dies within a few days (36). In less severe forms, infants show rachitic deformities of growth plates of long bones. Premature closure of the sutures may require surgical intervention to prevent brain damage (Figure 8-4). Alkaline phosphatase activity is low but calcium and phosphorus levels are normal. Large amounts of phosphoethanolamine are excreted in the urine. Use of steroids to prevent hypercalcemia and phosphate solution to improve mineralization have been suggested (37). More recently, enzyme replacement with intravenous infusion of alkaline phosphatase-rich plasma from patients with Paget bone disease has been reported (38). There may be improvement of the rickets with therapy, but frequent fractures and resulting deformity of the limbs may still limit growth severely.

**Table 8-5A. Newborn Skeletal Dysplasias (Lethal Chondrodystrophies) Clinical Features**

| Dysplasia (Inheritance) | Head and Neck | Chest and Trunk | Limbs | Skull |
|---|---|---|---|---|
| Achondrogenesis type I (AR) (Parenti–Fraccaro) | Round or oval face, membranous skull with multiple bone islands (type I); short neck | Short, round | Very short | Poorly mineralized, multiple bone plaques, face and skull proportinate |
| Campomelic dysplasias Long-limbed (AR) | Large calvarium, small flat face, low set ears, micrognathia | Small, narrow | Bowed femora and tibiae with dimple at maximum convexity | Enlarged, dolichocephalic; narrow shallow orbits ± Craniosynostosis |
| Short-limbed (NK) | Normocephalic or Craniosynostosis | | All short and bowed | |
| Chondrodysplasia Punctata (AR) | Flat face, depressed bridge and tip of nose ± cataracts | ± Ichthyosiform erythroderma | Proximal shortening | |
| Thanatophoric dysplasia (DL) | Large, bulging forehead; prominent eyes, depressed nasal bridge; wide fontanelles and sutures; ± clover-leaf skull | Small, narrow, pear-shaped thorax | Markedly short | Large calvaria, short base, small foramen magnum |

212

**Table 8-5B. Newborn Skeletal Dysplasias (Lethal Chondrodystrophies) Radiological Features**

| Dysplasia (Inheritance) | Ribs | Vertebrae | Pelvic Bones | Limb Bones |
|---|---|---|---|---|
| Achondrogenesis type I (AR) (Parenti–Fraccaro) | Thin, short, beaded | Absence of centers for vertebral bodies and sacrum | Short ilia, no pubic ossification | Extremely short; concave ends; multiple spurs |
| Campomelic dysplasias Long-limbed (AR) | Narrow and wavy; often 11 pairs | Hypoplastic cervical bodies, others flattened. Increased lumbar interpedicular distance | Tall, narrow; increased acetabular angles; vertical ischia, hypoplastic ischiopubic ramus | Long, slender, bowed femora and tibia |
| Short-limbed (NK) | 11 pairs | Mild flattening | Mild narrowing | Broad, angulated; widened metaphyses |
| Chondrodysplasia punctata rhizomelic (AR) | | Wide coronal clefts | Trapezoid ilia; stippling of ischiopubes | Stippled calcification in epiphyses, periarticular tissues |
| Thanatophoric dysplasia (DL) | Short, cupped and splayed anteriorly | Hypoplastic, inverted U-shaped (AP); marked flattening with notch-like central defect (lateral) | Small, short; flat spiculated acetabulae; small sacrosciatic notches | Short, bowed; metaphyseal flaring and spicule-like cupping |

Reproduced by permission from Sillence DO, Rimoin DL, Lachman R: *Pediatr Clin North Am* **25**:453, August 1978.
Abbreviations: AD = autosomal dominant, AR = autosomal recessive, NK = not known, DL = dominant lethal.

**Table 8-6A. Newborn Skeletal Dysplasias (Disorders of Bone Density) Clinical Features**

| Dysplasia (Inheritance) | Head and Neck | Chest and Trunk | Limbs | Skull |
|---|---|---|---|---|
| Hypophosphatasia (severe congenital) (AR) | Extremely soft, membranous skull, craniosynostosis | Soft collapsing thorax, respiratory distress | Short, flaccid, rachitic deformities | Decreased ossification of vault, base and face |
| Osteogenesis imperfecta Type I (AD) (blue sclerae) | Wide anterior fontanelle; distinctly blue-black sclerae | | ± Deformity due to fractures | Wormian bones |
| Type II (AR) (lethal crumpled bone) | Large, soft calvarium with multiple bone islands; narrow mid face; small mouth and chin; blue-black sclerae | Short trunk, soft chest collapsing with respiration | Short, bowed; bowing, broad horizontal thighs | Absent ossification of vault; Wormian bones; poor ossification of cranial base |
| Osteopetrosis (AR) (with precocious manifestations) | Square; frontal bossing; short upturned nose; ± optic atrophy | Short | Proportionate | |

**Table 8-6B. Newborn Skeletal Dysplasias (Disorders of Bone Density) Radiological Features**

| Dyplasia (Inheritance) | Ribs | Vertebrae | Pelvic Bones | Limb Bones |
|---|---|---|---|---|
| Hypophosphatasia (severe congenital) (AR) | Short, thin, wavy | Flattened, poorly ossified | Small; marginal ossification defects | Thin, ribbon-like; deep metaphyseal cupping; ossifcation defects in diaphyses |
| Osteogenesis Imperfecta | | | | |
| Type I (AD) (blue sclerae) | ± Fractures | | | Ostoporotic, mild type femoral bowing, ± fractures |
| Type II (AR) (lethal crumpled bone) | Continuously beaded (rosary appearance) | Flattened, irregular | Small | Short, broad crumpled long bones especially femora ± angulation |
| Osteopetrosis (AR) (with precocious manifestations) | Diffuse osteosclerosis | Diffuse osteosclerosis | Diffuse osteosclerosis | Diffuse osteosclerosis; flask-shaped ends of long bones |

Reproduced by permission from Sillence DO, Rimoin DL, Lachman R: *Pediatr Clin North Am* **25**:453, 1978.
Abbreviations: AD = autosomal dominant, AR = autosomal recessive.

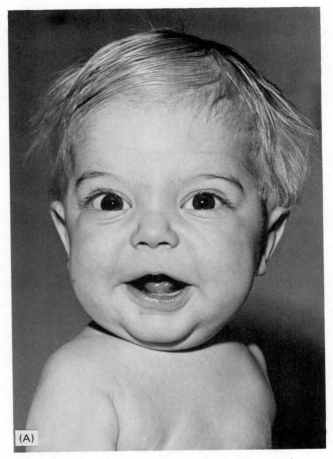

(A)

**Figure 8-4.** Infant with hypophosphatasia. In photo of face can be seen prominent eyes and frontal bossing (craniosynostosis). Metaphyseal flaring of rickets (widening of wrists and ankles) may be seen on full body view, as well as beginning dolicocephaly (craniosynostosis). (See also Figure 9–5.)

*Osteogenesis imperfecta* may also occur in a severe form in the neonatal period or in a less severe form later in childhood or adolescence. The bones are poorly mineralized, brittle, and fracture readily and repeatedly. Intrauterine fractures frequently occur and the affected infant is born with skeletal deformities due to the fractures which healed in abnormal position. Fractures also occur during birth and may lead to neonatal death. The sclerae of the eyes appear blue due to a defect in the formation of the outer white scleral covering. Many infants have ocular abnormalities including corneal opacities, keratoconus, and megalocornea. Deafness from otosclerosis is common in later life. Inconsequential trauma leads to

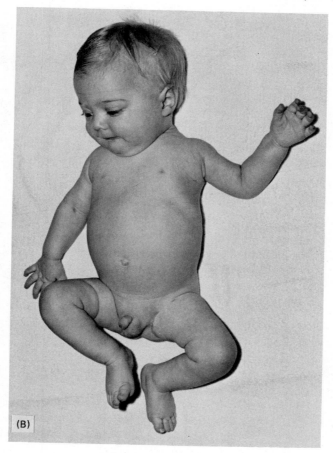

(B)

**Figure 8-4.** (Continued)

multiple fractures of the extremities. Callus formation is normal and healing is prompt, but bone formation is brittle and breaks again and again. Bizarre deformation can occur from the repeated breaking and healing cycle. Some improvement seems to occur after puberty (39).

Some *osteopetroses* can affect growth of infants but are more apt to become noticeable in childhood. *Exostoses* do not generally affect growth. *Dysostoses*, such as cleidocranial dysostosis or metaphyseal dysostosis, seldom affect growth in the neonatal period and will be introduced in the chapter on growth disorders in children.

### Inborn Errors of Metabolism

The inborn errors of metabolism most likely to affect the skeleton are the mucopolysaccharidoses, which produce a skeletal disturbance termed

**Table 8-7. Congenital Hypoplasia Syndromes With Associated Short Stature**

| Syndrome | Characteristics | Growth | Prognosis |
|---|---|---|---|
| Bloom syndrome (autos. rec. among Ukranian Jews) | Facial telangiectatic erythema, photosensitivity malar hypoplasia | Low birth weight, short stature | Feeding problems in infancy, frequent malignancies, chromosomal breakage |
| Coffin–Siris syndrome (unknown) | Hypoplastic (absent) 5th finger and toenails, coarse facies, sparse scalp hair with body hirsutism, Dandy–Walker brain malformation | Low birth weight, mild to moderate growth deficiency | Feeding problems, recurrent respiratory infections, mental deficiency |
| Cornelia de Lang syndrome (sporadic) | Bushy eyebrows, synophorys, long, curly eyelashes, low-pitched weak cry, small nose, anteverted nostrils, thin lip with midline beak, down curving mouth, micrographia, hirsutism, micromelia of hand and feet | Prenatal growth deficiency, delayed bone maturation, severe growth delay | Severe mental deficiency, sluggish and hypertonic, failure to thrive |
| De Sanctis–Cacchione syndrome (autos. rec.) | Microcephaly, photosensitivity erythroderma pigmentosa, and skin deterioration | Moderate to severe growth deficiency | Mental deficiency, spasticity, deterioration, seizures, early death |
| Dubowitz syndrome (autos. rec.) | Peculiar facies, infantile eczema, microcephaly | Low birth weight, delayed bone-age | Mild to moderate mental deficiency, hyperactivity |

| Hallermann–Streiff syndrome (autos. rec.) | Microphthalmia, congenital cataracts, small, pinched nose, hypotrichosis | Proportionate short stature | Feeding/respiratory problems, blind, normal intelligence |
|---|---|---|---|
| Johanson–Blizzard syndrome (unknown) | Microcephaly, hypoplastic alae nasae, hypothyroidism, deafness, pancreatic insuff. | Prenatal growth deficiency, hypothyroidism | Severe mental deficiency, improves with thyroxine therapy |
| Roberts syndrome (auto. rec.) | Microbrachycephaly, cleft lip, sparse hair, hypomelia, male cryptorchid | Prenatal growth deficiency, very severe growth deficiency | Severe mental deficiency, die in infancy |
| Seckel syndrome (autos. rec.) | Microcephaly, facial hypoplasia with prominent nose, low-set, malformed ears | Prenatal growth deficiency, severe growth defect | Moderate to severe mental deficiency, final height $3–3\frac{1}{2}$ feet, hyperkinetic |
| Silver–Russell syndrome (sporadic) | Asymmetry of limbs, short, curved 5th finger, triangular face with down-turned mouth | Prenatal growth defiency with short stature and delayed bone-age, short adult | Small in childhood delayed adolescence, hypoglycemia |

Adapted by permission from Smith DW: Patterns of malformation, in Vaughan VC, McKay RJ, Behrman RE (eds), *Nelson's Textbook of Pediatrics*, ed 11. Philadelphia, WB Saunders Co, 1979, pp 2035–2051.

Adapted by permission from Smith DW: *Recognizable Patterns of Human Malformations*, ed 3. Philadelphia, WB Saunders Co, 1982.

*dysostosis multiplex.* The effect of this skeletal dysplasia on growth is generally not seen until later in childhood. (See Chapter 9.) There are two *inborn errors of lipid metabolism* which closely resemble the mucopolysaccharides and affect skeletal growth in infancy:

*Gangliosidosis type 1* (Gm$_1$ or generalized Gangliosidosis) is a lysosomal disorder characterized by severe cerebral degenerative disease with onset soon after birth, coarse facial features resembling Hurler syndrome, and dysostosis multiplex radiographically. Activity of galactosidase in white blood cells and skin fibroblasts is deficient. Death usually occurs before 2 years of age.

*Mucolipidosis II* (I-cell disease) is also manifest within the first few months of life and is similar in appearance to Hurler syndrome. Coarse facial features and severe dysostosis multiplex by x-ray are usually evident at an early age. Characteristic inclusions are found in cultured skin fibroblasts and serum lysosomal enzyme levels are elevated. Death usually occurs in childhood from respiratory illness.

### Dysmorphic Syndromes

A number of dysmorphic syndromes are associated with growth deficiency. Many of them represent genetically determined hypoplasia syndromes, although the pattern of inheritance is not always evident. Postnatally, the children fail to show catch-up growth but tend to grow at an appropriate rate for their small birth size (10). A group of such disorders of "congenital hypoplasia" are listed in Table 8-7 in which, according to Smith, small stature is a particularly prominent manifestation (40).

The *Silver–Russell syndrome* with small but proportionate stature is the best known and most common of the dysmorphic syndromes. The syndrome was first described in 1953 by Silver in two children with short stature, low-birth-weight, and hemihypertrophy (41). The following year, Russell described five children with intrauterine growth retardation, characteristic facial appearance, and short arms (42). Two of Russell's subjects also had body asymmetry. Some still prefer to speak of the asymmetric (Silver) and or the nonasymmetric (Russell) variants, but since the growth patterns are identical, they will be treated as a single syndrome here.

Common features of the syndrome include short stature, triangular facies, downturned corners of the mouth, micrognathia, low-set ears, and cleft or high-arched palate (Figure 8-5). There is clinodactyly of the fifth finger, syndactyly of the second and third toes, and short arms and legs. Bone age is often retarded, but mental retardation is seen infrequently (43). Silver reported an elevation of urinary gonadotropins and early estrinization of vaginal mucosa (44), however, adolescent development usually occurs at the usual time (45). Excessive sweating, cafe-au-lait spots, and fasting hypoglycemia have been described as well. The etiology of Silver-Russell syndrome has not been decisively demonstrated. Most of

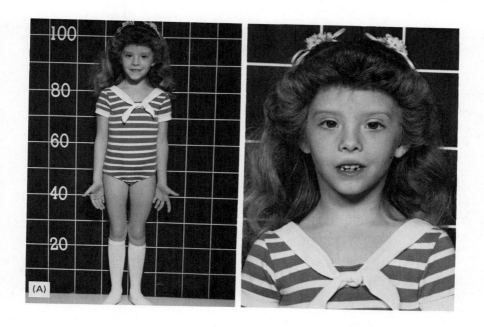

## SILVER–RUSSELL SYNDROME

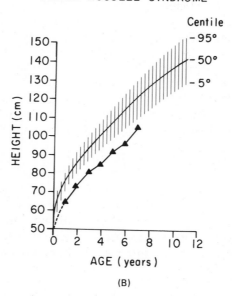

(B)

**Figure 8-5.** (A) Child with Silver–Russell syndrome (age 8) showing short stature, triangular shaped face, down-turned mouth, short arms, and clinodactyly. (B) Growth chart shows low-birth-weight and length (SGA) and near normal rate (velocity) of growth with persistent short stature through childhood.

the cases are sporadic, but Escobar et al. present a family with two half-sisters with Silver–Russell syndrome and suggest an autosomal dominant inheritance pattern (43).

Birth length and weight are usually small-for-gestational-age. The mean birth weight is between 1850–1900 g (43, 45). Growth proceeds at a normal rate but at 3–4 standard deviations below the mean. Catch-up growth is not characteristic (Figure 8-5). Bone age is delayed to about 70% of chronologic age but catches up at puberty, which occurs at about the usual time (45). Serum growth hormone levels have usually been normal, although there are occasional reports of growth hormone deficiency (46). Growth hormone fails to stimulate growth significantly in most children with Silver–Russell syndrome (47). Tanner and Ham reported a net gain of only 0.5 cm/y (48), not materially affecting the overall growth pattern (45). Predicted mature height suggests that youngsters with Silver–Russell syndrome will be short as adults.

Low birth weight (SGA) or prenatal onset of growth deficiency is characteristic of most of the infants with dysmorphic syndromes. Postnatal growth is variable, although children remain proportionately small, except in Robert's syndrome in which variable hypomelia occurs. Many of the syndromes are associated with mental deficiency, as well as characteristic malformation patterns (Table 8-7). The growth often appears related to the degree of mental deficiency (11).

In addition to the dysmorphic syndromes in which decreased, proportionate growth is one of the chief characteristics, there are a number of other syndromes in which growth deficiency of variable degree is associated, though not so conspicuously. These syndromes, together with their characteristic dysmorphic features, the effect on growth, and the prognosis are shown in Table 8-8. Details of the dysmorphic syndromes have been collected by Smith in *Recognizable Patterns of Human Malformations* (12), in which they may be identified by characteristic dysmorphic features.

### Extrinsic Growth Deficiency Disorders

Maternal size is the most important "natural" factor which influences size of the infant at birth. There are, however, other factors (maternal and fetal) which can also profoundly influence fetal growth and infant size at birth. Some of these were introduced in Chapter 2 while considering fetal growth patterns. We will now examine how some of these extrinsic factors can produce growth deficiency in a fetus with an otherwise normal growth potential.

#### Multiple Pregnancies (Crowding)

Multiple pregnancy carries with it a risk of premature labor, fetal transfusion syndrome, asphyxia neonatorum, hypoglycemia, neonatal death, cerebral palsy, small size for gestational age, long-term growth retardation, and low intelligence quotient (49). Aside from fetal transfusion syndrome,

**Table 8-8. Dysmorphic Syndromes With Associated Short Stature**

| Syndrome | Characteristics | Growth | Prognosis |
|---|---|---|---|
| Progeria | Senile-like appearance, alopecia, atrophy of subcutaneous fat | Deficient growth by 6 months, low rate of growth, severe by 1 year | Short life span, atherosclerosis, CAD by 14 years, normal intelligence |
| Cockayne syndrome | Senile-like appearance, retinal degeneration, impaired hearing, photosensitivity skin | Growth deficiency by late infancy | Mental deficiency, weakness |
| Rothmund–Thomson syndrome | Poikiloderma, skin erythema, telangiectasia, scarring, pigmented, depigmented and atrophic skin, cararacts, corneal dystrophy | Small stature, small hands and feet | Progressive skin disorder and cataracts in childhood |
| Rubenstein–Taybai syndrome | Broad thumbs and toes, down slanted palpebral fissures, hypoplastic maxilla | Short stature, delayed bone-age | Mental deficiency, respiratory infections, feeding difficulties |
| Menkes syndrome | Cerebral deterioration and seizures, twisted, fractured hair | Small at birth, short stature | Progressive CNS deterioration, death in infancy |
| Mechel–Gruber syndrome | Encephalocoele, polydactyly, polycytic kidney | Variable prenatal growth deficiency | Neonatal death |
| Prader–Willi syndrome | Hypotonia, obesity, small hands and feet | Small at birth, short in childhood | Hypotonic infant, mental deficiency, massive obesity |

**Table 8-8. (Continued)**

| Syndrome | Characteristics | Growth | Prognosis |
|---|---|---|---|
| Noonan syndrome | Turner-like syndrome with webbed neck, pectus excavatum, cryptocrchidism, pulmonary stenosis | Short stature | Mild mental retardation |
| Smith–Lemli–Opitz syndrome | Ptosis of eyelids, anteversion of nostrils, syndactyly of toes, hypospadias and cryptorchidism | Small at birth, failure to thrive | Moderate to severe mental deficiency |
| Aarskog syndrome | Hypertelorism, brachydactyly, shawl scrotum | Mild to moderate short stature, postnatal onset | Mild mental deficiency, reduced fertility |
| Robinow syndrome | Flat face, short forearm, brachydactyly, hypoplastic genitalia | Mild to moderate short stature | Normal intelligence |
| Williams syndrome | Prominent lips, hoarse voice, CHD, mild microcephaly | Mild prenatal growth deficiency, postnatal growth rate low | Fretful in infancy, behavioral problems, low IQ |
| Leprechaunism (Donahue syndrome) | Prenatal lack of adipose tissue, small face, thick lips, large ears, prominent eyes, body hirsutism, large phallus | Prenatal growth deficiency | Motor and mental retardation, severe failure to thrive, death in early infancy |

Adapted by permission from Smith DW: Patterns of malformation, in Vaughan VC, McKay RJ, Behrman RE (eds), *Nelson's Textbook of Pediatrics*, ed 11. Philadelphia, WB Saunders Co, 1979, pp 2035–2051.

Adapted by permission from Smith DW: *Recognizable Patterns of Human Malformations*, ed 3. Philadelphia, WB Saunders Co, 1982.

which can clearly affect the size of the twin receiving the smaller portion of the placental circulation, small size of the infant in multiple pregnancy seems related to crowding or uterine constraint (50). Restraint in growth within the uterus is, of course, seen in all infants as they approach term (See Chapter 2), but is quite pronounced in twinning and other multiple pregnancies. Added to this is the tendency for twins to be born prematurely; but growth is restricted even if corrected for gestational age. Fetal undergrowth in twins was noted in 24% of 262 twins reported by Manlan et al. (51) and in 60% of 17 sets of full-term twins reported by Miller and Merritt (52). The latter authors point out that in their series no other growth-retarding factors were noted in the pregnancies, suggesting that twinning alone (i.e., crowding) is responsible for the fetal growth retardation.

Postnatally, twins tend to grow a little more rapidly than normal, similar to singleton premature infants, but do not, in general, achieve complete catch-up growth (50). Twins are generally shorter and weigh less than singleton children at 5 years of age (53). Manlan et al., claim that high energy feedings in the neonatal period reversed the fetal growth retardation in 86% of 63 growth-retarded twin infants (51).

Long-term growth retardation is striking in twins dissimilar in size at birth. If one twin is at least 25% smaller than the co-twin at birth, the undersized twin remains smaller in height, weight, and head circumference throughout childhood and continues to be inferior in both growth and intelligence into adult life (54). The degree of effect on the intelligence of the smaller of twins is as yet undecided. Although some investigators report intellectual deficit in the smaller of twins, (54, 55), others report no difference (56). Capacity for catch-up growth is variable. Although, in general, catch-up growth is not complete, there have been reports of complete catch-up even in strikingly dissimilar twins (57). The reasons for the variability in catch-up growth are not known any better than the reason why twinning should have such a profound long-term effect on growth and possibly on intelligence. If it is, after all, a question of intrauterine nutrition, perhaps the suggestion of Manlan et al. to provide high energy food supplements in the immediate neonatal period may not be far from the mark (51).

## Intrauterine Growth Retardation

The term intrauterine growth retardation (IUGR) was suggested by Warkany to draw attention to a group of infants with low-birth-weight who were not born prematurely (2). Such infants were presumed to have suffered some insult in intrauterine life to prevent achievement of normal birth weight or birth length in utero. Such early growth failure had been recognized even earlier, and infants small at birth had been termed "ateliotic" (58) or "microsomic" (59). With growing interest in prematurity, all low-birth-weight infants came to be considered candididates for special observation and treatment. However, a closer look at the low-birth-weight infants showed that an appreciable number of infants with a birth weight under 2500 g were born at or near term (60). Measurements of weights and lengths at different gestational ages led to the recognition that an infant may be small or large for any gestational age (61, 62).

With the advent of ultrasound techniques, it became possible to follow the progress of an infant in utero without disrupting growth (63). Though the original concept of IUGR related to weight achievement versus gestational age, it is now feasible to detect fetal growth retardation from measurements of crown–rump length up to 12 weeks gestation (64), and biparietal head diameter (BPD) (65) or femur length (66), after the first trimester. From measurements of the BPD and abdominal perimeter (AP), it is possible to estimate fetal weight with reasonable accuracy. We can now extend the definition of intrauterine growth retardation to any infant falling below the 10th percentile for weight, length, or BPD for any gestational age, taking into consideration both size and time in uterus (65). By accepting all infants below the tenth percentile in our definition, we will include many normal small infants but will draw attention to those infants who are growing slowly within the uterus, and in such infants, we will be alerted to look for disorders which may influence postnatal health and growth.

Though "placental insufficiency" was blamed at first for the small infant size, it is now clear that obvious placental pathology accounts for only a small number of such small-for-date infants and many now prefer the more general term "fetal growth retardation" (FGR) to emphasize that whether the cause be fetal or uterine, the effect is on the fetus. In this review, the terms "intrauterine growth retardation" (IUGR) and "fetal growth retardation" (FGR) shall be used interchangeably.

We designate an infant with a birth weight less than 2500 g at birth as small (low-birth-weight), though there are cultures in which this definition would be inaccurate (67). Approximately 5–10% of live births and one-third of low-birth-weight infants are small for gestational age (68). Daikoku et al. estimate that in the United States 39,000 term infants per year weigh less than 2500 g and an additional 22,000 infants of preterm deliveries are born small for gestational-age (69).

If birth weight is accepted as the only criterion for fetal growth retardation, some infants who are short, but of normal weight will be excluded and thin babies of normal length will be included. The infant who is thin but of normal length suffers primarily from third trimester deprivation and experiences a rapid catch-up growth period in infancy, generally returning to the normal growth curve; infants short and of normal weight tend to be healthy but follow a retarded growth curve in infancy and childhood; the greatest morbidity and poorest growth achievements are seen in those infants who are both short and thin (52). Serial measurements by ultrasound have allowed recognition of two general patterns of growth in infants with IUGR. A low profile extending throughout pregnancy is seen in infants with early permanent loss of growth (cellular hypoplasia) (70, 71), while a late flattening of the growth curve (72) signals problems with the maternal-placental environment (65). Early flattening of the growth curve (before 35 weeks) carries a very high risk (94%) of IUGR (73).

### Causes of Intrauterine Growth Retardation

It is clear that fetal growth is dependent upon placental function (75) and that, in animals at least, a rather direct relationship can be shown between fetal size and placental function and size (74). Many conditions, however, such as maternal disease, drugs, or nutrition, may have an influence on placental physiology and substrate availability to the fetus while not producing obvious anatomical placental insufficiency. Fetal growth retardation may occur if there is abnormality of the placenta, of the fetus, or of the environment in which they interact (67). In the first group, the fetus has a normal growth capacity but, because of placental abnormality or insufficiency, growth of the fetus is curtailed. In the second group the fetus loses capacity for growth despite a normal uterine environment; this is seen in genetic disorders and fetal malformation syndromes. And in the last group, FGR is produced by intrauterine infections, maternal smoking or ingestion of alcohol or drugs (67). We present in the following discussion the division of factors associated with FGR as suggested by Miller and Merritt (52): (a) fetal factors, (b) medical complications of pregnancy, (c) maternal behavior or conditions during pregnancy, and (d) environmental factors (Table 8-9).

*Fetal Factors Associated with Intrauterine Growth Retardation.*    Chromosomal aberrations, skeletal dysplasias, congenital malformation syndromes, and inborn errors of metabolism which produce fetal or neonatal growth retardation have already been presented. (See Intrinsic Growth Disorders, in this chapter.) Most of these disorders represent primary growth disturbances originating within the fetus itself and are characterized by slow growth and small size for age throughout childhood. Growth patterns after infancy may also be affected by morbidity and mortality from congenital malformations.

*Maternal Medical Complications.*    Among maternal medical complications which can affect fetal growth are intrauterine infections with certain viruses and parasites, maternal diseases, especially those producing toxemia, abnormalities of uterus, placenta and cord, and some miscellaneous medical disorders (76) (Table 8-9).

*Intrauterine infections* (maternal infections) may affect fetal health and growth if the infectious agent is transferred by the placenta to the fetus and infects the fetus (75) or if the infection interferes with placental

## Table 8-9. Factors Associated with Fetal Growth Retardation

A.  Fetal Factors
 1.  Chromosomal Aberrations
 2.  Skeletal Dysplasia
 3.  Congenital Malformation Syndromes
 4.  Inborn Errors of Metabolism

B.  Maternal Medical Complications
 1.  Intrauterine Infections
  (a)  Rubella, CMV
  (b)  Toxoplasmosis, Syphilis, Varicella
 2.  Maternal Diseases
  (a)  Toxemia, Hypertension
  (b)  Severe Chronic Disease of Heart, Lung, Kidney, GI Tract, Thyroid or Adrenal Gland
 3.  Abnormalities of Uterus, Placenta or Cord
 4.  Miscellaneous Medical Disorders SLE, Anemia, Cancer, Leukemia, etc.

C.  Maternal Condition or Behavior During Pregnancy
 1.  Socioeconomic Status
  (a)  Lack of Prenatal Care
  (b)  Adverse Behavior Patterns
 2.  Maternal Nutrition
  (a)  Low Prepregnancy Weight
  (b)  Low Maternal Weight Gain
 3.  Extreme Maternal Age
  (a)  Before 17th Birthday
  (b)  After 35th Birthday
 4.  Maternal Medications and Drugs
  (a)  Cigarette Smoking
  (b)  Ethanol Ingestion
  (c)  Opiates, Hydantoin, Warfarin, Amenopterin
  (d)  Corticoids, Immunosuppressive Agents

D.  Environmental Factors
 1.  High Altitude
 2.  Exposure to High Dose or Radiation
 3.  Exposure to Toxic Substances

Derived with permission from Miller HC, Merritt TA: Abnormal factors affecting fetal growth, *Fetal Growth in Humans*. Chicago, Year Book Medical Publishers, 1979, p 26.

function. Most infections of the mother have no noticeable effect upon the fetus. Either the placenta is effective in screening out the organism or the fetus and placenta can successfully defend against the infectious agent (77). The organisms which most consistently affect fetal growth by intrauterine infection are the cytomegalovirus and rubella virus, although congenital toxoplasmosis and varicella have also been implicated (78, 79). Less commonly, malaria (Plasmodia), Chagas' disease (trypanosomiasis), and perhaps syphilis may also lead to IUGR (74). Malaria tends to cause prematurity while all the others can cause severe damage to the CNS of the fetus. It is possible that many infectious agents affect fetal growth in subtle ways undetectable by our current means of observation. Such a possibility is raised by the observation that many infants with FGR have elevated levels of IgM, which is present in prenatal infectious disease states (80).

*Cytomegalovirus* (CMV) is the most frequent of the congenital infections, although it has a low attack rate (76). Growth retardation is an uncommon event. Over 90% of babies infected with CMV in utero appear healthy and normal at birth, only 10% showing evidence of illness and intrauterine growth retardation (79). FGR occurs in babies with clinically obvious intrauterine infection suggested by hepatosplenomegaly, jaundice, hemolytic anemia, petechiae, thrombocytopenia, inguinal hernia, microcephaly, chorioretinitis, and periventricular calcification (76). Perhaps 10% of infected infants have obvious neurologic disability, 9% minimal brain dysfunction, and nearly 15% have sensory neural deafness and school failure (81).

Infection of the placenta with *rubella virus* with transmission to the fetus must occur during the first 16 weeks to produce major developmental abnormalities, including FGR. The risk of fetal damage with infection in the first month is 50%, in the second month 22%, and less than 10% thereafter (77). The rubella virus produces fetal damage by causing vascular insufficiency in organs, by damaging capillary endothelium, and by retarding cell division in the very young fetus at critical stages of organogenesis (79). About half the infants infected with rubella virus in utero develop IUGR. In the postnatal period, nearly 90% have hearing loss, 35% cataracts, and 10–40% mental retardation (82, 83). Immunity of the mother provides some protection to the fetus, although whether infection of an immune mother can still result in some fetal disease is still undetermined.

*Hypertensive disease*, with or without *toxemia*, is the most common maternal disease associated with fetal growth retardation. In a series reported by Low and Galbraith, severe preeclampsia, chronic hypertensive vascular disease, and chronic renal disease accounted for 76% of the small-for-gestational-age infants (84). Although it is not known for certain how hypertension or toxemia produce growth retardation, there is some indirect evidence that blood flow to the uterus and placenta is reduced in toxemic states. Localized infarction and fibrin deposition take place reducing the placental surface area for gas and nutrient exchange (85). In addition to toxemic states, chronic vascular hypertension, systemic lupus erythematosus with renal involvement, and nephropathies may lead to poor fetal growth (85).

Severe *maternal heart disease*, associated with cyanosis, may affect fetal growth. Oxygen saturation in the umbilical vein was reduced to 34–38% in three patients with cyanotic congenital heart disease studied by Novy et al. (86). Although there is an increase in hematocrit and a shift in the blood oxyhemoglobin dissociation curve, favoring delivery of oxygen to the fetus, it is presumed that fetal growth retardation in mothers with cyanotic heart disease is caused by inadequate delivery of oxygen to fetal tissues. Virtually all infants born to mothers with cyanotic heart disease are below the mean weight for gestational-age (85).

*Lesions of the placenta* which reduce the available surface area for exchange of nutrients have been associated with IUGR. The most common placental disorders associated with FGR are: (a) infarction and intervillous thrombosis of the placenta, (b) umbilical cord anomalies, (c) circumvallate placenta (85). Vascular anastomoses in monozygotic twin placentas has been mentioned in the section on multiple pregnancies. Chronic antepartum hemorrhage from premature separation of the placenta (*placentae previa*) is often associated with suboptimal growth, though growth seldom falls below the 10th percentile (87). *Anemia*, if profound and prolonged, may be responsible for some IUGR. Infants born to mothers with hemoglobinopathies may be small for gestational-age (88).

*Maternal Condition or Behavior during Pregnancy.*    Included here are maternal conditions or behavior which may involve an element of choice or which might be amenable to change with provision of adequate care and education.

1.   *Socioeconomic Status.*    Infants born to mothers of low socioeconomic circumstances weigh less on the average than infants from mothers living in better conditions. The cause of this relationship is difficult to identify. Offspring of mothers in poor health or poor physique have low-birth-weight and are born prematurely more often than those of mothers considered to be in good condition at the time of pregnancy (89). However, an extensive survey by Naylor et al. seeking a relationship between weight at birth and the following factors failed to identify any single factor which clearly affected weight at birth (90): (a) urban vs rural, (b) education of mother, (c) occupation of mother, (d) religion, (e) marital status, (f) housing density, (g) father present or absent, (h) education of father, (i) occupation of father, (j) family income, and (k) welfare help available.

Miller and Merritt suggest that low prepregnancy weight, low maternal weight gain during pregnancy, lack of prenatal care, cigarette smoking, and use of addicting drugs or alcohol during pregnancy have more direct relationship to fetal growth than socioeconomic status (52). Some of these factors could, of course, be influenced by socioeconomic status, however, the authors claim that mothers from low socioeconomic strata tended to choose behavior patterns which affected fetal growth adversely more often than did mothers from higher socioeconomic groups. For example, cigarette smoking was present in 60% of mothers from lower socioeconomic groups compared to only 15% in the highest group. "Significant differences were not observed in mean-birth-weights of infants born . . . to women in different socioeconomic circumstances, provided that they and their infants" . . . were free of other abnormal factors associated wtih fetal growth retardation (52).

Infants born to mothers of low socioeconomic status tend to have other natal and infancy problems more commonly as well, including prematurity, infections, lower intelligence, persistent growth deficiency, failure to thrive, and infant abuse. Whether low socioeconomic conditions are considered a primary or a secondary factor and whether one works to improve behavior patterns, to improve medical and nutritional care to poor mothers, or to change socioeconomic standards may not matter to the outcome, but it must be recognized that a large fraction of infants small-for-gestational-age will be born to mothers of low socioeconomic status and we must be prepared to identify correctible growth retarding factors.

2.  *Maternal Nutrition.*   Severe maternal malnutrition may cause a fall in birth weight but only rarely leads to an SGA infant (76). Malnutrition may play some role in fetal growth retardation seen in offspring of women of low socioeconomic status. Miller and Merritt emphasize low prepregnancy weight and low maternal weight gain as factors associated with fetal growth retardation (52). The health and nutritional status of the mother would seem to be the major determinants of these factors. Lechtig et al. demonstrated the importance of maternal nutrition by giving food supplements to pregnant women in rural Guatemala. Those who received food supplements gained weight better during pregnancy and gave birth to larger infants. A supplement of 10,000 kcal during the pregnancy resulted in an increase in birth weight of between 30–80 g (91). Maternal malnutrition must be severe and prolonged to affect the fetus perceptibly since the fetus is a very effective parasite. Nonetheless, severe acute malnutrition, such as that suffered during postwar starvation, does reduce birth weight of affected babies during the third trimester (92). Correction of starvation can lead to increases in infant weight of up to 300 g (93). Maternal malnutrition primarily affects the fetus during the last trimester, producing more reduction in weight than length (94), however; Winick claims that severe *prenatal malnutrition* can curtail cellular growth of the brain sufficient to cause irreparable damage (95). The concern for maternal nutrition and prevention of FGR should therefore extend to the prepregnancy period as well as throughout pregnancy.

3.  *Maternal Age.*   Extremely young or extremely old mothers run a greater than average risk of infants with fetal growth retardation. Miller and Merritt report a higher risk of both premature and small-for-gestational-age infants born to mothers under age 17, with the risk increasing inversely with the age of the teenage mother (52). On the other extreme, offspring of mothers over age 35 have increased risk of congenital malformations and Down's syndrome, and the risk of FGR is greater, as are, other complications of pregnancy (52).

**Table 8-10. Agents Known to Cause Intrauterine
Growth Deficiency in Humans**

| | |
|---|---|
| Cigarette smoking | Aminopterin |
| Alcohol (ethanol) | Heroin |
| Hydantoin (phenytoin) | Methadone |
| Trimethadione | Coumadin (warfarin) |

4. *Maternal Medication and Drugs.*   Many drugs or chemicals administered to a mother readily cross the placenta and affect the fetus. A spectrum of effects on the fetus may be seen, ranging from death of the developing organism to simple functional deficiencies. One can also see a variety of malformations of organs and tissues or intrauterine growth retardation. Agents known to cause intrauterine growth deficiency in humans are listed in Table 8-10.

5. *Cigarette Smoking.*   Cigarette smoking by the mother during pregnancy is the most frequently observed of the growth-retarding factors listed in Table 8-10 and is the most powerful known determinant of IUGR in the developed world (93). A mean decrease in birth-weight from 170–250 g can be expected in offspring of women who smoke during pregnancy (96), and birth length is about 1 cm less than in infants of mothers who do not smoke (97). The influence of smoking on growth seems to be greatest during the last 4 months of pregnancy. The number of cigarettes smoked daily which will clearly affect the infant's growth has not been determined unequivocally, but the effect on growth does seem to increase with increased consumption of cigarettes by the mother (98). As few as five cigarettes per day regularly throughout pregnancy has produced a significant decrease in birth weight (99). In the study of Miller and Merritt, the incidence of infants small-for-dates increased from 6.1% among nonsmoking mothers to 18.7% among infants of mothers smoking more than twenty cigarettes per day (52).

The mechanism by which intrauterine growth deficiency occurs in offspring of mothers who smoke during pregnancy is still somewhat controversial. A study by Cole et al. showed a lowering of the $pO_2$, suggesting intrauterine hypoxia as the cause of growth deficiency (100). A study by Nishimura et al. showed a strong teratogenic effect of nicotine independent of hypoxia (101). Some observors have pointed out the frequent relationship of smoking to low socioeconomic status and suggested that much of the effect on fetal size in the smoking mother may be nutritional deficiency. Cigarette smoking is found with a variety of other behavioral patterns associated with fetal growth retardation, however, cigarette smoking tends to be additive to these other factors. Miller and Merritt succeeded in isolating only cigarette smoking in their study and showed a reduction in birth weight and birth length attributable to cigarette

**Table 8-11. Incidence of Full-Term Short-for-Dates (SHFD) Infants Born to Mothers with Single and Combined Fetal Growth-Retarding Factors**

| Single Factors | Full-Term Infants | | | Combined Factors | Full-Term Infants | | |
|---|---|---|---|---|---|---|---|
| | Total No. | SHFD No. | % | | Total No. | SHFD No. | % |
| Cigarette smoking | 589 | 94 | 15.9 | | | | |
| LWG[a] | 111 | 12 | 10.8 | LWG[a] and smoking | 119 | 25 | 20.8 |
| Short maternal stature | 95 | 8 | 8.4 | Short stature and smoking | 41 | 13 | 31.7 |

Reproduced by permission from Miller HC and Merritt TA: Maternal Cigarette Smoking, in *Fetal Growth in Humans*. Chicago, Year Book Medical Publishers, Inc, 1979, pp 103–109.
[a] LWG, low weight gains (<227 g, ½ lb/week, trimesters 2 and 3). Cigarette smoking, one or more cigarettes per day throughout pregnancy. Short maternal stature (<155 cm, 61 in.). SHFD (birth length <5th percentile) See Appendix Tables A-1, A-2.

smoking alone (52). Table 8-11 from Merritt and Miller's study shows the incidence of small-for-dates full-term infants attributable to cigarette smoking alone and in combination with short mothers or mothers with low weight gain during pregnancy, both of which are common in mothers of low socioeconomic levels.

IUGR is not the only perinatal problem seen in infants of mothers who smoke. There is an increase in perinatal and neonatal mortality attributed to abruptio placentae, placenta previa, and prematurity (96). The magnitude of the mortality risk is pointed out by Stein and Susser, who claim that if 40% of pregnant women smoke cigarettes during pregnancy, a 25% increase in LBW infants could be expected leading to an excess perinatal mortality risk of 30% (93). Postnatal growth seems also to be affected by cigarette smoking (98). Follow-up has shown a small but definite decrease in size of children born to mothers who were heavy cigarette smokers (more than twenty cigarettes per day) (97). Data concerning long-term mental effects in children of mothers who smoke are less certain. Some degree of delay in reading and mathematics at age 7 has been suggested (100), but this effect is disputed by others (97).

6. *Alcohol Consumption.*    Ingestion of alcohol during pregnancy presents both potential for intrauterine growth retardation and teratogenesis (93). Heavy alcohol consumption by the pregnant mother results in increased fetal wastage or a pattern of malformations referred to as the *fetal alcohol syndrome* (102). This disorder is characterized by "severe prenatal-onset growth deficiency, developmental delay, and a variety of structural defects, including short palpebral fissures, multiple joint anomalies, and cardiac defects" (103). A reduction in birth weight and an

increased risk of FAS is seen in infants of mothers who ingest only a moderate amount of alcohol daily (104). Fisher et al. attribute FGR in the infant with fetal alcohol syndrome to selective fetal malnutrition brought about by injury to the placenta, induced by ethanol that could lead to a restriction of nutrients to the fetus (105). A rough dose–response relationship between amount of alcohol ingested and risk of abnormality in offspring has been suggested (103). Follow-up of children with FAS shows a low IQ related to severity of dysmorphic features, hyperactivity, and short attention span (76).

7. *Hydantoin Ingestion.* Ingestion of hydantoin during pregnancy is teratogenic and may give rise to a specific pattern of malformation termed the *fetal hydantoin syndrome* (106, 107). The disorder consists of prenatal growth deficiency, mental retardation, short nose with low nasal bridge, ocular hypertelorism, low set and/or abnormal ears, wide mouth with prominent lips and nail, and digital hypoplasia. In animals, a dose–response relationship has been shown but no figures are available for humans (103).

8. *Heroin and Methadone.* Offspring of heroin-addicted mothers have a high incidence of both prematurity and IUGR (108). The growth retardation of heroin addiction appears to be a direct effect on growing tissues and not a consequence of maternal and/or fetal malnutrition. Organ cell numbers are reduced in offspring of heroin-addicted mothers (103). Methadone has a similar, but less pronounced, effect on growth of infants (109). Teratogenesis is not seen with heroin or methadone. *Trimethadione, Coumadin,* and *Aminopterin* may be teratogenic and cause malformations and growth deficiency (12).

*Environmental Factors.* Infants born to mothers residing at very *high altitudes* are small, and the subsequent growth is less than that of matched controls who live at lower altitudes. Infants born and raised in villages high in the Andes of South America are smaller than their counterparts living at sea level (52). The presumed cause of IUGR is hypoxia, although red blood cell mass increases in the mother to compensate for the low $pO_2$ (73). Direct *radiation* to the pelvis may affect growth or be teratogenic. The severity of growth reduction is related to the time of exposure to radiation and the amount of radiation. Fetal wastage is the most common response to maternal uterine radiation. Some *environmental toxic substances,* such as mercury in the fisheries of Japan, have a teratogenic and growth retarding effect. Such exposures are difficult to prove in the individual and are seldom recognized unless there is widespread exposure or an epidemic of a new syndrome (110).

### Complications Associated with Intrauterine Growth Retardation
There is an increased risk in small-for-gestational-age infants of birth asphyxia, meconium aspiration syndrome, hypoglycemia, hyperglycemia,

hypocalcemia, and hypervisocosity syndrome in the immediate neonatal period (111, 65).

*Perinatal asphyxia* is the most common cause of death or neurologic sequelae in the SGA infant. The Apgar score is frequently low and the infant requires immediate resuscitation if death and serious CNS complications are to be prevented. During labor the SGA infant frequently passes meconium, which may be readily aspirated, resulting in a pneumonitis. The *meconium aspiration syndrome* may be recognized by staining of the amniotic fluid by meconium, respiratory distress shortly after birth, and coarse, patchy perihilar infiltrates on x-ray of the lungs. Immediate nasopharyngeal suction at the time of birth to remove meconium may prevent the aspiration.

The *immune system* of infants with IUGR is poorly developed. Leukocytes have decreased ability to destroy engulfed bacteria; opsonin activity is decreased; and levels of complement are low. IgM and IgA are low and cell mediated immunity is impaired. The latter deficiency is most pronounced in infants with IUGR who remain physically small throughout childhood (112).

Between 25 and 30% of infants with IUGR develop clinical *neonatal hypoglycemia*. At highest risk are those infants with fetal distress and low Apgar scores. Symptoms are nonspecific and include jitteriness, twitching, tachypnea, apnea, and convulsions. Infants who are symptomatic commonly have blood sugars less than 30 mg%. The liver glycogen stores in SGA infants are probably inadequate and rapidly depleted after birth: gluconeogenesis is sluggish, resulting in decreased capacity for new glucose production. There is increased glucose utilization because of large brain/liver ratio; increased utilization is exacerbated by neonatal disorders such as RDS, hypoxia, and thermal stress (113). Infants with IUGR should be fed as soon as they can tolerate breast or bottle. Some have even suggested i.v. glucose prophylactically in SGA infants weighing less than 2200 g (111).

Paradoxically, *hyperglycemia* or "transient neonatal diabetes" can also complicate the neonatal period of the infant with IUGR. Delayed maturation of the pancreatic islet cell produces a hyperglycemia without ketosis (114). Adequate hydration and small doses of insulin (0.25–0.5 u/kg/day) restore normoglycemia and eliminate symptoms. Complete recovery over a few weeks is usual.

*Hypocalcemia* occurs frequently in both premature and SGA infants. Secondary deficiency of magnesium is often also present. The hypocalcemia may be related to hypofunctional parathyroid tissue, or to increase in calcitonin secretion (115). Hypcalcemia may be prevented by prophylactic administration of oral calcium gluconate 500 mg/kg/24 hours (111) or continuous calcium infusion (116). If symptoms of neuromuscular irritability are present, intravenous calcium gluconate, 200 mg/kg, should be administered with continuous heart rate monitoring (111).

The hematocrit of infants with IUGR may exceed 65% increasing the likelihood of *hyperviscosity syndrome* and *necrotizing enterocolitis*. The syndrome is characterized by respiratory distress, cardiac failure and disturbed CNS function, such as jitteriness, lethargy, anorexia and convulsions. Treatment by partial exchange transfusion with fresh frozen plasma, reducing the hematocrit to 50–60% will relieve the symptoms and may prevent irreversible neurologic or gastrointestinal damage (111).

### Prognosis of Growth and Development in IUGR

The SGA infant who survives the neonatal period is at risk for poor growth, chronic medical problems, and central nervous system dysfunction (76). Although low-birth-weight infants who are appropriate for gestational age (AGA) usually catch up in length and weight sometime after infancy, SGA infants often do not, but tend to remain small throughout childhood (117–119). Infants who are in the lowest percentile for length at birth tend to show the slowest rate of catch-up growth, and poor catch-up growth is associated with greater risk of neurological or poor developmental sequelae (10). The most devastating of the outcomes are the developmental disabilities; chronic, nonprogressive disorders of CNS function resulting from damage to the developing brain. We see neurologic sequelae regularly in the rubella and fetal alcohol syndromes, less predictably in infants of toxemic mothers. The spectrum of developmental disabilities includes mental retardation, cerebral palsy, language disorders, learning disabilities, and visual and learning problems (76).

SGA infants have a higher incidence of long-term neurologic sequelae when compared to AGA infants (120). Delayed speech development is seen in about one-third (121). Others have reported neurologic handicaps to be no more frequent in SGA infants than in *premature* AGA infants. In both groups, 20–30% experience severe neurologic handicaps (122). The infant with IUGR who has delayed gross motor milestones may exhibit mild to moderate degrees of cerebral palsy. The same child may later have attention and behavioral problems and, at the time of school, be found to have a learning disability and attention deficit disorder (76). Because it is not always possible at birth to appreciate which SGA infants will do well or will have lack of catch-up growth and neurodevelopmental difficulties, all SGA infants should be carefully followed throughout infancy and childhood.

### Treatment and Prevention of IUGR

It is clearly impossible to prevent IUGR in cases where chromosomal aberrations or congenital malformation syndromes (including skeletal dysplasias) have marked the fetus from conception for growth retardation. Immunization of girls against rubella may prevent fetal infection with this virus but we have no way to prevent CMV infection or infestation with toxoplasmosis, nor do we have good ways to predict which infants will be severely affected. Exposure to toxoplasma may be reduced by avoiding cat excreta and ingestion of undercooked meat (77).

With some maternal health conditions such as hypertension, malnutrition or cigarette smoking, we can be forewarned of the high risk of IUGR. With ultrasound, biparietal head diameter, head circumference, and head/body ratios may be determined and fetal weight may be estimated. Some indication of risk for IUGR may be derived from low estriol excretion or low human placental lactogen levels, though neither is as accurate as ultrasound determinations. Responses of fetal heart rate to oxytocin or fetal movement and breathing activity, noted during ultrasound determinations, may give useful physiologic confirmation of fetal status (123). If IUGR is identified, every attempt should be made to improve the intrauterine environment. For example, stop mother's smoking, assure adequate nutrition for normal weight gain, and improve the uterine blood flow with bed rest. If the intrauterine environment cannot be changed appreciably, consideration should be given to early delivery, once there is evidence of pulmonary maturity (123).

Generally speaking, there are no manipulations of diet, drugs or hormones which are of much value in enhancing the growth of infants or children with IUGR. Currently, there is interest in the long-term effects of human growth hormone. Initial trials of hGH in children with IUGR were not very promising. No significant or sustained increase in growth rate could be demonstrated in children treated with hGH (48, 124). However, some initial acceleration of growth has been demonstrated on occasion with some sustained effect on growth over longer periods (125, 126). While it is clear that some children with IUGR respond to hGH, the growth acceleration is less than seen with hypopituitarism, and there is no reliable way to determine which children will benefit from hGH treatment (47). Availability of hGH from recombinant DNA offers the hope that controlled studies of hGH therapy in children with IUGR may become feasible soon.

## Congenital Endocrine Deficiencies and Inborn Errors of Metabolism

Though an inborn error of metabolism implies an "intrinsic" error in the developing fetus, most of the inborn errors do not affect fetal growth until after birth when the infant becomes dependent upon its own enzyme systems. The growth potential of tissues is basically normal if correction of the inborn error can be accomplished. Similarly, congenital endocrine deficiencies are operative upon an organism which, except for the "extrinsic" deficiency of hormone, is basically capable of normal growth. We have chosen to emphasize the neonatal or early infancy growth deficiency features of the congenital endocrine deficiencies and inborn errors of metabolism listed in Table 8-12.

**Table 8-12. Congenital Endocrine Deficiencies and Inborn Errors
of Metabolism Associated with Neonatal Growth Disturbances**

| | |
|---|---|
| Congenital hypothyroidism | Congenital adrenal hyperplasia |
| Congenital hypopituitarism | Glycogen storage diseases |
| Congenital absence of pancreas | Galactosemia |
| | Laron dwarfism |

## Congenital Hypothyroidism

Congenital hypothyroidism occurs in a little more than one in 4000 live births. Most of the infants (74%) have a primary thyroid dysgenesis while 13% have thyroid dyshormonogenesis with normal or enlarged thyroid glands. A smaller number 3–4% have pituitary–hypothalamic defects and the remaining 10% appear to have transient hypothyroidism (3). Most of the last three categories escape detection in infancy unless a newborn screening program provides the clue to the biochemical imbalance.

Though thyroxine seems to be essential for normal brain and skeletal development in utero, thyroid deficiency does not cause intrauterine growth retardation (127). Infants with congenital hypothyroidism are often heavier than normal at birth. Maenpaa found about one-third of infants with congenital hypothyroidism above the 90th percentile for both length and weight (128). A slightly prolonged gestational period may account for some of the increase in size at birth, but the infants are larger even when compared to infants of equal gestational-age.

*Clinical Presentation in Infancy.*    Congenital hypothyroidism is seldom evident at birth, though characteristic physiologic changes and growth failure begin in early infancy. While reporting clinical findings present by the first month of life in infants with congenital hypothyroidism, Lowrey et al. stressed the infrequency with which "classic myxedema" occurs within the first month (129). Most infants displayed a number of nonspecific findings, including feeding and respiratory difficulties, failure to gain weight, lethargy, and constipation (Table 8-13). In addition to constipation, lethargy, and frequent feeding and respiratory problems, Raiti et al. reported the occurrence of umbilical hernia, enlarged tongue, neonatal jaundice, altered cry and typical facies in from 25 to 70% of infants with hypothyroidism within the first 3 months (130). Smith et al. observed respiratory distress, poor feeding and lethargy in infants in the newborn nursery later diagnosed as having congenital hypothyroidism, but drew attention also to large posterior fontanelle, hypothermia, peripheral cyanosis, lag in stooling, abdominal distension and vomiting, prolonged icterus and edema of eyelids, labia, and feet (131) (Table 8-13).

Infants identified by neonatal measurement of serum thyroxine and/ or TSH have been reported retrospectively to exhibit a variety of signs or

**Table 8-13. Congenital Hypothyroidism Signs and Symptoms in the Newborn Period 0–1 Month**

| Signs/Symptoms | Lowrey et al. (%) | Smith et al. (fraction) | LaFranchi (%) | Illig (fraction) |
|---|---|---|---|---|
| | | *Frequency Noted* | | |
| Feeding difficulties | 62 | 6/15 | 24 | 8/14 |
| Respiratory difficulties | 58 | 5/15 | | |
| Lethargy | 37 | 4/15 | 32 | 5/14 |
| Constipation | 34 | 5/15 | 40 | <20% |
| Failure to gain weight | 45 | | | |
| Prolonged icterus | | 11/15 | 28 | 11/14 |
| Large post. fontanelle | | 5/15 | 12 | 7/14 |
| Mottled skin (cyanosis) | | 5/15 | 24 | <20% |
| Abdomen distention | | 7/15 | 20 | |
| Hypothermia | | 5/14 | 8 | |
| Umbilical hernia | | | 28 | <20% |
| Hypotonia | | | 36 | 3/14 |
| Edema | | 8/15 | | |
| Prolonged gestation | | 7/15 | | |
| Large tongue | | | 20 | <20% |
| Hoarse cry | | | 20 | <20% |
| Dry skin | | | 20 | <20% |

symptoms of hypothyroidism within the first few weeks of life. LaFranchi reports constipation, lethargy, prolonged jaundice, and poor feeding to be the most common symptoms occurring early (132). Most common signs included hypotonia, umbilical hernia, skin mottling, large anterior fontanelle, macroglossia, hoarse cry, distended abdomen, dry skin, and jaundice (132) (Table 8-13). Illig reports similar observations in the nursery in fourteen infants discovered by neonatal TSH elevation to have congenital hypothyroidism. The most common findings were prolonged jaundice, feeding problems, large posterior fontanelle, decreased activity, and muscular hypotonia. Enlarged tongue, hoarse cry, dry cool skin, constipation, and umbilical hernia were noted less frequently (133) (Table 8-13).

Reports are generally in agreement that a minority of infants with congenital hypothyroidism will present with classic myxedema; that is, puffy face, flattened nasal bridge, large protruding tongue, hoarse cry, protruberant abdomen with umbilical hernia, cold, mottled skin with jaundice, and delayed reflex relaxation (Figure 8-6). However, subtle physiologic changes may be recognized even within the first few days of life. The large open posterior fontanelle and "scooped-out" appearance

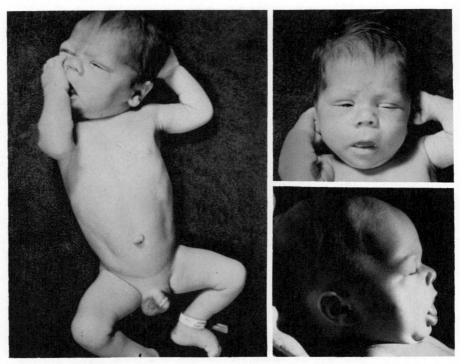

**Figure 8-6.** Infant with congenital hypothyroidism showing dull facial expression (lethargy) with puffiness of eyes and face, open mouth with protruding, enlarged tongue, short extremities, and umbilical hernia; features commonly seen in a hypothyroid infant in first few months of life.

of the nasal bridge have been emphasized (134), as has the prenatal lag in skeletal maturation with epiphyseal dysgenesis (131). Smith claims that careful examination of the infant in the newborn nursery may allow identification of some physiologic aberrations in essentially all infants with congenital hypothyroidism (131).

Growth deficiency in the untreated infant with hypothyroidism is characterized by failure to gain weight, slow growth of limbs (there is retention of infantile body proportions), and delayed skeletal maturation (127). Ordinarily, by birth, epiphyseal centers of the distal femur and proximal tibia, as well as the cuboid of the foot, are present. In congenital hypothyroidism these centers are characteristically missing and if present, are ragged with scattered foci of calcification (epiphyseal dysgenesis). Evidence suggesting that neurologic deficits and mental deficiency are less common in infants receiving adequate thyroxine therapy before 3 months of age (130) has prompted a continued interest in recognition of hypothyroidism in the earliest neonatal period.

*Newborn Screening: Diagnosis of Congenital Hypothyroidism.*    The availability of screening programs for detection of congenital hypothyroidism has reduced the anxiety, if not also the necessity, of clinical identification of congenital hypothyroidism in the neonatal period (135). Measurement of thyroxine ($T_4$) on a filter paper spot of blood collected within 3–5 days after birth is the most common screening test for hypothyroidism currently being used. Thyrotropin (TSH) is measured from the same blood spot if $T_4$ is found to be low. A diagnosis of congenital hypothyroidism is made if low $T_4$ and high TSH are found from the filter paper blood determinations and confirmed by recall testing. All infants with congenital thyroid aplasia or hypoplasia, and most of those with inadequately functioning ectopic tissue, will be detected by this means. A thyroid scintiscan with $Tc^{99m}$ or $I^{123}$ may be necessary to identify those with ectopic tissue or hypoplastic thyroids, but this may be deferred until after the neonatal period to a time when there is less danger of brain damage from prolonged absence of thyroid.

Infants with goiter at birth may not all have a low $T_4$. Sometimes the thyroid dyshormonogenesis is partial in infancy. TSH will usually be elevated, however, and thyroidal uptake of $I^{123}$ will be high. Special tests will be necessary to discover the specific cause of goitrous hypothyroidism. Infants with low $T_4$ but normal TSH pose a problem in diagnosis. Some of these represent benign deficiency of thyroxine-binding globulin (TBG). A blood spot TBG determination has been suggested to discover this normal variant (136), however, it seems unlikely that such a measurement will become routinely available. Either TBG measurement or $T_4/T_3U$ ratios may be used to detect benign deficiency of TBG.

Premature infants, especially those with respiratory distress syndrome and sick infants under stress in the newborn intensive care unit, display low $T_4$ and $T_3$ levels with normal TSH. This seems to be a transient decrease in iodothyronines with complete spontaneous recovery occurring in 2–4 weeks, but sometimes taking as long as 20 weeks. The significance of the low $T_4$ and $T_3$ is not yet known, but there may be some actual physiologic advantage to low $T_3$ values in a sick premature infant; the intellectual development of sick premature infants who survive appears to be excellent (137).

A small number of infants (1 in 60,000) will have pituitary-hypothalamic deficits with mild hypothyroidism. Occasionally deficits in other pituitary function may result in neonatal hypoglycemia and demand immediate attention, but for the most part, extensive testing of pituitary function may be safely deferred until after the neonatal period, at which time TRH stimulation of TSH may identify a TSH deficiency.

Transient neonatal hypothyroidism is being recognized with increasing frequency from screening tests for hypothyroidism. When a history of maternal ingestion of an antithyroid substance such as PTU or iodide can be elicited, the diagnosis can be made with some assurance and the baby watched without therapy. However, if no known predisposing cause can be identified, infants with low $T_4$ and high TSH must be treated as others with congenital hypothyroidism. Unless the thyroid gland is palpated or identified by scan, the potentially normal function may never be discovered.

*Treatment of Congenital Hypothyroidism.*    The *treatment* of choice for congenital hypothyroidism is L-thyroxine given orally once daily. The average starting dose is 8–10 μg/kg/day, reducing gradually by 6 months to 7–8 μg/kg/day. Adequacy of therapy is monitored by $T_4$ and TSH measurements and the clinical status of the infant. During infancy, TSH may remain at levels up to 20 μU/mL during physiologic replacement of thyroxine. Thereafter, with adequate therapy TSH should suppress to levels under 10 μU/mL. $T_4$ levels are normally higher in infancy than in later childhood and levels of 8–16 μg/dL are not uncommon in a well-treated infant.

The amount of medication is changed as often as needed during the first 2 years of life to assure optimal thyroxine therapy. The goals of therapy should be normal velocity of growth and skeletal maturation, freedom from physiologic stigmata of hypothyroidism, normal neurologic and mental development, and suppression of TSH to normal (138). TSH probably represents the most sensitive biochemical indicator of adequate physiologic replacement of thyroxine. The average dose of thyroxine required from 6 months to 2 years of life is 5–7 μg/kg/day. After 2 years, the average need for thyroxine drops to about 4–5 μg/kg/day, and after 3 years, 3–4 μg/kg/day should suffice. Too vigorous therapy will result in hyperactivity, restlessness, high resting pulse, sweating, poor sleep habits, and poor weight gain. Persistent overtreatment may result in premature craniosynostosis and delayed neurologic development (139). Inadequate therapy may be recognized by continued lethargy, hypotonia, constipation, dry skin and hair, slow development, suboptimal growth with retention of infantile body proportions, and delayed skeletal maturation.

*Response to Therapy: Prognosis.*    With optimal thyroxine therapy, full recovery of physiologic aberrations of hypothyroidism can be expected. There should be clearing of jaundice, improvement in constipation, replacement of lethargy and hypoactivity with normal activity and alertness, restoration of normal skin and hair texture (there may be temporary loss of coarse hair with eventual replacement with hair of normal texture), loss of hoarse voice, and reduction in size of tongue. Growth rate (both length and weight) should be normal and there may be catch-up growth in limb length with restoration of body proportions to normal. Skeletal maturation should progress at a normal rate and may be used to monitor long-range adequacy of therapy (138).

It is clear from the reported observations of intellectual achievement in hypothyroid infants that those treated before 3 months of age have significantly higher average intelligence quotients (130, 140, 141). It is equally clear that neurologic damage incurred in utero or in early infancy from thyroid deficiency is essentially irreversible and does not improve materially even with optimal thyroxine therapy thereafter. Neurologic sequelae such as tremor, spasticity, and hyperactive reflexes may be seen as products of thyroid deficiency and appear more commonly with more severe mental impairment (132). It is known that thyroxine crosses the human placenta very slowly. It follows then, that the infant with thyroid aplasia is essentially without thyroid hormone throughout intrauterine life. Infants with identifiable hypoplasia or ectopic functioning rests of thyroid tissue fare better intellectually than do those with total aplasia, but there still remains a great deal of variability in intellectual impairment among those with no identifiable thyroid tissue at birth, beginning treatment at the same time postnatally. One may speculate that those who do better may have had some thyroid tissue in utero for a time and were robbed of that tissue by atrophy later in utero, but we have no proof of this. Breast-fed infants may receive enough thyroxine through breast milk to attenuate some of the problems of congenital hypothyroidism (142). Human breast milk has been reported to contain widely varying amounts of thyroxine and tri-iodothyronine and, though suboptimal, enough apparently in some instances to prevent some of the otherwise progressive brain damage and mental deficiency. Growth has been restored nearly to normal though skeletal maturation remains grossly delayed (142).

It is clear that early diagnosis and early treatment with optimal amounts of thyroxine is the most sound means available at the moment to assure normal growth and prevent progressive mental impairment in congenital hypothyroidism (143). Screening identification in the newborn period plus alert, appropriate action by primary care physicians may result in substantial reduction in morbidity of hypothyroidism and help answer our questions about how vulnerable the infant is to thyroid deficiency in utero.

## Congenital Hypopituitarism

Congenital hypopituitarism is a rare neonatal problem, due either to a hypothalamic defect or to pituitary apalasia or hypoplasia. Congenital absence of the pituitary gland is found in infants with anomalies of the anterior part of the head such as trigonocephaly or septo-optic dysplasia (144). Absence of pituitary or hypothalamic trophic hormones does not generally affect intrauterine growth appreciably and the infant's length and weight are nearly normal at birth (145). However, microphallus is commonly seen in the male newborn, suggesting a need for pituitary gonadotropins in regulating the development (though not sex determination) of the male genitalia of the fetus. Absence of ACTH and possibly hGH may also lead to profound hypoglycemia in the neonatal period.

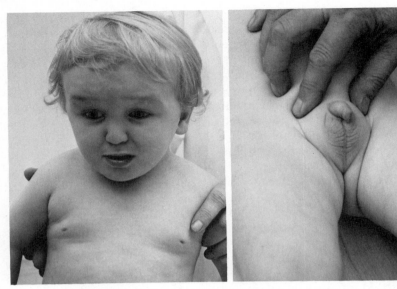

**Figure 8-7.** Infant with congenital hypopituitarism and micropenis. Choanal atresia and cleft palate present at birth with hypoglycemia, seizures, and hypothyroidism presenting in neonatal period. Short stature (<5th percentile) and micropenis being treated with hGH and testosterone.

The combination of neonatal hypoglycemia and microphallus in a male infant is recognized as a common presentation of congenital hypopituitarism (146). Optic hypoplasia in infancy may provide the clue to other anterior brain anomalies including absence or hypoplasia of the pituitary (Figure 8-7).

Though there is no intrauterine growth retardation in infants with congenital hypopituitarism, postnatal growth becomes increasingly dependent upon thyroid and growth hormone and failure to provide replacement therapy will result in progressive lack of growth with characteristics of both growth hormone and thyroid deficiency. Neonatal hypoglycemia may demand immediate attention and may not be controlled until cortisol, thyroid, and human growth hormone replacement are provided. The microphallus usually responds well to 25 mg of injectable testosterone enanthate monthly for 3–4 months (147).

### Congenital Absence of Pancreas
Insulin is a primary anabolic hormone during fetal life. Congenital absence of the pancreas leads to severe intrauterine growth retardation. The placenta is relatively impermeable to insulin and therefore, the infant is dependent for insulin in utero on its own pancreatic islet cells. Lack of insulin in utero results in decreased production of both DNA and protein,

suggesting that insulin may have a primary role in regulating normal growth of the fetus (148).

## Congenital Adrenal Hyperplasia

(Inborn Error of Cortisol/Aldosterone Synthesis) A number of enzyme defects occur in the adrenal gland, leading to inborn errors of cortisol synthesis which result in underproduction of cortisol and/or aldosterone and overproduction of androgens. The lack of cortisol results in negative feedback stimulation of ACTH, which at high levels stimulates adrenal hyperplasia and overproduction of adrenal androgens unaffected by the enzyme block. Although there is minimal effect on fetal growth from cortisol synthesis defects, the excess adrenal androgens do affect fetal development of the external genitalia, producing virilization of the female. At birth, the female infant has ambiguous genitalia, which with appropriate tests of genetic sex pattern, x-ray or ultrasound identification of internal genital structures, and biochemical evidence of adrenal enzyme deficiency (17-OH-progesterone elevation), can be shown to be those of a virilized, but normal, female.

If the enzyme deficiency results in complete block in synthesis of cortisol and aldosterone, the infant suffers from acute adrenal insufficiency within the neonatal period. Such infants fail to thrive, becoming rapidly lethargic and emaciated; vomiting and anorexia contribute to weight loss and dehydration. Severe, rapid dehydration leads to hypovolemia, vascular collapse and death. Recognition of the syndrome in the neonatal period is essential to prevent progression to dehydration, shock and death. In the female, the ambiguous genitalia should provide the clue, but in a male infant the effects on the external genitalia may be minimal or not noticeable. Recognition depends on knowing that adrenal insufficiency can be a cause of failure to thrive and rapid dehydration in infancy. Excess androgen from the adrenal may accelerate somatic and skeletal growth and produce virilization of children. These effects of the adrenal on growth and sexual development will be discussed in more detail in Chapter 10.

## Glycogen Storage Disease

Enzyme defects in glycogen metabolism can lead to defects in availability of glucose. In many of these inborn errors of metabolism, glycogen storage and release is faulty, giving rise to a spectrum of syndromes variously affecting growth in the infant and child. Only two of the twelve currently identified glycogen storage diseases produce noticeable growth defects, though two others produce a failure to thrive, often ending in death in infancy.

Type I, glucose-6-phosphatase deficiency, the first described and the most common of the glycogen storage diseases, is characterized by stunted growth, enlarged liver and kidneys, "doll face" (chubby cheeks), tendency to hypoglycemia and lactic acidosis, which may contribute to slow growth, hyperlipidemia, hyperuricacidemia, gout, and bleeding. The metabolic problems tend to become less severe as patients grow older.

Type XI has no known enzyme defect, but there is liver storage of glycogen and extreme stunted growth. Growth hormone levels are normal but growth is reduced to the level of subjects with pituitary deficiency. There is a tendency to acidosis, hyperlipidemia, generalized aminoacidemia, galactosuria, glucosuria, and phosphaturia. Affected children develop florid rickets in early life unless treated with Vitamin D and phosphate supplements. Correcting the rickets has minimal effect on the growth.

Type II, lysosomal acid-alpha-glucosidase deficiency, is characterized by abnormal glycogen in liver, muscle, and heart leading eventually to cardiac failure, failure to thrive, and death in infancy.

Type IV, amylo-1, 4-1, 6 transglucosidase deficiency (brancher enzyme deficiency) is characterized by early hepatosplenomegaly, cirrhosis, ascites, and liver failure with failure to thrive and death in early childhood (149, 150).

### Galactosemia

Galactosemia is an inborn error of galactose metabolism caused by deficiency of galactose-1-phosphate uridyl transferase. In early infancy, children with galactosemia have feeding difficulties and poor weight gain associated with jaundice, hepatomegaly, vomiting, lethargy, irritability, convulsions, cataracts, ascites (liver cirrhosis), and mental retardation. Damage to the liver and brain is progessive and may become rapidly irreversible.

Diagnosis is suggested by reducing substance (galactose) in the urine of an infant which does not react to glucose oxidase. The enzymatic defect may be demonstrated in the erythrocytes, forming the basis for a newborn spot blood screening test. Galactose must be excluded from the diet early in infancy to avoid severe cirrhosis, poor growth, cataracts, and mental retardation. With good dietary control, the prognosis is generally good. Deficiency of galactokinase may also produce galactosemia, but cataracts are the only noticeable defect and growth is not affected (151).

### Laron Syndrome

Children with Laron syndrome resemble those with hypopituitarism (see Chapter 9), but have normal levels of human growth hormone and are unresponsive to human growth hormone administration. Low somatomedin activity has been demonstrated in children with Laron growth deficiency (152). It is speculated that children with Laron syndrome lack human growth hormone receptors and fail to produce somatomedin in response to human growth hormone. Most infants with Laron syndrome have been small at birth, suggesting that the deficiency of somatomedin in utero is more critical than human growth hormone deficiency and suggesting a role for somatomedin in regulation of fetal growth, apart from its response to human growth hormone. At the moment, there is no effective therapy of Laron syndrome. Treatment will have to await availability of somatomedin for administration to humans.

## GROWTH EXCESS DISORDERS OF INFANCY

Compared to factors which cause growth deficiency in infancy, there are only a few which cause growth excess. The intrinsic disorders include large-for-gestational-age infants with congenital anomalies and chromosomal disorders. Extrinsic factors causing excess growth include infants of diabetic mothers, a few with nesidioblastosis, and infants with neonatal hyperthyroidism. Most LGA infants represent normal large infants or infants of mothers with diabetes or gestational diabetes (73).

### Intrinsic Excess Growth Disorders
### Large-for-Gestational-Age Infants with Congenital Anomalies
#### Beckwith–Wiedemann Syndrome

Infants with the syndrome of exomphalos, macroglossia, and gigantism (Beckwith–Wiedemann syndrome) are large for gestational-age and frequently born prematurely. Birth weights have averaged 4 kg and birth length 52.6 cm (12). The infants have large muscle mass and thick subcutaneous fat deposits. The most consistent congenital anomalies are macroglossia, omphalocele, unusual ear creases, and visceromegaly (153, 154). Pancreatic islet cell hyperplasia often leads to neonatal hypoglycemia, requiring treatment with diazoxide or hydrocortisone for several months. Apnea, cyanosis, and seizures are frequently seen soon after delivery. The large tongue may produce respiratory embarrassment and feeding difficulties and partial glossectomy may be required (155). Affected individuals who survive infancy are generally healthy, though mental deficiency has occurred in some (153, 155). Early postnatal growth may be slow, but thereafter the children tend to grow rapidly, following approximately the 90th percentile. Skeletal maturation is advanced (12). The cause of the syndrome is not known. It is usually sporadic, occurring more commonly in females and, in the 100 reported cases, there have been three sibships (12).

#### Sotos' Syndrome

Infants with "cerebral gigantism" (Sotos' syndrome) are large at birth with an average weight of 3.9 kg and an average length of 55.2 cm. Respiratory and feeding problems occur frequently in the newborn period. Thereafter, the children appear to be generally healthy. Growth is rapid throughout childhood and associated with accelerated skeletal maturation (156, 157). Because of the accelerated skeletal maturation some of the children achieve a normal adult height (Figure 8-8). Associated anomalies include large

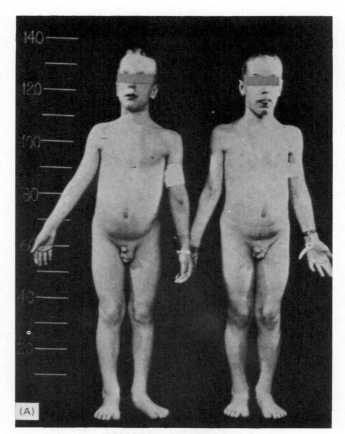

CEREBRAL GIGANTISM

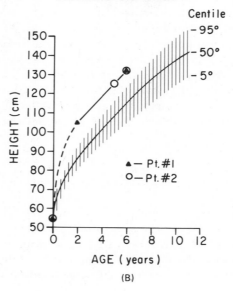

(B)

hands and feet, macro-dolichocephaly, coarse facial features and prognathism (acromegalic features) without evidence of excess human growth hormone. Most of the children have exhibited moderate to severe mental deficiency with delayed development and poor coordination (clumsiness and awkwardness) (156–158). Recently cataracts have been described (159). No specific and consistent endocrine or hypothalamic aberrations have been detected yet. Human growth hormone and insulin levels are normal. Attention was directed originally to the pituitary, however, no consistent abnormalities have been found (156–158). Hook and Reynolds suggest the possibility of increased sensitivity to human growth hormone in utero which has some appeal because of their acromegalic features (157); however, human growth hormone excess would not explain the mental deficiency nor the accelerated bone maturation.

### Weaver's Syndrome
The syndrome described by Weaver et al. in two boys is characterized by macrosomia, accelerated skeletal maturation, camptodactyly and unusual facies (wide face, flat occiput, ocular hypertelorism, large ears, and micrognathia) (160). The infants are large at birth and grow rapidly throughout infancy. The etiology is unknown.

### Marshall's Syndrome
Two infants reported by Marshall et al. displayed accelerated linear growth and skeletal maturation of prenatal onset. They were underweight for length, failed to thrive postnatally, and died in infancy of pneumonia (161). Associated defects include dolichocephaly with shallow orbits and broad middle phalanges.

## Extrinsic Excess Growth Disorders
### Infants of Diabetic Mothers
Infants of diabetic mothers (IDM) or mothers with gestational diabetes are heavier than infants of normal mothers from about 32 weeks gestation onwards. Those who survive until late pregnancy are large-for-gestational-age at birth. Much of the increase in size is attributable to increase in body fat. The infants are also longer than average at birth. The head may appear small due to the fat accumulation in the face, neck, and torso (Figure 8-9). There is no excess accumulation of fluid; the fluid loss

---

**Figure 8-8.** Twins with cerebral gigantism reported by Hook and Reynolds. Photo of twins (A) shows large size, normal body proportions, and slightly acromegalic features. Intelligence borderline—normal levels of hGH and adrenal androgens. Growth chart (B) shows identical birth length in normal range with rapid growth beginning in infancy and remaining above 97th percentile through childhood. (Reproduced by permission from Hook EB, Reynolds JW: Cerebral gigantism. *J Pediatr* **70**:900, 1967.)

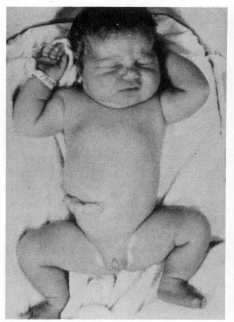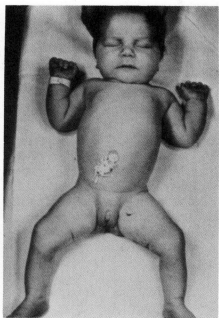

**Figure 8-9.**    Infant of diabetic mother, showing in the left-hand panel large size, exhausted, and surfeited appearance at birth. After a few days, as seen in the right-hand panel, there is loss of fullness to the face. Infants of diabetic mothers generally exhibit a neonatal lag-down growth pattern. (Reproduced by permission from Farquahr JW: The infant of the diabetic mother. *Clin Endocrinol Metab* **5:**237, 1976 (March).)

immediately after birth is generally no different in IDM than in the normal infant. The normal large, fat baby does not differ in appearance from the infant of a diabetic mother, though there may be physiologic evidence of immaturity in the neonatal period in the IDM (73).

The description of the IDM by Farquahr captures best the combination of excessive size and immaturity in the immediate newborn period: "They convey a distinct impression of having had such a surfeit of both food and fluid pressed upon them by an insistant hostess that they desire only peace so that they may recover from their excesses" (162) (Figure 8-9).

Infants of diabetic mothers often die unexpectedly late in pregnancy, sometime after the 36th week. For this reason, early delivery is often necessary. The degree of immaturity because of early delivery contributes to the severity of neonatal problems which include temperature instability, respiratory distress syndrome, irritability, apneic episodes, spontaneous thrombosis of renal and adrenal veins, jaundice, and dehydration. In general, the IDM may be expected to function appropriately for gestational age but not as a full-term baby (163). In addition to general evidence of immaturity at birth, the IDM often experiences hypoglycemia immediately after birth. A precipitous fall in blood sugar is often seen just after birth in the IDM. The hypoglycemia has been attributed to excess insulin from the baby's pancreas stimulated by maternal hyperglycemia (164). Infant hyperinsulinemia may also contribute to the macrosomia in late fetal life. Islet cells of the infant have been noted to be full of insulin. High insulin levels are present in the neonatal period (165), and insulin release in response to glucose load is more brisk and higher in IDM than in infants of normal mothers (166), however, direct proof of excess anabolic activity from hyperinsulinism has yet to be shown. Blood glucose levels in IDMs generally follow those of the mother. If mother's levels are kept under tight control just before birth, there appears to be less problem with blood sugar fluctuations in the infant during the neonatal period (4). It appears that the heavier the baby or the higher the maternal glucose level at delivery, the further the blood glucose will fall (4). Blood sugar levels stabilize after a few hours, and the IDM seems to tolerate profound and prolonged hypoglycemia surprisingly well. The danger of brain damage and the necessity for preventive treatment remain controversial (167, 168).

Hypocalcemia is also often seen in the immediate neonatal period, contributing to hyper-irritability, tremor, twitching and jitteriness. Neonatal tetany may be seen anytime within the first few days of life, generally persisting for a little more than a week. It is generally attributed to immature parathyroid function (4).

The surfeited, obese, and immature appearance of IDM at birth usually shows regression within a week or two and, in general, growth thereafter follows a normal course reflecting the genetic patterns of the parents (Figure 8-9). However, a few studies have suggested that subsequent obesity affects a high proportion of IDM and seems to be directly related to the birth weight of the infant (169, 170). Whether this is related to fat cell accumulation in late fetal life or genetic and environmental factors after birth has not been determined (4).

## Insulin Excess Disorders

In addition to infants of diabetic mothers and of gestational diabetes, excessive size at birth may also be seen in other conditions of *excess insulin production*, such as infants with *nesidioblastosis* or *islet cell hyperplasia*. These conditions must be kept in mind in considering infants with hypoglycemia and excessive size in the neonatal period.

## Fetal Hyperthyroidism

Although a very rare phenomenon, hyperthyroidism in the fetus may result in accelerated growth in length and accelerated skeletal maturation which frequently leads to premature closure of cranial sutures. Despite increased length at birth, the infants with hyperthyroidism are generally thin with limited subcutaneous fat and even decreased muscle mass. In addition to the changes in length and skeletal maturation, evidence for hyperthyroidism is generally present, including irritability, tachycardia, tachypnea, goiter, stare, and so on. Diagnosis may be confirmed by elevation of $T_4$ and/or $T_3$ RIA.

Neonatal hyperthyroidism occurs most commonly in infants of mothers hyperthyroid during pregnancy. Thyroid stimulating immunoglobulins from the mother cross the placenta to stimulate growth and overactivity of the infant's thyroid gland. Evidence of thyrotoxicosis and accelerated skeletal maturation are evident at birth. The process is self-limiting, however, resolving spontaneously as the immunoglobulins are eliminated. Treatment in the neonatal period to reduce the hypermetabolism and its effects on circulation (e.g., heart failure) may be necessary. Subsequent growth after the hyperthyroidism is controlled is at a normal rate but the acceleration of skeletal maturation is irreversible.

## REFERENCES

1. Elwood JM: The end of the drop in twinning rates? (Letter). Lancet 1(8322):470, 1983.
2. Warkany J, Monroe BB, Sutherland BS: Intrauterine growth retardation. Am J Dis Child 102:249, 1961.
3. Fisher DA, Dussault JH, Foley TP, et al.: Screening for congenital hypothyroidism: Results of screening one million North American infants. J Pediatr 94:700–705, 1979.
4. Farquhar JW: The Infant of the diabetic mother. Clin Endocrinol Metab 5:237–264, March, 1976.
5. Meredith HV: Body weight at birth of viable human infants, a worldwide comparative treatise. Hum Biol 42:217–264, 1970.
6. Robson JRK, Larkin FA, Bursick JH, et al: Growth standards for infants and children: A cross-sectional study. Pediatrics 56:1014, 1975.
7. Thomson AM, Billewiez WZ, Hytten FE: The assessment of fetal growth. J Obstet Gynecol (Br Commwlth) 75:903, 1968.
8. Holmes GF, Miller HC, Hassanein E, et al: Postnatal somatic growth in infants with atypical fetal growth patterns. Am J Dis Child 131:1078, 1977.
9. Ounsted M: Trajectories of growth. Am J Dis Child 131:1076, 1977.
10. Manser JI: Growth in the high risk infant. Clin Perinatology 11(Feb):19, 1984.
11. Smith DW: Growth deficiency dysmorphic syndromes. Postgrad Med J 54(2):147–154, 1978.
12. Smith DW: Recognizable Patterns of Human Malformations, ed 3. Philadelphia, WB Saunders Co, 1982.
13. Lacey KA, Parkin JM: The causes of short stature: A community study of children in Newcastle–upon–Tyne. Lancet 1:42, 1974.
14. Smith DW, Wilson AC: The Child with Down's Syndrome. Philadelphia, WB Saunders Co, 1973.
15. Tolksdorf M, et al: Clinical aspects of Down's syndrome from infancy to adult life. Hum Genetics 2(Suppl):3, 1981.
16. Boehncke H, Lenz W: Ullrich–Turner Syndrom bei zwei Schwestern. Zeitschr Kinderhkd 85:197, 1961.

17. Tho PT, McDonough PG: Gonadal dysgenesis. *Pediatr Ann* **3**(Dec):56–70, 1974.

18. Ullrich O: Ueber typische Kombinationsbilder multipler Abartungen. *Ztschr Kinderhkd* **49**:271, 1930.

19. Ullrich O: Turner's syndrome and status Bonnevie-Ullrich: A synthesis of animal phenogenetics and clinical observations on a typical complex of developmental anomalies. *Am J Hum Genet* **1**:179, 1949.

20. Benson PF, Cough MH, Polani PE: Lymphagiography and chromosome studies in females with lymphoedema and possible ovarian dysgenesis. *Arch Dis Child* **40**:27, 1965.

21. Matthies F, Macdiarmid WD, Rallison ML, et al: Renal anomalies in Turner's syndrome, types and suggested embryogenesis. *Clin Pediatr* **10**:561, 1971.

22. Rimoin DL: The Chondrodystrophies, in *Advances in Human Genetics*, ed 5. New York, Plenum Press, 1975, pp 10–118.

23. Rimoin DL: Skeletal dysplasias. *Clin Orthop* **114**:2–179, 1976.

24. Sillence DO, Rimoin DL, Lachman R: Neonatal dwarfism. *Pediatr Clin North Am* **25**:453, 1978.

25. Rimoin DL, Horton WA: Short stature. *J Pediatr* **92**:697, 1978.

26. Murdoch JL, Walker BA, Hall JG, et al: Achondroplasia—A genetic and statistical survey. *Ann Hum Genet* **33**:227, 1970.

27. Friedman WA, Mickle JP: Hydrocephalus in achondroplasia: A possible mechanism. *Neurosurgery* **7**:150, 1980.

28. Nehme AE, Riseborough EJ, Tredwell SJ: Skeletal growth and development of the achondroplastic dwarf. *Clin Orthop* **116**:8, 1976.

29. Okerlaid F, Danks D, Mayne V, et al: Asphyxiating thoracic dystrophy. *Arch Dis Child* **52**:758, 1977.

30. McKusick VA: Dwarfism in the Amish. *Trans Assoc Am Physicians* **78**:151–168, 1964.

31. Walker BA, Murdoch JL, McKusick VA: Hypochondroplasia. *Am J Dis Child* **122**:95, 1971.

32. Wynne-Davies R, Walsh DK, Gormley J: Achondroplasia and hypochondroplasia: Clinical variations and spinal stenosis. *J Bone Joint Surg (Br)* **63B**:508, 1981.

33. Fryne JP, et al: Cartilage–hair hypoplasia. *Acta Paediatr Belg* **33**:265, 1980.

34. Gruhn JG, Gorlin RJ, Langer LO: Dyssegmental dwarfism—A lethal anisospondylic camptomicromelic dwarfism. *Am J Dis Child* **132**:382, 1978.

35. Nissenbaum M, Chung SMK, Rosenburg HK, et al: Thanatophoric dwarfism—Two case reports and survey of the literature. *Clin Pediatr* **16**:690, 1977.

36. Wolff C, et al: Hypophosphatasia congenita letalis. *Eur J Pediatr* **138**:197, 1982.

37. Bongiovanni AM, Album MM, Root AW, et al: Studies in hypophosphatasia and response to high phosphate intake. *Am J Med Sci* **255**:163, 1968.

38. Whyte MP, Valdes R, Ryan LM, et al: Infantile hypophosphatasia: Enzyme replacement therapy by intravenous infusion of alkaline phosphatase-rich plasma from patients with Paget bone disease. *J Pediatr* **101**:379, 1982.

39. Spranger J: Osteogenesis imperfecta 1982. *Prog Clin Biol Res* **104**:223, 1982.

40. Smith DW: Patterns of Malformation, in Vaughan VC, McKay RJ, Behrman RE (eds), *Nelson's Textbook of Pediatrics*, ed 11. Philadelphia, WB Saunders Co, 1979, Chapter 29, pp 2035–2051.

41. Silver HK, Kiyasu N, George J, et al: Syndrome of congenital hemihypertrophy, shortness of stature and elevated urinary gonadatrophins. *Pediatrics* **12**:368, 1953.

42. Russell A: A syndrome of intrauterine dwarfism recognizable at birth with craniofacial dysostosis, disproportionately short arms and other abnormalities, five examples. *Proc R Soc Med* **47**:1070, 1954.

43. Escobar V, Gleiser S, Weaver DD: Phenotypic and genetic analysis of the Silver-Russell syndrome. *Clin Genet* **13**:278–288, 1978.

44. Silver HK: Asymmetry, short stature and variations in sexual development. *Am J Dis Child* **107**:495–515, 1964.

45. Tanner JM, Lejarraga H, Cameron N: The natural history of Silver-Russell syndrome: A longitudinal study of 39 cases. *Pediatr Res* **9**:611–623, 1975.

46. Nishi Y, Kawaguchi S, Nakanishi Y, et al: Silver-Russell syndrome and growth hormone deficiency. *Acta Paediatr Scand* **71**:1035, 1982.

47. Ad Hoc Committee on Growth Hormone Usage: Growth hormone in the treatment of children with short stature. *Pediatrics* **72**:891, 1983.

48. Tanner JM, Ham TJ: Low birthweight dwarfism with asymmetry, Silver's syndrome: Treatment with human growth hormone. *Arch Dis Child* **44**:231, 1969.

49. Marivate M, Norman RJ: Twins, *Clin Obstet Gynecol* **9**(Dec):723, 1982.

50. Smith DW: *Growth and Its Disorders.* Philadelphia, WB Saunders Co, 1977, p 84.

51. Manlan G, Scott KE: Contribution of twin pregnancy to perinatal mortality and fetal growth retardation: Reversal of growth retardation after birth. *Can Med Assoc J* **118**:365, 1978.

52. Miller HC, Merritt TA: *Fetal Growth in Humans.* Chicago, Year Book Medical Publishers, 1979, pp 25–30, 57–63, 103–109, 143–147.

53. Chamberlain R, Davey A: Physical growth in twins, post mature and small-for-dates children. *Arch Dis Child* **50**:437, 1975.

54. Babson SG, Phillips DS: Growth and development of twins dissimilar in size at birth. *N Engl J Med* **289**:937, 1973.

55. Kaelber CT, Pugh TF: Influence of intrauterine relations on the intelligence of twins. *N Engl J Med* **280**:1030–1034, 1969.

56. Fujikura T, Froelich LA: Mental and motor development in monozygotic twins of dissimilar birth weights. *Pediatrics* **54**:884, 1974.

57. Buckler JMH, Robinson A: Matched development of a pair of monozygotic twins of grossly different size at birth. *Arch Dis Child* **49**:472, 1974.

58. Gilford H: Ateleiosis: A form of dwarfism. *Practitioner* **70**:797, 1903.

59. Ballantyne JW: in *Manual of Antenatal Pathology and Hygiene: The Embryo.* Edinburgh, W Green & Sons, 1904.

60. Gruenwald P, Dawkins M, Hepner R: Chronic deprivation of the fetus. *Sinai Hosp J,* Baltimore, **11**:51, 1963.

61. Lubchenco LO, Hansman C, Boyd E: Intrauterine growth in weight, length and head circumference as estimated from live births at gestational ages 26 to 42 weeks. *Pediatrics* **37**:403, 1966.

62. Usher R, McLean F: Intrauterine growth of live born Caucasian infants at sea level: Standards obtained from measurements in seven dimensions of infants born between 25–44 weeks of gestation. *Pediatrics* **74**:901, 1969.

63. Sabbagha RE: Intrauterine growth retardation: Avenues of future research in diagnosis and management by ultrasound. *Semin Perinatol* **8**:31, 1984.

64. Robinson HP, Fleming JEE: A critical evaluation of sonar crown-rump length measurements. *Brit J Obstet Gynecol* **82**:702, 1975.

65. Chervenak FA, Jeanty P, Hobbins JC: Current status of fetal age and growth assessment. *Clin Obstet Gynecol* **10**:423, 1983.

66. Hadlock FP, Harris RB, Deter RL, et al: Fetal femur length as a predictor of menstrual age: sonographically measured. *Am J Radiol* **138**:649, 1982.

67. Tambyraja RL, Ratnam SS: The small fetus: Growth-retarded and preterm. *Clin Obstet Gynecol* **9**:517, 1982.

68. Anderson NG: A 5-year survey of small for dates infants for chromosomal abnormalities. *Aust Paediatr* **12:**19, 1976.

69. Daikoku NH, Johnson JW, Graf C, et al: Patterns of intrauterine growth retardation. *Obstet Gynecol* **54:**211, 1979.

70. Winick M: Cellular changes during placental and fetal growth. *Am J Obstet Gynecol* **109:**166, 1971.

71. Campbell S: The assessment of fetal development by diagnostic ultrasound. *Clin Perinatol* **1:**507, 1974.

72. Crane JP, Kopta MM, Welt SI, et al: Abnormal fetal growth patterns: Ultrasonic diagnosis and management. *Obstet Gynecol* **50:**205, 1977.

73. Tropper PJ, Fox HE: Evaluation of antepartum fetal well-being by measuring growth. *Clin Perinatol* **9:**271, 1982.

74. Battaglia FC: Intrauterine growth retardation: An invitational symposium, *J Reprod Med* **21:**283, 1978.

75. Benirschke K: General considerations on growth retardation. *Sem in Perinatol* **8:**52, 1984.

76. Allen MC: Developmental outcome and follow-up of the small for gestational age infant, *Sem in Perinatol* **8:**123, 1983.

77. Alford CA, Pass RF: Epidemiology of chronic congenital and perinatal infections in man. *Clin Perinatol* **8:**397, 1981.

78. Klein JO, Remington JS, Marcy SM: An introduction to infections of the fetus and the newborn infant, in Remington JS, Klein JO (eds), *Infectious Diseases of the Fetus and Newborn Infant.* Philadelphia, WB Saunders Co, 1976, pp 1–32.

79. Knox GE: Influence of infection on fetal growth and development. *J Reprod Med* **21:**352, 1978.

80. Yeunge CY, Hobbs JR: Serum-gamma-G globulin levels in normal premature, post-mature, and "small-for-dates" babies. *Lancet* **1:**1167, 1968.

81. Hanshaw JB, Sheiner AP, Moxley AW, et al: School failure and deafness after "silent" congenital cytomegalovirus infection. *N Engl J Med* **295:**468, 1976.

82. Cooper LZ: Congenital Rubella in the United States, in Krugman S (ed), *Infections of the Fetus and Newborn Infant.* Chicago, Year Book Medical Publishers, 1975, p 1.

83. Menser MA, Dods L, Harley JD: A twenty-five year followup of congenital rubella. *Lancet* **2:**1347, 1967.

84. Low JA, Gailbraith RS: Pregnancy characteristics of intrauterine growth retardation. *Obstet Gynecol* **44:**122, 1974.

85. Resnik R: Maternal diseases associated with abnormal fetal growth. *J Reprod Med* **21:**315, 1978.

86. Novy MJ, Peterson EN, Metcalfe J: Respiratory characteristics of maternal and fetal blood in cyanotic congenital heart disease. *Am J Obstet Gynecol* **100:**821, 1968.

87. Hibbard BM, Jeffcoate TNA: Abruptio placentae. *Obstet Gynecol* **27:**155, 1966.

88. Faikpui EZ, Moran EM: Pregnancy in the sickle hemoglobinopathies. *J Reprod Med* **11:**28, 1973.

89. Thomson AM, Billewizc WZ: Nutritional status, maternal physique, and reproductive efficiency. *Proc Nutr Soc* **22:**55, 1963.

90. Naylor AF, Myrianthopoulos NC: The relation of ethnic and selected socioeconomic factors to human birth weight. *Ann Hum Genet* **31:**71, 1967.

91. Lechtig A, Delgado H, Lasky RE, et al: Maternal nutrition and fetal growth in developing societies. *Am J Dis Child* **129:**434, 1975.

92. Smith CA: The effect of wartime starvation in Holland upon pregnancy and its outcome. *Am J Obstet Gynecol* **53:**599, 1947.

93. Stein ZA, Susser M: Intrauterine growth retardation: Epidemiological issues and public health significance. *Semin Perinatol* **8:**5, 1984.

94. Villar J, Blizan JM: The timing factor in the pathophysiology of the intrauterine growth retardation syndrome. *Obstet Gynecol Survey* **37:**499, 1982.

95. Winick M: Fetal malnutrition and growth processes. *Hosp Pract* **5**(May):33, 1970.

96. Landesman-Dwyer S, Emanuel I: Smoking during pregnancy. *Teratology* **19:**119, 1979.

97. Hardy JB, Mellitis DD: Does maternal smoking during pregnancy have a long-term effect on the child? *Lancet* **2:**1332, 1972.

98. Naye RL: Influence of maternal cigarette smoking during pregnancy on fetal childhood growth. *Obstet Gynecol* **57:**18, 1981.

99. Russell CS, Raylor R, Maddison RN: Some effects of smoking in pregnancy. *J Obstet Gynecol Br Commwlth* **73:**742, 1966.

100. Cole PV, Hawkins LH, Roberts D: Smoking during pregnancy and its effect on the fetus. *J Obstet Gynecol (Br Commwlth)* **79:**782, 1972.

101. Nishimura H, Nakai K: Developmenal anomalies in offspring of pregnant mice treated with nicotine. *Science* **127:**877, 1958.

102. Jones KL, Smith DW: Recognition of the fetal alcohol syndrome in early infancy. *Lancet* **2:**999, 1973a.

103. Jones KL, Chernoff GF: Drugs and chemicals associated with intrauterine growth deficiency. *J Reprod Med* **21:**365, 1978.

104. Kruse J: Alcohol use during pregnancy. *Am Fam Pract* **29:**199, 1984.

105. Fisher SE, Atkinson M, Burnap JK, et al: Ethanol-associated selective fetal malnutrition: A contributing factor in the fetal alcohol syndrome. *Alcoholism: Clin Exp Res* **6:**197, 1982.

106. Hanson JW, Myrianthopoulos NC, Harvey MAS, et al: Risks to the offspring of women treated with hydantoin anti-convulsants, with emphasis on the fetal hydantoin syndrome. *J Pediatr* **89:**662, 1976.

107. Hanson JW, Smith DW: The fetal hydantoin syndrome. *J Pediatr* **87:**285, 1975.

108. Stone ML, Salerno LJ, Greene M, et al.: Narcotic addiction in pregnancy. *Am J Obstet Gynecol* **109:**716, 1971.

109. Zelson C, Lee SJ, Casalino M: Neonatal narcotic addiction. *N Engl J Med* **289:**1216, 1973.

110. Nishimura H, Tanamura T: *Clinical Aspects of the Teratogenicity of Drugs.* New York, American Elsevier Publishing Co, 1976, pp 276–280.

111. Bard H: Neonatal problems of infants with intrauterine growth retardation. *J Reprod Med* **21:**359, 1978.

112. Chandra RK: Impairment of immunity in children with intrauterine growth retardation. *J Pediatr* **95:**157, 1979.

113. Hay WH: Fetal and neonatal glucose homeostasis and their relation to the small for gestational age infant. *Semin Perinatol* **8:**101, 1984.

114. Pagliara AS, Karl IE, Kipnis DM: Transient neonatal diabetes—Delayed maturation of the pancreatic beta cell. *J Pediatr* **82:**97, 1973.

115. David L, Anast CS: Calcium metabolism in newborn infants—The interrelationship of parathyroid function and calcium, magnesium and phosphorus metabolism in normal, "sick" and hypocalcemic newborns. *J Clin Invest* **54:**287, 1974.

116. Salle BL, David L, Chopard JP, et al: Prevention of early neonatal hypocalcemia in low birth weight infants with continuous calcium infusion: Effect on serum calcium, phosphorus, magnesium, and circulating immunoreactive parathyroid hormone and calcium. *Pediatr Res* **11:**1180, 1977.

117. Babson SG: Growth of low birthweight infants, *J Pediatr* **77:**11, 1970.

118. Beck GJ, Vanderberg BJ: The relationship of the rate of intrauterine growth of low birthweight infants to later growth. *J Pediatr* **86:**504, 1975.

119. Fitzhardinge PM, Steven EM: The small-for-date infant I. Later growth patterns. *Pediatrics* **49:**671, 1972.

120. Koops BL: Neurologic sequelae in infants with intrauterine growth retardation. *J Reprod Med* **21:**343, 1978.

121. Fitzhardinge PM, Steven EM, Paul MH: The small-for-date infant II. Neurological and intellectual sequelae. *Pediatrics* **50:**50, 1972.

122. Hommers M, Kendall AC: The prognosis of very low birthweight infants. *Dev Med Child Neurol* **18:**745, 1976.

123. Hobbins JC, Berkowitz RL, Grannum PAT: Diagnosis and antepartum management of intrauterine growth retardation. *J Reprod Med* **21:**319, 1978.

124. Grunt JA, Enriquez AR, Daughaday WH: Acute and long-term responses to hGH in children with idiopathic small-for-dates dwarfism. *J Clin Endocrinol Metab* **35:**157, 1972.

125. Lanes R, Plotnick LP, Lee PA; Sustained effect of human growth hormone therapy on children with intrauterine growth retardation. *Pediatrics* **63:**731–735, 1979.

126. Lenko HL, Leisti S, Perheentupa J: The efficacy of growth hormone in different types of growth failures: Analysis of 101 cases. *Eur J Pediatr* **138:**241, 1982.

127. Fisher DA: Intrauterine growth retardation: Endocrine and receptor aspects. *Semin Perinatol* **8:**37, 1984.

128. Maenpaa J: Congenital hypothyroidism—Etiological and clinical aspects. *Arch Dis Child* **47:**14, 1972.

129. Lowrey GH, Aster RH, Carr EA, et al.: Early diagnostic criteria of congenital hypothyroidism. *Am J Dis Child* **96:**131, 1958.

130. Raiti S, Newns GH: Cretinism—Early diagonsis and its relation to mental prognosis, *Arch Dis Child* **46:**692, 1971.

131. Smith DW, Klein AM, Henderson JR, et al: Congenital hypothyroidism—Signs and symptoms in the newborn period. *J Pediatr* **87:**958, 1975.

132. LaFranchi SH: Hypothyroidism. *Pediatr Clin North Am* **26:**33, 1979.

133. Illig R: Congenital hypothyroidism. *Clin Endocrinol Metab* **8:**49, 1979.

134. Lightner ES: Congenital hypothyroidism: Clues to an early clinical diagnosis. *J Fam Pract* **5:**527, 1977.

135. Levy HL, Mitchell ML: The current status of newborn screening. *Hosp Pract* **17**(Jul):89, 1982.

136. Robertson EF, Wilkins AC, Oldfield RK, et al: Blood spot thyroxine-binding globulin: A means to reduce recall rate in a screening strategy for neonatal hypothyroidism. *J Pediatr* **97:**604, 1980.

137. Klein AH, Foley B, Kenny FM, et al: Thyroid hormone and thyrotropin responses to parturition in premature infants with and without the respiratory distress syndrome. *Pediatrics* **63:**380, 1979.

138. Redmond GP: Therapy of congenital hypothyroidism in the era of mass screening. *Semin Perinatol* **6:**181, 1982.

139. Weichsel ME: Thyroid hormone replacement therapy in the perinatal period—Neurologic considerations. *J Pediatr* **92:**1035, 1978.

140. Klein AH, Meltzer S, Kenny FM: Improved prognosis in congenital hypothyroidism treated before age three months. *J Pediatr* **81:**912, 1972.

141. MacFaul R, Grant DB: Early detection of congenital hypothyroidism. *Arch Dis Child* **52:**87, 1977.

142. Bode HH, VanJonack WJ, Crawford JD: Mitigation of cretinism by breast feeding. *Pediatrics* **62:**13, 1978.

143. Hulse JA, Grant DB, Jackson D, et al: Growth development, and reassessment of hypothyroid infants diagnosed by screening. *Br Med J* **284**:1435, 1982.

144. Brewer DB: Congenital absence of the pituitary gland and its consequences. *J Pathol Bacteriol* **73**:59, 1957.

145. Gluckman PD, Grumbach MM, Kaplan SL: The neuroendocrine regulation and function of growth hormone and prolactin in the mammalian fetus. *Endocrine Rev* **2**:363, 1981.

146. Lovinger RD, Kaplan SL, Grumbach MM: Congenital hypopituitarism associated with neonatal hypoglycemia and microphallus: Four cases secondary to hypothalamic hormone deficiencies. *J Pediatr* **87**:1171–1181, 1975.

147. Lee PA, Mazur T, Danish R, et al: Micropenis: Criteria, etiologies and classification. *Johns Hopkins Med J* **146**:156, 1980.

148. Lemmons JA, Ridenour R, Orsini EN: Congenital absence of the pancreas and intrauterine growth retardation. *Pediatrics* **64**:255, 1979.

149. Hug G: Glycogen storage diseases, in Vaughan VC, McKay RJ, Behrman RE (eds), *Nelson's Textbook of Pediatrics*, ed 11. Philadelphia, WB Saunders Co, 1979, pp 531–544.

150. Green HL: Glycogen storage disease. *Semin Liver Dis* **2**:291, 1982.

151. Komrower GM: Galactosemia thirty years on: The experience of a generation. *J Inherit Metab Dis* **5**(supp 2):96, 1982.

152. Laron Z: Deficiencies of growth hormone and somatomedins in man. *Spec Top Endocrinol Metab* **5**:149, 1983.

153. Beckwith JB: Macroglossia, omphalocele, adrenal cytomegaly, gigantism and hyperplastic visceromegaly. *Birth Defects* **5**:188, 1969.

154. Filippi G, McKusick VA: The Beckwith–Wiedemann syndrome. *Medicine* **49**:279, 1970.

155. Irving I: Exomphalos with macroglossia: A study of eleven cases. *J Pediatr Surg* **2**:499, 1967.

156. Sotos JF, Dodge PR, Muirhead D, et al: Cerebral gigantism in childhood: A syndrome of excessively rapid growth with acromegalic features and a nonprogressive neurologic disorder. *N Engl J Med* **271**:109, 1964.

157. Hook EB, Reynolds JW: Cerebral gigantism: Endocrinological and clinical observations of six patients including a congenital giant, concordant monozygotic twins and a child who achieved adult gigantic size. *J Pediatr* **70**:900, 1967.

158. Abraham JM, Snodgrass GJAI: Sotos' syndrome of cerebral gigantism. *Arch Dis Child* **44**:203, 1969.

159. Yeh H, Price RL, Lonsdale D: Cerebral gigantism and cataracts. *J Pediatr Opth* **15**:231, 1978.

160. Weaver DD, Graham CB, Thomas IT, et al: A new overgrowth syndrome with accelerated skeletal maturation, unusual facies, and camptodactyly. *J Pediatr* **84**:547, 1974.

161. Marshall RE, Graham CB, Scott CR, et al: Syndrome of accelerated skeletal maturation and relative failure to thrive: A newly recognized clinical growth disorder. *J Pediatr* **78**:95, 1971.

162. Farquhar JW: The infant of the diabetic mother. *Arch Dis Child* **34**:76, 1959.

163. Priestley BL: Neurological assessment of infants of diabetic mothers in the first week of life. *Pediatrics* **50**:578, 1972.

164. Hollingsworth DR: Endocrine and metabolic homeostatis in diabetic pregnancy. *Clinic Perinatol* **10**:593, 1983.

165. Francois R, Picaud JJ, Tuitton-Ugliengo A, et al: The newborn of diabetic mothers. *Biol Neonate* **24**:1–31, 1974.

166. Baird JD, Farquhar JW: Insulin-secreting capacity in newborn infants of normal and diabetic women. *Lancet* **1**:71, 1962.

167. Haworth JC: Neonatal hypoglycemia: How much does it damage the brain? *Pediatrics* **54**:3, 1974.

168. Pildes RS, Cornblath M, Warren I, et al: A prospective controlled study of neonatal hypoglycemia. *Pediatrics* **54**:5, 1974.

169. Farquhar JW: Prognosis for babies born to diabetic mothers in Edinburgh. *Arch Dis Child* **44**:36, 1969.

170. Verdy M, Gagnon MA, Cannon D: Birth weight and adult obesity in children of diabetic mothers. *N Engl J Med* **290**:576, 1974.

# 9
# Growth Disorders in Children

Most parents recognize growth of children as an indicator of health and well-being and become concerned if they perceive alterations in the growth patterns of their children. The question of growth aberration is dealt with many times daily by every practitioner caring for the health of children, although many children seen for "growth problems" are not truly abnormal but represent variants of normal.

In this chapter, we will discuss normal variants of growth in children, as well as those disorders of growth deficiency and growth excess occurring in childhood outlined in Table 9-1. Disorders of growth with prenatal onset, in which a growth disturbance is evident by the time of birth, have been described in Chapter 8. The growth disturbances which begin in infancy and that continue to cause growth deficiency in childhood will be reviewed here briefly. Delayed and accelerated pubertal growth will be discussed in detail in Chapter 10. The division of growth disturbances into age periods was made for convenience of presentation. Acknowledging the continuous nature of growth, overlap among age periods is inevitable although we hope it will not be too disturbing or confusing.

## NORMAL VARIANTS

Most children suspected of growth aberrations are, in actuality, variants of the normal population, lying at the extremes for height and weight, being larger or smaller than average, or experiencing early or late maturing patterns. In a community study of short children in Newcastle–upon-Tyne, Lacy and Parkin found normal variants in 82% of the children whose heights were less than the 3rd percentile and in 50% of the children whose heights were more than 3 standard deviations below the mean (1). Horner and colleagues found that over 50% of children seen for short stature in a university endocrine clinic had constitutional

**Table 9-1. Growth Disorders in Children**

A. *Normal Variants*
   1. Familial short stature
   2. Constitutional delayed growth
   3. Familial tall stature
   4. Constitutional accelerated growth
B. *Disorders of Growth Deficiency*
   1. Intrinsic growth disorders
      (a) Chromosomal imbalance syndromes
      (b) Skeletal dysplasias
      (c) Mucopolysaccharidoses (storage diseases)
      (d) Congenital malformation syndromes
      (e) Intrauterine growth retardation
   2. Extrinsic growth disorders
      (a) Nutritional disorders
      (b) CNS and psychosocial disorders
      (c) Systemic disorders
      (d) Endocrine disorders
      (e) Metabolic disorders
      (f) Iatrogenic disorders
C. *Disorders of Excessive Growth in Childhood*
   1. Intrinsic disorders
      (a) Chromosomal disorders
      (b) Genetic disorders
      (c) Congenital malformation syndromes
   2. Extrinsic disorders
      (a) Endocrine disorders
      (b) Iatrogenic–endocrine disorders
      (c) Nonendocrine disorders

short stature (2), a figure very similar to that seen in our own clinic (Table 7-1).

## Familial Short Stature

Although most short parents are not surprised if their children are small, it is surprising how many want to "make sure there isn't something we can do about it" or react with dismay to the statement that the child is "off the growth chart".

Initial history should include accurate heights of both natural parents, checked, if possible at the time of examination of the child. If the height of the child is appropriate for mid-parent height (see mid-parent height "target formula" of Tanner in Chapter 6 or the Tables of Garn and Rohmann in the Appendix) and if serial measurements show him or her to be making appropriate progress and the child is generally healthy, nothing more than the history, physical exam, and adjustment for mid-parent height need be done. Estimate of the level of osseous maturation may be desirable to show tempo of growth and maturation, and to provide some reassurance about ultimate height (See Chapter 6). When both parents are small, the children will also be likely to be small, although there is a tendency to approach the mean height for the population (3).

Children with familial short stature grow proportionally for their age throughout childhood, although they remain in the lower population percentiles, and they experience pubertal growth and development at the usual time. There is no therapy which will increase eventual height of children with familial short stature. Anabolic steroids may accelerate the rate of growth and maturation but will not increase eventual stature (4) and may, if used excessively, compromise eventual stature (5).

## Constitutional Delayed Growth

A child with a slow tempo of growth is expressing variation in biologic maturation which is inherent in the growth process. The slowly maturing child will take longer to complete the growth process. Time of adolescence and final height achievement will be delayed. Because he or she is biologically slower, the child with constitutional delayed growth appears younger and smaller than children of his or her own age. Although occurring with equal frequency in boys and girls, delayed growth and maturation seems to pose more social and psychologic problems for boys and hence, more boys than girls are seen in growth clinics with this complaint. Concern about constitutionally small boys may be a function of the social setting, being more likely in suburban than urban centers (6). The need to be like peers is more pressing at the time of adolescence and delay in adolescent growth spurt and sexual development becomes a serious concern to the boy with constitutional delayed growth.

Size at birth is usually normal in such children, although shortly after birth, growth deceleration occurs. The growth shifts are similar to those described by Smith et al. for normal children seeking their genetically determined growth channels within the first year or two of postnatal growth (7), but in children with constitutional delay, the lag-down growth is more severe and more prolonged (2). Although there is considerable individual variation in timing and duration of the early lag-down growth, most children resume normal growth velocity by 3 years of age (2).

Throughout childhood, growth in children with constitutional delay proceeds at a normal rate. Though often below the 3rd percentile, the growth pattern parallels the growth curves (Figure 9-1). Osseous maturation (bone-age) is usually delayed by 2–3 years and is consistent with height achievement (bone-age is approximately equal to height age). Unusual shortness or bone-age out of proportion to height should prompt further study. A child who has both short parents and constitutional delayed growth may be quite short throughout childhood, and adjustments

hood, the child with human growth hormone deficiency may have a similar lag-down growth pattern but growth does not resume at a normal rate after age 3 but tends to continue to lag down after age 3 with continued deceleration of osseous maturation as well.

Most of the extrinsic growth disorders listed in Table 9-4 may present as slow growth and delay in osseous maturation and must be distinguished from constitutional delayed growth by typical physical or laboratory features. Children with chronic renal insufficiency, mild hypothyroidism, or hypopituitarism may be difficult to identify without further laboratory testing. Examination of the urine for specific gravity, albumin and sediment, and a serum BUN or creatinine may be necessary to exclude renal insufficiency. Serum $T_4$ and TSH will serve to distinguish mild hypothyroidism. There is no simple test to distinguish hypopituitarism from constitutional delayed growth. Frasier emphasizes a normal growth rate as being most helpful in identifying the growth pattern of constitutional delayed growth (6). If there is still question, a screening test for growth hormone may be performed. (See Chapter 7.) A positive response is usually seen in children with constitutional delayed growth, but Illig and Prader have reported some preadolescent slow maturing children whose response became normal only after priming with estrogen or testosterone (8). It is difficult to demonstrate the normal state in every instance and careful clinical judgement may be necessary to avoid unnecessary and expensive endocrine testing in every child with short stature.

Constitutional delayed growth is a physiologic variant of normal growth and requires no treatment. Given enough time, puberty, with its growth spurt, occurs naturally and height achievement is consistent with genetic expectations. However, it is acknowledged that small size and physical immaturity for age may produce a psychologic impact on a child which may deserve consideration of intervention. Boys in particular sense a marked disadvantage in being smaller, weaker, and appearing younger than their peers. This feeling of inadequacy intensifies as peers enter puberty and the subject remains in the slow-growing prepubertal state. This can lead to withdrawal, depression, acting out, or other undesirable behavior with danger of deep, lifelong psychologic wounds.

Reassurance of the normal nature of the growth pattern and a prediction of normal eventual height (see Chapter 6) may be all that is necessary in most youngsters. This can be achieved by showing the family the constant growth rate on growth charts and the ultimate height achievement expected because of the delayed bone-age. A prediction of adult height can be made from height, bone age, and chronologic age. (See Chapter 6.) The accuracy of the Bayley–Pinneau height prediction tables has been reported to be acceptably accurate if the bone age is near normal, but adult height may be overestimated in children with bone age retarded more than 2 SD below their chronologic age (9). If simple reassurance is not successful, psychological counseling may be needed to help the child to a better self-image and to help the family to cope with their feelings about small size and slow maturation.

If reassurance and counseling are insufficient to alleviate the feelings of inadequacy in the child, use of an anabolic steroid may be considered. Testosterone or its derivatives (anabolic steroids) do accelerate growth and may induce adolescence if the child's "biologic" (skeletal) maturation is close to the usual age of puberty (10). It must be borne in mind, however, that use of anabolic agents in dosages adequate to accelerate growth may also accelerate skeletal maturation (5). The response to anabolic steroids seems to depend upon both dosage and age of the subject. Children with a skeletal-age of less than 9 or 10 have a high risk of rapid skeletal maturation and consequent reduction in final height. Children with a skeletal-age of over 10 seem to have about equal acceleration of height and skeletal maturation (11, 12).

To achieve growth acceleration, an anabolic steroid such as oxandrolone or fluoxymesterone in a low to moderate dosage may be used. Oxandrolone may be given in a dosage of 0.1–0.25 mg/kg of body weight per day or fluoxymesterone 5–10 mg/day depending upon the size of the child. The effects on growth, osseous maturation, and on sexual maturation should be monitored every few months. Liver toxicity is occasionally seen with anabolic steroids and hepatic tumors with high doses. Careful observation for hepatotoxicity should be part of follow-up examinations. Frasier suggests that "therapy by discontinued if there is no catch-up growth in a 6 month period of observation, if epiphyseal maturation advances out of proportion to the change in chronologic age, or if unacceptable virilization in induced" (6). In our experience, acceleration of skeletal maturation is apt to occur with higher dosage of anabolic steroids, but lack of acceleration of growth is often seen at lower, safer dosages (5). It is difficult to get the desired effect without undesirable side effects. If both growth acceleration and advancement of puberty are desired, the effects may be obtained more surely with injections of testosterone (see Chapter 10, Management of Delayed Puberty), but neither testosterone nor human chorionic gonadotropin are appropriate to induce acceleration of growth alone (6).

Though anabolic steroids are capable of accelerating growth in children with constitutional delayed growth, ultimate height will not increase. Psychological relief in helping the child to achieve his growth potential at an accelerated rate must always be weighed against the possibility that skeletal maturation will be accelerated and ultimate adult height will be less. A recent prospective study of testosterone treatment of constitutional delay of growth and development in male adolescents (ages 14–17 years) reports a modest increase in *predicted* adult height after a brief course of testosterone enanthate (13), but a later study of boys with short stature treated with an oral androgen (stanozolol) suggests that the predicted adult height after androgen therapy may be overly optimistic and that the actual adult height achieved is statistically identical to pretreatment predicted adult height (9). Both studies seem to agree, however, that short-term therapy with androgens does not reduce adult height achievement. Testicular growth is suppressed during the treatment period with anabolic steroids, but ultimate growth and function of testes appears to be satisfactory (4). Thyroxine therapy has no salutary effect on the growth pattern of constitutional delayed growth (6). Although a brief course of testosterone (or oral androgen) appears to be an effective, safe means of promoting growth in select male adolescents (13), the best single treatment remains patience to allow natural growth at the natural time.

Currently, there is a great deal of interest in the efficacy of growth hormone (hGH) therapy in children with familial short stature and constitutional growth delay (14), but there is, as of this writing, insufficient information to determine whether such children are suitable candidates for hGH therapy. It has been suggested that some children with slow growth rates who secrete normal amounts of hGH in response to provocative stimuli may produce a biologically inactive hGH (15, 16, 17). A somatomedin response to short-term hGH administration was suggested as an indicator of probable long-term growth response to hGH therapy (16), although others have found no such correlation (18, 19). Most of the youngsters chosen for hGH therapy have had growth rates below 5 cm/yr and would not fit our usual definition of constitutional delay of growth, but their response to therapy, though irregular and unpredictable, does raise the question of subtle abnormalities of hGH secretion or action, including "partial GH deficiency" (20, 21). It is clear that hGH treatment does increase the growth rate in some short, normal children (16–19), but the only reliable test of its efficacy at the moment is a trial of hGH over several months. Treatment of "normal" children should be approached with circumspection, realizing that we do not know of the side effects of hGH when used in pharmacologic doses. Based on observations of acromegaly in adults, it is possible that high dosage therapy with hGH could produce insulin resistance and transient diabetes mellitus, accelerate atherogenesis, and produce hypertension (14). Carefully controlled studies should define the potential for the use of hGH in non-GH-deficient short children (14). Before prescribing growth hormone for children with ill-defined short stature, the pediatrician should balance the perceived need for growth and the possible psychologic benefits against the cost of the hormone, the risk of harm and the emotional burden if the treatment should fail (20).

## Familial Tall Stature

Children with *familial tall stature* are often large at birth (in length as well as weight) and grow rapidly from infancy on. Throughout childhood, these children are larger than average, following the growth curve at above the 95th percentile. There is no disproportion of growth or any specific health problem. Puberty usually occurs at at the appropriate time,

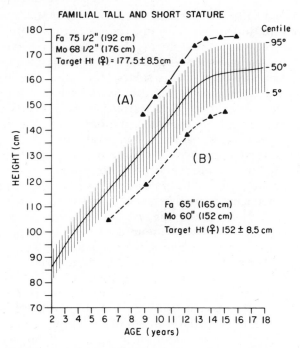

**Figure 9-2.** Growth patterns of familial tall (A) and short (B) stature. Subject A, father 192 cm (75.5 inches), mother 176 cm (68.5 inches), with target height of 177.5 ± 8.5 cm. Pubertal development began at age 12, menses at age 13½; final height, 177 cm. Subject B, father 165 cm (65 inches), mother 152 cm (60 inches), with target height of 152 ± 8.5 cm. Pubertal development began at age 11, menarche at age 13. At age 15 BA = CA, height is 148.5 cm (58½ inches), pubertal development Tanner stage 4. Predicted mature height 152 cm.

although it may be delayed or accelerated, characteristic of the family pattern. Osseous maturation is appropriate for chronologic age and ultimate or predicted mature height is appropriate for mid-parent height percentiles. (Figure 9-2).

Height is usually viewed as an advantage and most tall parents are pleased when their children are tall. A premium is placed on tall boys for some athletic games. However, in the same societies many tall girls feel awkward, undesirable, or socially excluded when their height greatly exceeds that of their peers. If social pressures seem likely to create sufficient psychological problems for the girl, intervention therapy may be considered to prevent achievement of excessive height. The decision to offer such therapy is based upon (a) the predicted mature height of the girl, (b) the current age and pubertal status of the girl, and (c) the level of concern of the family (particularly the mother) and of the girl.

We generally discourage intervention therapy in familial tall stature unless the girl's height is likely to approach or exceed 72 inches. Although for some families even this is an acceptable height; for other families, concern is voiced at much lower height predictions. The ideal age for intervention therapy in girls is before puberty or at least before menarche. Since the therapy involves acceleration of pubertal development, we have not generally encouraged therapy before age 10 (skeletal-age). Therapy after establishment of menses offers very little prospect of substantial height reduction. In our series, treatment after age 13 produced a height reduction of less than 2½ cm (1 inch) which was not statistically significant (22). Similar results are reported by others (23–25). The ultimate decision in favor of treatment must be made by the family who alone can judge the degree of concern for social and psychological handicaps which might affect the child with excessive height. Their decision should only be made with full understanding of the nature and cost of the therapy, the probable results of therapy, and the risk of undesirable side effects. Some investigators have raised doubts over whether the benefits outweigh the risks of high-dosage estrogen administration (26). We agree that limitation of excessive height in girls remains controversial, but prefer to let the family judge the need for intervention while generally counseling a conservative approach.

Many estrogen therapy regimens have been suggested to limit excessive height in a girl. Zachmann suggested ethinyl estradiol 0.3 mg/day (27) while Andersen et al. used injectable estradiol valerate, 10 mg/wk (28). We perfer to use a conjugated estrogen (Premarin) which allows a variety of dose levels, though in earlier trials we did use estradiol valerate (22). Beginning with 0.625 mg/day, we increase the daily level at 3 month intervals until we can see a clear accelerating effect on osseous maturation. This usually requires daily administration of 1.25–5.0 mg. We often see an initial growth spurt in height and weight, thereafter, height velocity slows and osseous maturation continues to accelerate. Once the maintenance dosage is established, we add a progestational agent, medroxyprogesterone, 10 mg daily for 6 days at monthly or 6-week intervals to allow menses at regular intervals and to prevent endometrial hyperplasia. Treatment is continued until no further linear growth is observed in at least two 3-month intervals and the osseous maturation approaches adult level (16 year level or more). This usually requires 18–36 months of estrogen therapy (Figure 9-3). In our experience, this regimen has achieved a height reduction of approximately 5 cm, ranging from less than 2 to more than 11 cm (22). Others report an average height reduction ranging from 2.9 to 4.6 cm (23, 27, 28).

When the medication is discontinued, a small amount of residual growth does occur, representing final vertebral growth. This amounts to approximately 1.0 cm (or ½ inch) (23). Spontaneous menses are usually established within the first 3 months after stopping the medication, although we have

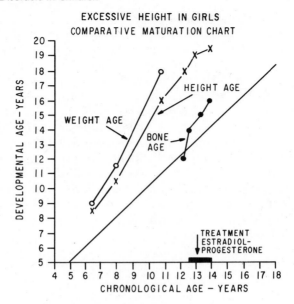

**Figure 9-3.**  Tall girl (familial tall stature) treated with estrogen to avoid excessive height. Predicted mature height (PMH) = 185 cm (73 inches); actual height achieved after therapy 179 cm (70½ inches).

seen a few girls who take longer. Residual problems in reproductive potential have been reported. In a follow-up survey of twenty girls approximately 10 years after therapy we found no girls who were experiencing fertility problems (22).

With use of estrogens, weight gain is common, and perhaps even universal as is nausea at high estrogen levels. Headaches, menstrual spotting, and leg cramps also occur. Fortunately, very few serious side effects have been reported yet in girls treated for limitation of excessive height. The risk of long-term hypothalamic suppression and "functional" sterility is unknown, but risk of thromboembolism does increase with higher dosages of estrogen and progestin. The Center for Disease Control reports no increase in breast cancer among young women using estrogens (oral contraceptives) (29), however, there may be an increased risk of cervical carcinoma (30) and a small risk of liver neoplasms (31). We recommend regular breast examinations and pap smears for all girls who have undergone estrogen therapy.

In contrast to tall girls, boys with familial tall stature do not often express concern over their potential height. There are some who desire to know how tall they will be, and though the standards for height prediction are often inaccurate at extremes, a reasonable estimate can usually be made. Some families consider heights well over 6 feet to be a disadvantage for boys as well as for girls, and some desire therapy with androgen to limit such height perceived as excessive.

The efficacy of testosterone and of low-dose estrogen in limiting excessive height in boys has been reported by several authors (32–34). In boys with a predicted mature height of 195–200 cm (6½ feet), Zachmann et al. achieved an average reduction of 5.4 cm (2.25 inches) by using depo-testosterone injections of 500–1000 mg intramuscularly monthly (33). Growth velocity was accelerated initially in those under 14 years of age at the time of treatment, but the greatest height reduction was achieved in this group. In the low-dose estrogen-treated group, there was instant growth inhibition, probably because of the effect of estrogen on somatomedin activity (34). Development of secondary sexual characteristics was stimulated in younger boys by testosterone therapy (33); mild reversible gynecomastia occurred in boys given ethinyl estradiol, 0.05 mg/day (34). The major side effects noted were atrophy or inactivation of the testes. During treatment with testosterone, the testicles remain small and, in those already in puberty, may even decrease in size, presumably the consequence of testosterone suppression of gonadotropins (33). Spontaneous recovery of testicular growth occurred in all instances, although in a few recovery required up to 5 years (32–34).

Whether testosterone therapy for limiting excessive height should be considered depends on both psychological pressures and physiologic or pubertal status of the boy. Diminishing effect on ultimate height can be expected if the pubertal growth spurt has already passed its peak (after a skeletal maturation level of 14 years). If severe psychologic disadvantages are perceived to be likely because of excessive height, treatment should be considered before the peak pubertal height velocity has been reached.

## Constitutional Accelerated Growth

The child with accelerated growth and maturation tends to be large-for-age but appropriate for the level of skeletal maturation. That is, bone-age equals height-age throughout childhood. The pubertal growth spurt and sexual maturation occur early, corresponding roughly to skeletal maturation level. Final height attainment is not excessive but is consistent with mid-parent height (Figure 5-2).

Children with a constitutional accelerated growth tend to be stocky in build. Because of his larger size and increased strength during childhood and early adolescence, the boy performs well athletically and often assumes the leadership role among his peers. The girl with accelerated growth and early maturity may be self-conscious about her size, early adolescent development, and early menarche. There is no effective treatment of naturally occurring accelerated growth. It may be desirable to consider birth control measures in the girl who achieves reproductive potential at an early age before social or emotional maturity has been achieved.

### Table 9-2. Intrinsic Growth Disorders in Childhood

A. *Chromosomal Imbalance Syndromes*
  1. Down's syndrome
  2. Turner's syndrome
B. *Skeletal Dysplasias*
  1. Osteochondrodystrophies
     (a) Metaphyseal dysplasias
     (b) Spondyloepiphyseal dysplasias
     (c) Multiple epiphyseal dysplasias
     (d) Dyschondrosteosis
  2. Osteochondrodysplasia with osteopetrosis
  3. Albright hereditary osteodystrophy
C. *Dyostosis Multiplex* (storage diseases)
D. *Congenital Malformation Syndromes*
  1. Silver–Russell syndrome
  2. Cockayne's syndrome
  3. Progeria
  4. Noonan's syndrome
  5. Aarskog's syndrome
E. *Intrauterine Growth Retardation*

## DISORDERS OF GROWTH DEFICIENCY

When we speak of *intrinsic* disorders of growth deficiency, we imply that growth potential is limited by genetic, chromosomal, or intrauterine factors over which we have little control. Such limitations of growth potential are seen in chromosomal imbalance syndromes, skeletal dysplasias, congenital malformation syndromes, and some intrauterine growth retardation. By *extrinsic* growth disorders, we imply that growth potential is basically normal, but that growth is impeded by factors over which we may have control and that removal of such growth-limiting factors may lead to resumption of normal growth. We see extrinsic factors affecting growth in childhood in nutritional deficiencies, psychosocial disorders, systemic illnesses, endocrine deficiencies, some metabolic disorders, and medicinal use of hormones.

### Intrinsic Growth Disorders

Many of the intrinsic growth disorders exhibit growth retardation in infancy and have been introduced in Chapter 8. There are some with an intrinsic defect which present more commonly with growth failure in late infancy or in childhood, and others which have characteristic growth patterns through childhood which deserve emphasis (Table 9-2).

## Chromosomal Imbalance Syndromes

Down's syndrome is characterized during childhood by short stature and slow growth (35). Skeletal maturation, delayed during childhood, accelerates at puberty, and final height is achieved by about 15 years of age. Muscle tone tends to improve as the child grows older but mental deficiency worsens. Many children with Down's syndrome tend to become "chunky"; weight increases faster than height (Figure 8-1). Hypothyroidism, generally associated with lymphocytic thyroiditis, occurs commonly and may contribute to slow growth and delayed skeletal maturation. Adolescent sexual development is incomplete in boys, who are infertile; however, girls may menstruate and be fertile. Adult height is very short and is related somewhat to parental height (36).

Most of the remaining chromosomal excess syndromes associated with growth failure do not survive into childhood. Those children who survive have characteristic dysmorphic features and persistent growth failure. (Note: Klinefelter's syndrome will be discussed among growth excess disorders.)

Turner's syndrome may be recognized at birth if the infant is small for gestational-age, has the characteristic lymphedema of the feet and hands, and cutis laxa (loose folds of the skin of the posterior neck) (see Figure 8-2). However, the most consistent features of the syndrome are short stature and gonadal dysgenesis, neither of which may be evident in the newborn. It is imperative, therefore, to bear in mind the possibility of Turner's syndrome when considering the cause of short stature and/or sexual infantilism in a girl at any age. The clinical syndrome of small stature, sexual infantilism, webbed neck, and cubitus valgus in females was described by Turner in 1938 (37). Subsequently, high levels of urinary gonadotrophins directed attention to primary ovarian failure. In 1954 these patients were discovered to have negative sex chromatin (38) and in 1959 to have a 45 XO chromosomal pattern (39).

Characteristic features of Turner's syndrome (Figure 9-4) include the following: small stature which occurs in nearly 100% and may be evident at birth; ovarian dysgenesis present in over 90%, varying from complete absence of any germinal tissue (streak ovary) to hypoplastic but partially functional tissue; lymphedema present in over 80% and usually evident in the newborn period, often with some residual puffiness of the fingers and toes in later childhood; shield-shaped chest and mild pectus excavatum, present in over 80% with widely spaced nipples which may be inverted or hypoplastic; prominent low set ears present in over 80%; narrow high palate and small mandible present in 50–80%; low posterior hair line present in 80% with webbing of the skin of the neck (pterygium colli) present in over 50%; cubitus valgus present in over 70%, medial tibial exostosis 60%, short fourth metacarpal or metatarsal 50%; dysplastic nails—narrowed, deep-set or hyperconvex 50–70%; horseshoe kidney or other kidney malposition with

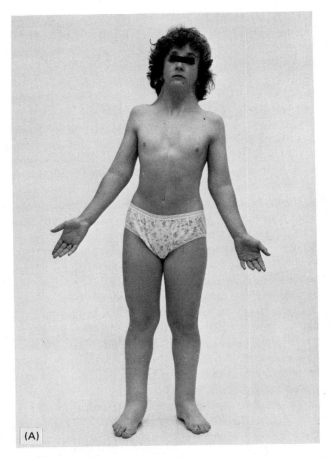

(A)

**Figure 9-4.** Turner's syndrome in girl at age 14. (A) Note lack of sexual development, cubitus valgus, webbing of neck, (B) low posterior hairline (surgical scar from scoliosis surgery), ptosis, low set ears, shield shaped chest, pectus excavatum, widely spaced nipples, and pedal edema. (C) Growth along or below the 5th percentile during childhood with lack of pubertal growth spurt despite therapy with Anavar and sex steroids.

duplication of renal collecting systems 60%; *bone dysplasia* with coarse trabeculation in metaphysis of long bones 50%; excessive *pigmented nevi* 40–50%, *telangiectasis* of skin and gut (GI bleeding) and *cutis laxa* approximately 20%, *distal palmer axial triradii* approximately 40%; perceptive *hearing impairment* 50% with frequent *otitis media* and 5% full deafness; *cardiac defects* 20%, most commonly coarctation of the aorta (36, 40–42).

The diagnosis of Turner's syndrome may be suspected in any short girl, but the suspicion is considerably enhanced by the presence of some

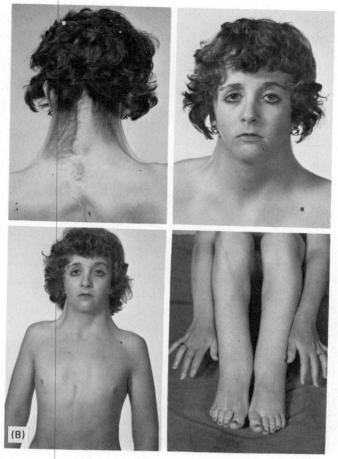

(B)

**Figure 9-4.** (Continued)

of the major somatic anomalies common in Turner's syndrome (Figure 9-4). Diagnosis is confirmed by a chromosomal karyotype demonstrating an X chromosome deletion (XO), a mosaic pattern (XO/XX) or isochrome formation with partial X deletion. The serum or urine gonadotropins are elevated. Even in mid-childhood, levels of gonadotropins are above the usual childhood levels and rise to "menopausal" levels at the usual time of adolescence. Linear growth proceeds slowly throughout childhood at about 50–75% of normal velocity, and there is characteristically no pubertal growth spurt (43). Skeletal maturation is moderately delayed. Final height is almost always under 150 cm (60") with a mean of 142 cm (56") (44, 45). The height achieved seems to be related somewhat to mid-parent height, taller subjects with Turner's syndrome coming from taller parents (36).

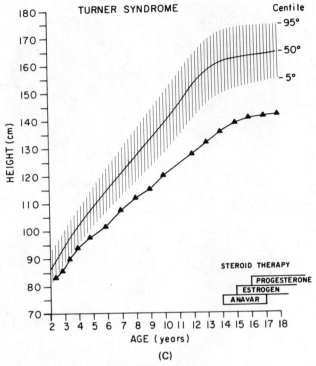

(C)

**Figure 9-4.** (Continued)

Patients treated with estrogens grow fairly constantly until full height is achieved at 16–19 years of age (44, 45). Despite the delay in skeletal maturation, there is no late growth spurt even when sex hormones are used in treatment (25); sex steroids merely speed the attainment of the predetermined growth potential. There is no difference in height achievement between XO and mosaic Turner phenotypes (44, 45). Children with Turner's syndrome are generally healthy, happy, and well-adjusted. Frequent ear infections may require placement of tympanic tubes, although hearing may be impaired also for other reasons. Cosmetic surgery is desirable for severe webbing of the neck (Figure 9-4), although a completely normal appearance is still difficult to achieve. Keloid formation of the scar is common. Plastic repair may also improve the appearance of the inner canthal folds, ptosis of the eyelids, and protruding ears. Kidney anomalies are usually positional and do not affect kidney function. Cardiac surgery is occasionally needed to correct the coarctation of the aorta or other congenital heart defects. Lymphocytic thyroiditis with hypothyroidism is common in Turner's syndrome and should be watched for throughout childhood and adolescence. Both thyromegaly and hypothyroidism may appear insidiously and not be noticed by relatives or medical practitioners.

By and large, youngsters with Turner's syndrome are of average intelligence; some have specific learning disabilities which may require special educational attention. Short stature can create some psychological problems. In our experience, however, most youngsters adapt well to their size and sexual infantilism. Youngsters with Turner's syndrome do not require hormonal therapy until the time of puberty, when they should receive appropriate sex hormones to stimulate the appearance of secondary sex characteristics.

There is no therapy which will alter the growth pattern materially through childhood. The short stature is unrelated to any known endocrine deficiency. Growth hormone levels are usually normal as are levels of somatomedins, although there are reports of growth hormone deficiency in Turner's syndrome. Initial reports of hGH therapy in Turner's syndrome showed minimal acceleration of growth (46), but later trials suggest the possibility that such patients might benefit from hGH in combination with or without anabolic steroid therapy (47, 48). Sex steroids administered at the usual time of puberty do not seem to alter eventual height (32), although some investigators have claimed some advantage from use of anabolic steroids given 12–18 months before beginning sex hormone therapy (49, 50). We generally offer hormonal therapy in our clinics when the child is near the usual age for puberty and is socially and psychologically ready for puberty. (See treatment of Turner syndrome in Chapter 10.)

The remaining chromosomal deficiency syndromes have persistent growth failure if they survive infancy. They are recognized by their dysmorphic features. Their growth patterns after infancy can be judged from the information supplied in Table 8-3 or by consulting the description of the individual syndrome in Smith's *Recognizable Patterns of Human Malformation* (36).

## Skeletal Dysplasias

Skeletal dysplasias are characterized by disproportionate growth of extremities versus trunk and usually may be recognized in childhood from the clinical picture and characteristic radiographic appearance. Most of the skeletal dysplasias affect growth either in utero or in early infancy and have been discussed in Chapter 8 where terms used to describe skeletal dysplasias are presented. We will discuss here the growth disturbances resulting from metaphyseal chondrodysplasias, spondyloepiphyseal and multiple epiphyseal dysplasias, dyschondrosteoses, osteopetroses, and Albright hereditary osteodystrophy (Table 9-2).

## Osteochondrodysplasias

A *metaphyseal chondrodysplasia* is an intrinsic disorder of skeletal development characterized radiographically by irregularity, widening, and frag-

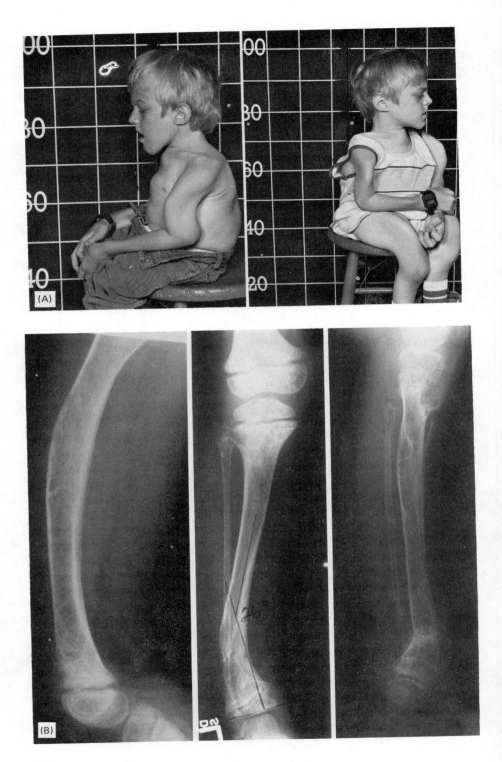

mentation of the metaphyses of long bones with disturbed histologic structure of the metaphysis. The chondrodysplasias must be distinguished from rickets, scurvy, or trauma in which the growth potential of cartilage and bone is normal (51).

*Hypophosphatasia* is the only metaphyseal chondrodysplasia with a recognizable inborn error of metabolism. A deficiency of alkaline phosphatase allows accumulation of pyrophosphate which interferes with normal tissue calcification. The presentation of this disorder in infancy has been described in Chapter 8. If the infant survives the first year of life, spontaneous improvement occurs. Hypercalcemia, which may initially require steroids, becomes less acute with age and may be controlled with a phosphate solution (52). Craniosynostosis and premature shedding of teeth may require neurosurgical or dental attention. In the case we have been following through childhood, fractures of the legs and arms have occurred with very mild trauma producing severe shortening and malformation of the limbs (Figure 9-5). Both liver and bone alkaline phosphatase are low, while intestinal phosphatase may be normal or elevated. Excretion of phosphoethanolamine is increased. Clinically normal heterozygotes can be identified by low serum alkaline phosphatase and urinary excretion of phosphoethanolamine. The disorder is inherited as an autosomal recessive trait. There is extreme variability in presentation of symptoms varying from neonatal death from respiratory failure to a mild tarda from with almost no skeletal disturbance (51).

*Classic metaphyseal chondrodysplasia*, first described by Jansen, (53) is inherited as an autosomal dominant disorder. Tubular bones are severely shortened with striking metaphyseal irregularities by x-ray especially marked in the distal femur and proximal tibia. Epiphyses and diaphyses are broad and short. With fusion of the epiphyses the metaphyseal irregularities tend to disappear, however, the bones remain short and deformed. There may be later sclerosis and hyperostoses of the skull. Despite severe shortening of the bones, general health remains good (51).

*Schmid-type of metaphyseal chondodysplasia*, transmitted also as an autosomal dominant disorder, is a relatively benign condition with a much milder dysplasia than the Jansen form (54). Affected individuals reach an adult height of 130–160 cm and can expect a normal life span. The metaphyseal irregularities are most marked in the proximal rather than the distal femur and there is usually insufficient deformity to justify osteotomy. The radiologic changes may be confused with vitamin D resistent rickets or traumatic metaphyseal damage in the "battered child" (51).

Metaphyseal chondrodysplasias also occur in combination with deficiencies of the immune system and malabsorbtion. A *deficiency of adenosine*

**Figure 9-5.** Hypophosphatasia in boy at age 13 (A) showing shortening and deformity of extremities, sternal and chest deformity, and dolicocephaly. (B) X-rays of femur and lower leg show severe deformity from fractures and osteomalacia.

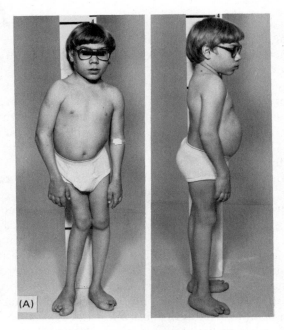

(A)

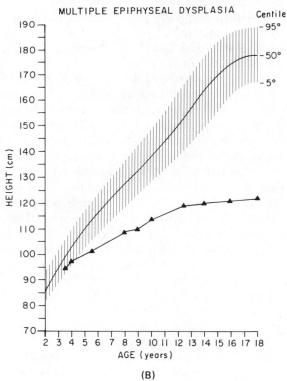

MULTIPLE EPIPHYSEAL DYSPLASIA

Centile

- 95°
- 50°
- 5°

HEIGHT (cm)

AGE (years)

(B)

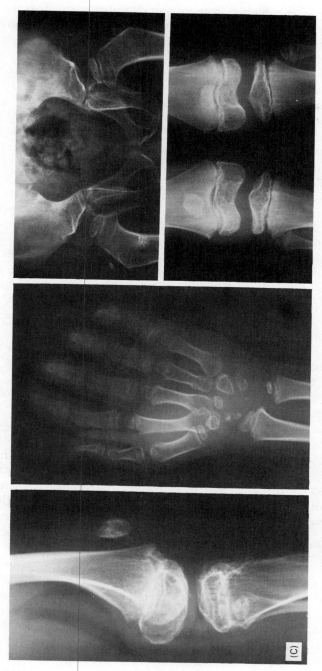

**Figure 9-6.** Multiple epiphyseal dysplasia (age 16). (A) There is limitation of movement of hips, genu valgus deformity, and deformity of hands and feet. (B) Extreme limitation of statural growth beginning in early childhood. Normal pubertal development without growth spurt at age 14. (C) X-rays display dysplastic epiphyses in hands, hips, and knees.

*deaminase* appears to be a feature common to chondrodystrophies associated with immune deficiency states. They are characterized by failure to thrive, chronic diarrhea with malabsorbtion, chronic or recurrent pneumonia, and candidiasis and other infections, along with short stature. The skin is thickened and the hair is sparse. X-rays show metaphyseal changes and flaring and cupping of the costo-chondral junctions (51). In the *Schwachman–Diamond syndrome*, malabsorption and neutropenia are associated with metaphyseal chondrodysplasia. The bone disorder is mild and respiratory infection is common (55, 56). In cartilage–hair hypoplasia (see Chapter 8) the metaphyseal chondrodysplasia is associated with defects of blood cells, the immune system and the hair. Death from chicken pox has been common (57).

*Spondyloepiphyseal dysplasia* tarda is a hereditary disorder usually transmitted as an X-linked trait although autosomal recessive and autosomal dominant transmissions have also been suggested. Short stature becomes apparent after age 5–10 years. Pain in the back or pain and stiffness in weight-bearing joints may be the first clinical signs of the disorder. There is shortening of the trunk and neck so that final height achievement is only 52–62 inches (36). X-rays show narrowing of intervertebral spaces and calcification of intervertebral discs. The femoral neck is short and femoral disc is flattened. Progressive degenerative joint disease occurs in weight-bearing joints of adults.

*Multiple epiphyseal dysplasia* is an autosomal dominant or recessive skeletal dysplasia characterized by late ossifying, small, irregular, mottled epiphyses, pain and limitation of motion in the hips or other weight-bearing joints, and short stature (58). The epiphyses are symmetrically involved, have irregular outlines, are often fragmented or stippled, and ossification centers are small (Figure 9-6). There may be metaphyseal irregularity; phalanges and metacarpals are short. Spine and skull are usually normal though some vertebral bodies may be blunted and flat (36). Slow growth and waddling gait may be evident by early childhood. Pain and stiffness of joints, particularly the hips, may also begin in childhood but is more common in adulthood. The joint involvement resembles osteoarthritis. Mild to moderate shortness of stature is usual, most affected persons achieving a height of 145–170 cm, although on occasion the shortness and joint limitation can be severe (58).

We have observed a family with three children affected with multiple epiphyseal dysplasia. The parents and two siblings are normal, suggesting an autosomal recessive inheritance pattern. The multiple epiphyseal dysplasia has been associated with infancy-onset diabetes mellitus, ectodermal dysplasia, mild chronic anemia, a defect in white blood cell migration, and chronic azotemia leading to end stage renal failure. The multiple epiphyseal dysplasia resembles that described in the literature, however, the shortness is more severe (Figure 9-6). We have not been able to find any unifying link between the multiple epiphyseal dysplasia and the other features of the disorder. Nor have we found reports of other similar cases and presume it may represent a new autosomal recessive syndrome (59).

*Dyschondrosteoses* produce shortening by affecting growth of diaphyses of long bones. *Leri–Weill dyschondrosteosis* is characterized by short forearm and bowing of the radius (Madelung deformity), partial dislocation of ulna, and short lower leg. It is an autosomal dominant disorder with variable short stature, adult height ranging from 135 cm to normal (36, 60). *Langer mesomelic dyschondrosteosis syndrome* is characterized by short, deformed forearms and lower legs (mesomelia), hypoplasia of fibula, and small mandible. It is transmitted as an autosomal recessive trait and heterozygotus individuals have mild to moderate shortness of stature wtih Madelung deformity (36, 61).

*Osteochondrodysplasias with Osteopetrosis.* The mechanism by which osteo-petrosis or osteosclerosis interferes with long bone growth is uncertain but several osteopetrosis syndromes display small stature. *Maroteaux–Lamy pyknodysostosis syndrome* is an autosomal recessive disorder characterized by short stature, general skeletal osteosclerosis (increased bone density), and frequent fractures (62). The head is brachycephalic with frontal bossing; there is delayed closure of the sutures and hypoplasia of facial bones. Tooth eruption may be delayed and teeth deformed. The acromial end of the clavicle is dysplastic, nails are flattened and grooved, and distal phalanges are tapered. Orthopedic correction of fractures may prevent lower limb deformity. The French painter, Toulouse-Lautrec, is said to have had pyknodysostosis and short stature because of multiple fractures of the lower extremities (36).

*Cleidiocranial dysostosis* is characterized by mild to moderate shortness of stature, partial to complete aplasia of the clavicle, late ossification of cranial sutures, and delayed eruption of teeth (63). Brachycephaly occurs with bossing of bones of the skull, giving the skull a "hot-cross-bun" appearance. Teeth are often aplastic or have enamel hypoplasia; there may be super-numery teeth. Facial bones are hypoplastic and sinuses may be absent. Mentality is usually normal but hearing may be reduced. A narrow thorax may cause respiratory distress in infancy and a narrow pelvis may prevent vaginal delivery in the pregnant mother (36).

*Albright hereditary osteodystrophy* is an X-linked, dominant disorder char-acterized by short stature, short metacarpals, rounded face, hypocalcemia and mineral deposits in subcutaneous tissues and basal ganglia. Albright first suggested the name pseudohypoparathyroidism because of low serum calcium and tetany, suggestive of hypoparathyroidism which failed to respond to parathyroid extract (64). Since then, many cases of the syndrome, without hypocalcemia, have been described under the name of pseudopseudohypoparathyroidism, prompting a change in name to one more descriptive of the syndrome, since in the form without hypocalcemia there is no parathyroid disorder (65).

**Table 9-3. Growth Limitation in Mucopolysaccharidoses**

| Syndrome | Type | Growth Limitation | Age at Onset | Dysostosis Severity |
|---|---|---|---|---|
| Hurler's | I-H | Severe[a] | 6–18 mo | + + + + |
| Scheie's | I-S | Mild | Childhood | + + |
| Hunter's | II | Moderate | 2–4 yr | + + + |
| Sanfilippo's | III,a,b | Moderate | After 1–3 yr | + + |
| Morquio's | IV | Severe | After 1–3 yr | + + + + |
| Maroteaux–Lamy | VI | Mild/severe | After 1–3 yr | + +/+ + + + |
| Glucuronidase def | VII | Moderate[a] | After 1st yr | + + + |

[a] Growth may be accelerated during the first year of life.

Children with Albright hereditary osteodystrophy are short, stocky, and moderately obese. Their final height usually ranges from 137 cm (54 in.) to 150 cm (60 in.), although height can be normal. Mental dullness is common with a mean IQ of 60. The face is rounded, dentition is delayed, and enamel hypoplasia is common. The metacarpals and metatarsals, especially the fourth and fifth, are shortened, giving the clenched fist the characteristic "knuckle-knuckle-dimple-dimple" appearance. Cone-shaped epiphyses are seen roentgeniographically. Calcification occurs in basal ganglia and in subcutaneous tissue, and exostoses of long bones are common. Hypocalcemia in childhood may be associated with seizures or tetany. Serum parathyroid hormone (PTH) levels are normal or high suggesting an end-organ unresponsiveness to PTH. Vitamin D in large doses (25,000–100,000 units/day) may be necessary to correct the hypocalcemia and prevent tetany or seizures. The hypocalcemia sometimes ameliorates spontaneously with age (36, 66).

### Mucopolysaccharidoses (Storage Diseases)

With the exception of generalized gangliosidosis and mucolipidosis II (see Chapter 8), growth is normal during infancy in children who have mucopolysaccharidoses, oligosaccharidoses, or mucolipidoses. Growth becomes noticeably affected at various ages in early childhood in these disorders (Table 9-3). Though they are diverse in their presentation, their severity, and their enzyme deficiencies, the skeletal dysplasia, termed *dysostosis multiplex* is remarkably uniform; only the skeletal changes of Morquio's syndrome are characteristic enough to make the diagnosis from radiographic features alone (67). The mucopolysacchridoses (MPS), currently divided into seven groups, are characterized biochemically by storage of dermatin, heparitin, or keratan sulfate and by specific enzyme defects.

*Hurler's syndrome* (MPS type I-H) is an autosomal recessive disorder characterized by coarse faces, severe mental retardation, stiff joints, and corneal opacity. Deceleration of growth can usually be seen between 6–

18 months. Growth during the first year of life may actually be rapid, but ultimate height seldom exceeds 110 cm (36). Delay in development and mental deficiency is usually evident in the latter half of the first year. Coarsening of facial features, noisy breathing with frequent respiratory infections, and limited hip mobility may be evidenced in the first 6 months. Death usually occurs in childhood from respiratory or cardiac failure (68).

Children with *Scheie's syndrome* (MPS type I-S) have the same enzyme defect as do those with Hurler's syndrome, however, the effects on growth, skeleton, and brain are much less pronounced (36). The face does not resemble "gargoylism", but a broad mouth and full lips are characteristic. Corneal opacification occurs early. Joint limitation of hands leads to claw deformity but mentality is usually normal and growth disturbance is mild (69).

*Hunter's syndrome* (MPS type II) is an X-linked disorder with appearance of clinical features around 2–4 years. Coarse facial features, growth deficiency, stiff joints, and clear cornea characterize this syndrome. Growth deficiency begins at around 2 years of age and there is gradual decline in growth rate throughout the early childhood years (36). In the juvenile type, mental deterioration begins in early childhood and progresses to severe mental deficiency and death in later childhood. In an adult-type, mental deficiency is usually mild and survival into middle age is possible. Adults may reach a height of 120–150 cm (70).

*Sanfilippo's syndrome* (MPS type III A and B) is an autosomal recessive disorder which appears to be the most common of the mucopolysaccharidoses. It is characterized by mild coarsening of the faces and stiffness of joints and severe mental deficiency (71). Growth is normal or accelerated for 1–3 years, followed by slow growth and deterioration of mental function. Most have long survival time (36).

*Morquio's syndrome* (MPS type IV) is an autosomal recessive disorder characterized by mildly coarse facial features, corneal clouding, severe kyphosis, and knock-knee deformities. There is severe limitation of growth beginning between 1 and 3 years. Growth ceases in later childhood with achievement of a final height of only 80–115 cm (36). Marked flattening of the vertebrae leads to short neck and trunk and kyphoscoliosis. Defects in the vertebrae may lead to respiratory insufficiency or cord compression. Early in the disease there is flaring of the lower rib cage, prominent sternum (carinatum), frequent URI's and otitis media, and growth deficiency. Later corneal clouding and severe deformities develop. Mentality is usually normal (72).

*Maroteaux–Lamy syndrome* (MPS type VI) is characterized by coarse faces, stiff joints and cloudy cornea but mental deterioration does not occur. Growth deficiency usually begins a little later than with Hurler's syndrome, and the skeletal and joint manifestations and the corneal opacification are generally somewhat less pronounced (36, 73).

*Glucuronidase deficiency* (MPS type VII) is characterized by variable mental deficiency, accelerated growth during the first year of life but progressive short stature thereafter, hepatosplenomegaly, skeletal deformity of thorax and spine, frequent pulmonary infections, and granular inclusions in leukocytes (74).

*Oligosaccharidoses or mucolipidoses* are characterized by specific enzyme defects leading to storage or excretion of oligosaccharides, gangliosides, glycopeptides, mucopolysaccharides, and glycolipids. Infants affected with $GM_1$-gangliosidosis and mucolipidosis-2 exhibit intrauterine growth retardation. (See Chapter 8.) The remainder of the oligosaccharidoses and mucolipidoses present in later infancy or early childhood with dysostosis multiplex, growth deficiency, and physical features suggesting Hurler's Syndrome such as coarse facial features, joint limitation, corneal clouding, and mental deficiency. The oligosaccharidoses and mucolipidoses can only be distinguished from mucopolysaccharidoses by lack of mucopolysaccharides in the urine and by identification of specific enzyme defects (67).

The term *dysostosis multiplex* is used to denote the skeletal changes which occur in the mucopolysaccharidoses and mucolipidoses. The skeletal changes are remarkably uniform and unique for disorders of complex carbohydrate metabolism, although they vary in severity and distribution among the disorders. Widening of the ribs appears to be one of the earliest signs of dysostosis multiplex. The bodies of the vertebrae remain immature and are ovoid in shape. Anterior wedging of the vertebrae may produce a gibbous deformity. The ilia are hypoplastic. The metacarpals are short, wide, and pointed proximally. The phalanges are bullet-shaped. There may be expansion of the shafts of short tubular bones and coarsened irregular bone structure. In some forms of the disorder, there is thickening of the calvarium and premature closure of the cranial sutures (67).

In a child with elevated mucopolysaccharides, severe dysostosis multiplex would suggest either Hurler's or Maroteaux–Lamy syndrome. Less severe bone changes would be found in Hunter's syndrome and mild defects in Sanfilippo- and Scheie-type mucopolysaccharidosis or in the mucosulphatidoses. In a child with normal mucopolysaccharides in the urine, severe dysostosis multiplex is seen in GM-gangliosidosis, other beta-galactosidase deficiencies and in mucolipidoses 2 and 3. Boney changes are moderately severe in mucolipidosis type 1 and mild in other oligosaccharidases and mucolipidoses.

In Morquio's syndrome, the bone changes are characteristic enough to allow diagnosis to be made from the radiologic features. Vertebral bodies are flattened and pointed anteriorly. At the dorsal-lumbar junction backward displacement of the malformed vertebral bodies leads to gibbous formation which may cause spinal cord compression. Pelvic hypoplasia is severe and associated with dysplasia of the femoral head and severe coxavalga, which leads to the marked knocked-knee deformity seen in Morquio's syndrome. In the hands, there is diaphyseal constriction of short tubular bones. Hypoplasia of the odontoid process leads to atlantoaxial instability, which may lead to spinal cord compression in the cervical area. Prophylactic spinal fusion has been advocated (67).

### Congenital Malformation Syndromes

Dysmorphic syndromes commonly associated with growth deficiency are listed in Tables 8-7 and 8-8. Many are born small for gestational-age, suggesting an intrauterine growth retardation or "congenital hypoplasia" (43). Characteristically, such children exhibit postnatal growth deficiency as well. Catch-up growth does not occur. The velocity of growth may be nearly normal throughout childhood, although height achievement is well below the mean for a normal population. Each dysmorphic syndrome has a somewhat characteristic growth pattern and expectations for growth are best derived from growth data for the specific syndrome (36). Growth characteristics of Silver-Russell syndrome are described in Chapter 8 and displayed in Figure 8-5. Such a pattern of growth is characteristic of syndromes of congenital hypoplasia (75).

A few of the dysmorphic syndromes present with growth disturbances later in infancy or childhood. These include the following relatively rare syndromes: Progeria syndrome; Cockayne's syndrome; Noonan's syndrome; Aarskog's syndrome.

*Progeria (Hutchinson–Gilford syndrome)* is a sporadically occurring disorder characterized by a senile appearance with alopecia, thin skin, skeletal hypoplasia or dysplasia, growth failure, and early death from coronary artery disease. Birth-weight is often low, although not strikingly so. Growth failure becomes severe after the first year. Hair may be lacking at birth or may be lost sometime within the first 18 months with degeneration of hair follicles. The skin becomes thin and subcutaneous fat tissue is lost in infancy. Deficient skeletal growth becomes evident by 6–18 months and velocity of growth is reduced to about one-half to one-third of normal (36). Coxavalaga deformity of the hips occurs and distal phalanges and clavicle may undergo degeneration. Dentition eruption is delayed. Artherosclerosis especially of coronary arteries, aorta and mesenteric arteries occurs as early as five years of age and is the usual cause of death. Life span is shortened to an average of 14 years (76–78).

*Cockayne's syndrome* is an autosomal recessive disorder characterized by senile appearance, growth failure, mental retardation, retinal degeneration, impaired hearing, and photosensitivity of the skin (36, 79). Although growth and development may be normal during infancy, growth deficiency with loss of subcutaneous fat (failure to thrive) usually becomes evident by age 4. The trunk is relatively short with a tendency to kyphosis. Human growth hormone levels are normal (80). Progressive mental deterioration, weakness, tremor, and unsteady gait become evident by early childhood. The affected children assume a cachectic appearance, emphasized by optic atrophy and blindness, cataracts, and joint contractures (81). At death, extensive atheromata, vascular calcification, and other evidence of pre-mature aging are seen. A recent report of emphysema and alpha-1 antitrypsin deficiency in a 5 year old with Cockayne's syndrome suggest that even the lungs show evidence of premature aging (82).

*Noonan's syndrome* is a familial disorder of unknown etiology character-ized by short stature, mental retardation, webbing of the neck, pectus excavatum, variable gonadal dysplasia, and pulmonary artery stenosis (83). Noonan's and Turner's syndromes share a number of physical features, including short stature, epicanthic folds, ptosis of eyelids, low set ears, webbed neck, low posterior hairline, shield chest, cubitus valgus, and congenital heart disease (84). Patients with Noonan's syndrome, however, are more likely to have mild mental retardation, pectus excavatum, and a variety of congenital heart lesions, particularly pulmonary artery stenosis, and the chromosomal karyotype is normal (84). Small penis, cryptorchid-ism, and delayed puberty is common in boys with Noonan's syndrome, with complete gonadal failure in some (36, 85).

*Aarskog's syndrome* is an X-linked dominant disorder, characterized by mild to moderate short stature, hypertelorism, brachydactyly, and a "shawl" malformation of the scrotum (86). Growth deficiency usually becomes evident at from 1 to 3 years and may be associated with delayed skeletal maturation and delayed adolescence. The face is round with hypertelorism, small nose, broad philtrum, and maxillary hypoplasia. Fingers are short with clinodactyly of the fifth finger. The scrotum forms a "shawl" at the base of the penis. Testes are undescended (36, 86, 87).

### Intrauterine Growth Retardation

Any growth disturbance beginning in utero seems to have the capacity to affect postnatal growth and size achievement as well. Infants with intrinsic prenatal growth disturbances such as chromosomal disturbances (trisomy 21), skeletal dysplasias (achondroplasia), or dysmorphic syndromes (Silver–Russel syndrome) are characteristically small for gestational-age at birth (IUGR) and remain small throughout childhood. Their size achievement in childhood and as adults seems to be programmed by the intrinsic defect or congenital hypoplasia (43). Growth retardation in utero from extrinsic or secondary factors seems also to be able to affect not only size at birth but postnatal growth as well. The postnatal growth pattern is variable but complete catch-up growth is not frequently seen. Infants of normal length but low-birth-weight appear to be an exception. Rapid weight gain after birth in this group usually results in a normal postnatal growth pattern (88); however, most infants small for gestational-age because of intrauter-ine growth disturbance related to placental or maternal growth restricting factors remain small throughout childhood (89) and, although experienc-ing a pubertal growth spurt, tend to remain below the mean size for their expected growth (Figure 9-7).

The cause or causes of postnatal growth deficiency in children with intrauterine growth retardation from extrinsic factors is not well understood. It may be that any factor affecting growth during a "critical period" of growth may result in hypoplasia of critical tissues that influence subsequent rates of growth and final height achievement. Whatever the cause, children with intrauterine growth retardation frequently exhibit a pattern of slow growth throughout childhood which must be borne in mind when considering the growth deficiency of a child with proportionate but slow growth.

Treatment of intrauterine growth retardation (IUGR) with hGH has yielded responses varying from no growth to nearly 8 cm/yr, reflecting perhaps the different causes of IUGR (46, 90). The response has been transient in some, but prolonged in others (46, 90); there is enough evidence that some children with IUGR benefit from therapy to encourage further trials of hGH treatment in this group of youngsters with intrinsic short stature (14, 91).

## Extrinsic Growth Disorders

When we speak of an extrinsic growth disorder in childhood, we imply that the tissues responsible for growth of the individual (primarily the skeletal system) have normal potential for growth but are impeded in growth by an "extrinsic" factor, secondarily limiting growth. It is further implied that if the extrinsic factor or factors can be removed, "catch-up growth" and a subsequent normal growth pattern can be realized. The extrinsic disorders which affect the growth of the child and have their onset after birth are listed in Table 9-4. Disorders of nearly every organ system of the body may adversely affect growth of the child. Those disorders affecting linear or total growth of the child are emphasized in this chapter. In Chapter 11 a discussion of failure to thrive will highlight those disorders affecting weight more than linear growth.

### Nutritional Disorders

Chronic malnutrition retards growth and is the most ubiquitous and preventable cause of short stature in the world. In industrialized societies, chronic protein-calorie undernutrition is quite rare and more likely associated with gastrointestinal or central nervous system disorders interfering with food utilization.

Though often a product of inadequate economic means or disrupted social situation, the underfed infant may simply be the victim of ignorance of the infant's needs, leading to inadequate calories offered. The underfed infant is usually fretful, and if weighed and measured serially fails to make expected progress. (See Chapter 11.) Catch-up growth can be expected to occur with solution of the feeding problem.

Acute protein-calorie undernutrition affects primarily weight gain from which rapid catch-up growth can be expected, but chronic protein-calorie

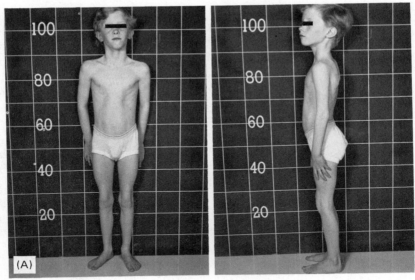

**Figure 9-7.**   Child with *intrauterine growth retardation* born prematurely (34 weeks gestation), small placenta with poor vascular supply, birth weight 600 g (1 lb 5 oz), birth length 29 cm (11½ inches), SGA despite prematurity. Some initial catch-up growth is seen in early infancy, but the child remains small and frail (A) into childhood and grows slowly, remaining well below the 5th percentile into childhood for both height (B) and weight (C).

*undernutrition*, especially if occuring in early childhood, has a pronounced effect on linear growth, bone maturation, and intellectual development. Winick and Rosso report that severe malnutrition in infancy can curtail normal increase in brain cellularity and lead to faulty brain growth and development (92). In a study by Stock and Smythe, undernutrition early in infancy produced irreversible intellectual impairment evidenced by small OFC, deficits in visual–motor perception, and low intellectual scores through childhood and adolescence (93). The first 2 years of life constitute the period of most rapid postnatal brain growth and represent both a "critical" period most susceptible to undernutrition and the period in which "catch-up" brain growth must occur if permanent damage is to be avoided (93). Malnutrition after 2 years of age seems to have less effect on brain growth and intellectual achievement.

Catch-up growth usually occurs when undernutrition is corrected, although the catch-up growth is limited to usual periods of growth (93, 94). If undernutrition in infancy is corrected there is apparently no long term effect of protein-calorie malnutrition on either bone age or cortical bone thickness (95). McCance and Widdowson, however, observed a permanent deficit in size when nutritional deficiency was induced during

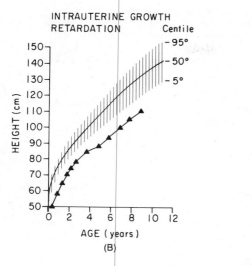

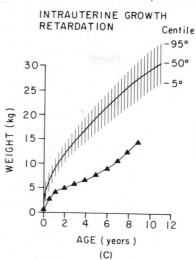

**Figure 9-7.** (Continued)

"critical periods" of growth, despite provision subsequently of an adequate diet (96). This failure to achieve catch-up of physical growth after malnutrition is echoed by others (97, 98). Davis et al. have recently suggested that short stature in many children may be associated with prolonged deficiency in caloric intake, associated with "poor appetite" or disorders in eating habits (99). The concept of short stature arising in segments of our society which are deprived socially, economically, and nutritionally is echoed by Lacey and Parkin, who consider short stature a "social disorder" (1).

The causes of short stature in malnutrition may be explained by the effects of undernutrition on both cellular growth factors and on their endocrine regulation. Both a reduction in cell size (100) and in cell number (92) have been shown to be a consequence of chronic undernutrition. Transient decrease in growth hormone production (101) and failure to respond to growth hormone (102) have been reported. In marasmic infants, Parra et al. have reported reduced caloric expenditures, low muscle glycogen, and adaptive endocrine mechanisms to preserve muscle composition (103). In severe protein deficiency, levels of growth hormone are elevated but somatomedin levels are low. Although protein deficiency seems to be more effective in reducing somatomedin activity, there is a decrease in somatomedin activity with protein-calorie malnutrition as well (104). When protein is inadequate, somatomedin, even when present, cannot adequately stimulate cartilage growth (104).

In severe *diabetes insipidus* (DI) there is a striking retardation of growth, especially noteworthy in nephrogenic DI. As a child with DI increases

**Table 9-4. Extrinsic Growth Disorders
in Childhood**

A. *Nutritional Disorders*
   1. Malnutrition (environmental)
   2. Gastrointestinal disorders
B. *CNS/Psychosocial Disorders*
   1. Mental deficiency
   2. Deprivation syndrome
C. *Systemic Disorders*
   1. Cardiovascular disorders
   2. Pulmonary disease
   3. Renal disease
   4. Anemia (chronic)
   5. Chronic infections
   6. Hepatic insufficiency
   7. Collagen–vascular disorders
D. *Endocrine Disorders*
   1. Hypothyroidism
   2. Hypopituitarism
   3. Cushing's syndrome
E. *Metabolic Disorders*
   1. Rickets, renal tubular acidosis
   2. Diabetes mellitus
   3. Hypercalcemia, hypokalemia
F. *Iatrogenic Disorders*
   1. Glucocorticoid excess
   2. Anabolic steroids

food intake, there is an increase in solute load, with increase in polyuria and polydypsia. Subjects with DI appear to voluntarily limit their food intake to decrease the obligate polyuria. This generally leads to inadequate caloric intake (105). Improvement in growth occurs with adequate vasopressin therapy in those patients with DI who are sensitive to vasopressin.

*Zinc deficiency* has been recognized recently to be a factor contributing to poor growth and delayed sexual maturation in humans in a number of Near East and Mediterranean countries (106, 107) and in subjects with sickle cell disease (108), malabsorption, infection, or liver disease (106, 109). Anorexia, growth retardation, skin lesions, hypogonadism, lethargy, delayed healing, and increased susceptibility to infections are some common features of nutritional deficiency of zinc (106). In adolescents, delayed puberty may be noted; after zinc sulfate supplementation, a growth spurt and accelerated genital development occur. Combined zinc and growth hormone deficiency has been described which responded to zinc supplementation, suggesting a possible permissive role for zinc in growth hormone secretion or activity (110).

At present there is no specific test for zinc deficiency. Plasma and hair zinc concentrations are generally lower than "normal" in zinc deficiency states, but the critical test for zinc deficiency is a definitive clinical response to zinc supplementation under controlled conditions. Specific changes in growth, skin, and gonads have been regularly seen in treated zinc-deficient subjects (106). A daily supplemental dosage of 40 mg of zinc sulfate will usually provide adequate zinc. Segments of our population which are protein deficient may need higher zinc intake especially during infancy and adolescence (111). Solomens et al. suggest caution in indiscriminate use of zinc supplement in growth-retarded children, but agree that in children or adolescents who display a plateau in growth, zinc deficiency might be entertained as a possible cause (109).

Failure of growth in most *gastrointestinal diseases* is manifested by weight loss more than lack of general growth, and may be better discussed as failure to thrive (see Chapter 11), however, a few disorders such as regional enteritis may produce growth failure without obvious intestinal manifestations (112). Gastrointestinal disorders likely to be associated with growth failure include (a) chronic intestinal obstruction, including Hirschsprung's aganglionosis of the colon; (b) malabsorption disorders such as cystic fibrosis of the pancreas or celiac disease; and (c) inflammatory bowel disease, most prominently regional enteritis (Crohn's disease) and ulcerative colitis. The failure of growth in children with intestinal disease may result from anorexia, inadequate digestion or malabsorption of food, or continuous loss of nutrients from diarrhea. The common denominator is inadequate calories accepted or retained, resulting in undernutrition.

*Intestinal obstruction* may produce vomiting or intermittent constipation and diarrhea, as well as inadequate food intake, depending on the level of obstruction. Vomiting and rapid weight loss demand immediate attention, but low obstruction (Hirschsprung's disease) may produce a more indolent failure to grow with abdominal distention, constipation, and intermittent diarrhea. Identification and correction of the intestinal obstruction are usually followed by restoration of normal nutritional intake and full catch-up growth.

*Malabsorption,* whether due to deficiency of pancreatic enzymes, lack of intestinal enzymes, or villous atrophy, gives rise to bulky, foul smelling stools and undernutrition. In *cystic fibrosis,* to undernutrition produced by a deficiency of pancreatic enzymes must be added progressive deterioration of pulmonary function which may contribute substantially to growth failure. In the absence of severe pulmonary disease the undernutrition may be controlled satisfactorily with pancreatic enzyme replacement. In *celiac disease,* intolerance to wheat gluten produces atrophy of intestinal villi, resulting in severe and chronic malabsorption. The abdomen becomes prominent and subcutaneous tissue depots become thin, giving the child a wasted, pot-bellied appearance (Figure 11-2). Removal of wheat gluten from the diet results in disappearance of the malabsorption syndrome and catch-up growth. In his original description of the "catch-up" growth phenomenon, Prader described the rapid return to normal growth pattern of the child with treated celiac disease (113). Occult celiac disease, demonstrable only by intestinal biopsy, is also said to produce short stature (114).

Growth retardation and delay in sexual maturation occur in approximately 20% of children with chronic regional *ileitis* (Crohn's disease) (115) and rarely may be the presenting and most prominent complaint (112). Although endocrine deficiencies and steroid therapy have been implicated as factors contributing to the growth failure seen in Crohn's disease, nutritional deficiency appears to be the most consistent finding (116). Circulating thyroxine levels have been reported to be normal or low, but plasma TSH is normal (115). Growth hormone production is normal and, although release is subnormal with certain stimuli, growth patterns are not changed by administration of human growth hormone (117). Somatomedin activity is responsive to the nutritional state (104). Corticosteroid therapy may contribute to the growth delay of regional enteritis, but delayed linear growth usually precedes treatment with corticosteroids. The use of alternate day corticosteroids controls the inflammatory process, permits improved nutrition, and may restore a near normal growth pattern (118).

Perhaps the most eloquent proof of the role of undernutrition in the genesis of growth failure in regional ileitis is the catch-up growth which occurs when the undernutrition is corrected by medical/nutritional or surgical therapy. When the caloric intake is increased to approximately 80 cal/kg/day with a protein intake of 1.6 g/kg/day, both above the usual adolescent requirement, a reversal of the growth failure occurs (119). Medical therapy or surgical resection are equally effective in promoting optimal growth if adequate nutrition is thereby assured (115).

*Ulcerative colitis* produces growth failure by mechanisms similar to those of regional ileitis. The effects of colectomy on reversal of growth arrest have not been uniform. Some growth acceleration has occurred after colectomy but ultimate catch-up growth has been disappointing (115). Drug therapy, such as sulfasalazine and corticosteroid enemas, reduces mucosal inflammation and promotes mucosal healing. Alternate day steroid therapy usually allows growth to approach normal rates (118). As with chronic regional ileitis, medical or surgical therapy is only successful in restoring growth to normal if adequate nutrition can be assured by therapy. A medical/nutritional regimen promotes an improved growth velocity which is comparable to that reported after surgical resection or total parenteral nutrition (115). Oral nutrition may require supplementation with IV nutritional therapy and on occasion by total parenteral nutrition (hyperalimentation). Total parenteral nutrition has not been as effective in ulcerative colitis as in Crohn's disease (120).

## CNS and Psychosocial Disorders

The role of the central nervous system in control of growth is not yet well understood, however, it is clear that serious damage to the brain or to specific areas of the brain may affect growth of animals and humans.

Children with *mental deficiency* tend to be shorter and lighter than children of normal intelligence of the same age. There even appears to be a linear relationship—the least intelligent being the smallest—although there is considerable individual variation. The growth in mentally defective children proceeds at a slower rate for a longer period of time, but ultimate size is still small compared to normal subjects (121, 122).

Mosier et al. have shown that radiation damage of the central portion of the brain of rats produces stunting of growth which is not a result of pituitary deficiency (123). Growth impairment occurs only if the damage is bilateral and includes the area of the hypothalamus and surrounding midbrain structures. It may be that in mentally deficient children there is deficient elaboration or release of hypothalamic substances as suggested by Castells et al. (124), but in the radiation damaged rats, thyroxine and human growth hormone were ineffective in restoring growth (123). This argues rather eloquently for some as yet unexplained role of the hypothalamus or adjacent central nervous system midbrain structures in controlling growth which is separate from its pituitary regulatory function.

Some mentally deficient children may be small because of the nature of their cerebral deficit—the same factors which produce the dysmorphic syndrome may produce both mental deficiency and growth deficiency, as in Seckel's growth retardation (microcephaly) or in Down's syndrome (trisomy-21). It is difficult at times to separate undernutrition from mental deficiency, but when dysmorphic or chromosomal syndromes and malnutrition are allowed for, there is still significant growth retardation related only to mental deficiency.

Tumors in the area of the diencephalon produce a *diencephalic syndrome* characterized by emaciation, with weight low for length. In this syndrome growth hormone levels are normal and caloric deficiency does not seem severe enough to explain the growth deficiency (125).

Severe emotional disturbances (anorexia nervosa) or emotional deprivation (psychosocial deprivation) regularly result in growth deficiency. *Anorexia nervosa* generally affects children near the age of adolescence and affects weight more severely than length. A state of functional "hypopituitarism" is often noted as a part of the syndrome of emaciation and anorexia. A more detailed description of this disorder will be found in Chapter 11 on Failure to Thrive. The mechanisms of growth failure in anorexia nervosa are similar to those found in children with psychosocial deprivation.

*Psychosocial deprivation* describes an environmental—behavioral disorder characterized by shortness of stature, unusual eating habits, delay in sexual maturation and emotional and psychological deprivation. It represents a form of child neglect or psychological child abuse, sometimes associated with physical abuse (126). Children with psychosocial deprivation are symetrically small with height and head circumference reduced proportionally, but with weight usually low for height. Skeletal maturation is delayed, corresponding roughly to height-age. There may be soft lanugo body hair, sparse scalp hair, and a prominent abdomen, commonly seen in children suffering from malnutrition (101, 126). Most investigators agree that the children are often the victims of systematic food restriction (127).

A reversible hGH deficit has been described in psychosocial dwarfism. Growth hormone levels are usually low and unresponsive to hypoglycemia or arginine (101). A slow wave sleep deficit has recently been described in four children with psychosocial dwarfism, leading to the speculation that the functional deficit of hGH may be a consequence of lack of stage IV sleep (128). Frasier and Rallison report a girl with psychosocial dwarfism, not only unable to secrete growth hormone in response to hypoglycemia or arginine, but also growth-unresponsive after administration of growth hormone. Removal from an emotionally deprived home resulted in rapid return of normal growth hormone levels and catch-up growth without human growth hormone supplementation (129). The return of pituitary function to normal upon correction of the deprivation has been regularly observed, giving rise to the synonym of "reversible hyposomatotropism" for the disorder (101).

The growth failure in psychosocial deprivation probably represents a form of environmental malnutrition. It is probable that nutritional and emotional deprivation results in low somatomedin activity which prevents growth even with growth hormone administration. Whitten and coworkers succeeded in isolating food intake without changing the pattern of emotional deprivation and seem to have convincingly shown the importance of food deprivation in growth failure and in the reported bizarre eating habits of the deprived child (127).

Catch-up growth has usually been gratifying if the deprivation did not begin in earliest infancy or if correction of the emotional deprivation is not delayed until adolescence. Even then, catch-up growth does occur, though full growth potential may not be achieved. Improvement in intellectual performance can be expected also, but realization of full intellectual potential depends upon early recognition and correction of the psychosocial deprivation (130).

## Systemic Disorders

Many chronic diseases of children may interfere with normal growth. The severity of the growth failure is related to both the degree to which normal physiology is compromised by the illness and the duration of the illness. Early recognition and correction is usually followed by catch-up growth, however, if the growth failure is severe or prolonged, complete catch-up is not realized.

## Cardiovascular Disease

Growth retardation occurs with an increased frequency in children with all types of congenital heart disease (CHD) (131). In a series of 890 children with a variety of congenital heart lesions, Mehrizi and Drash noted that over half fell below the 16th percentile and 27% were below the 3rd percentile on growth charts for both height and weight, weight being affected slightly more than height (132). Growth failure is more common in children with heart lesions which cause cyanosis (132, 133) and in those with large left to right shunts especially with pulmonary congestion (133). Mehrizi and Drash found the greatest degree of retardation in children with cyanotic heart disease in which both vessels arise from the right ventricle, or in complete transformation of the great vessels (132).

Growth retardation in ventricular septal defects (VSD) with pulmonary hypertention is more severe than in VSD with normal pulmonary pressure (134). Complicated atrial septal defects (ASD) may produce severe growth retardation but simple ostium secundum defects do not affect growth (132). Growth in children with patent ductus arteriosus (PDA) is generally retarded (131), but the cause of the growth retardation is frequently attributed to factors other than the PDA (135, 136). Severe coarctation of the aorta in infancy produces growth failure but milder forms in later life seldom do (131). Children with CHD frequently have extra-cardiac anomalies or a dysmorphic syndrome which may contribute to growth retardation (133–36).

Correction of the cardiovascular defect permits catch-up growth toward normal (Figure 9-8). Success of catch-up growth is related to (a) age at which correction is accomplished, (b) achievement of normal cardiovascular physiology, and (c) the underlying cause of the congenital defect. Early surgical intervention allows the best catch-up growth (131). Greatest improvement in growth has been reported after correction of pulmonary stenosis while the least has been seen after correction of coarctation of the aorta (132). When correction of the defect fails to correct the hypoxemia, growth failure is not appreciably improved (133).

## Respiratory Disease

Since oxygen is required for normal growth and the lungs represent the only source of oxygen, it seems self-evident that disease of the lung will cause growth failure, but in many lung diseases it is difficult to separate the effect on growth of chronic hypoxemia from other contributing factors. Growth is clearly deficient in the child with *cystic fibrosis* who has severe

CONGENITAL HEART DISEASE

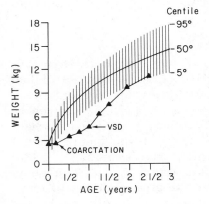

**Figure 9-8.** Infant of normal weight at term birth. Congestive heart failure at 3 weeks from *coarctation* of aorta and *VSD*. Repair of coarctation at 2 months with improvement in growth, but through the first year failed to achieve normal growth. VSD with pulmonary hypertension repaired at 13 months with subsequent catch-up growth. (Courtesy of Dr. Mark Boucek.)

obstructive lung disease, but the child with cystic fibrosis also has chronic lung infection and maldigestion from a pancreatic defect. One cannot attribute the growth failure to hypoxemia without considering the roles of malnutrition and infection as well. Growth failure in chronic *bronchiectasis* may well represent at least an equal effect of infection and hypoxemia. Only in *chronic, partial airway obstruction* such as that seen in the Robin anomaly or obstructive sleep apnea do we approach pure hypoxemia as a cause of growth failure (137), but even here, whether the growth deficiency is related to inadequate caloric intake, excessive caloric expenditure from labored breathing, or hypoxemia is not known (137). Improvement of both airway and food intake are necessary to achieve better growth.

*In children with asthma,* growth deficiency and delayed maturation may result from either chronic hypoxemia or corticosteroid therapy. Growth is delayed in 6–10% of children with asthma, related generally to severity of the disease (138), although Ferguson et al. found impaired linear growth associated with the atopic state and not the severity of the asthma (139). If the asthma requires intermittent steroid therapy, the number of growth-retarded children increases and if continuous steroids are required up to 50% suffer from growth retardation (138, 140). In a child with severe asthma growth may be adversely affected by respiratory insufficiency, dietary inadequacy, chronic or recurrent infections, and by drugs required to control the asthma (138).

Catch-up growth can be achieved during remission from the asthmatic symptoms providing corticosteroid therapy can be reduced or discontinued. Persistence of asthma tends to slow or prevent full catch-up growth (140). If corticosteroids are not required, the delay in growth is temporary and does not affect ultimate height, although the weight spurt of adolescence is delayed and some remain thin into adulthood (141). If the severity of the asthma requires continuous use of corticosteroids, the recovery of growth potential is less likely and permanent stunting of growth may occur (140).

## Renal Disease

Growth deficiency may be the initial complaint leading to discovery of renal disease. It is characteristic not only of glomerular disease, but of diseases of the proximal tubule (142) and of nephrogenic diabetes insipidus as well. With the success of hemodialysis and renal transplantation, growth failure has become the "single most important problem in the clinical management of uremic children" (143). Reduction in statural height is greatest in children with congenital renal disease, in those with kidney anomalies, or in inherited renal disorders, but height is below the 3rd percentile in approximately one-third to one-half of all uremic children and velocity of growth is below the 3rd percentile in over half. Puberty is usually delayed as is skeletal maturation (143, 144) (Figure 9-9).

Growth failure is symmetric except for the deformity produced by renal osteodystrophy which in some children contributes appreciably to the short stature (145). Although superficially resembling rickets, renal osteodystrophy is histologically and biochemically a distinct disorder. In chronic renal failure, metabolism of Vitamin D to $1,25(OH)_2D$ is decreased resulting in decreased intestinal absorption of calcium, limited skeletal remodeling, and decreased endochondral bone formation at the epiphyses. Hypocalcemia and hyperphosphatemia lead to elevation of parathyroid hormone (PTH), which promotes osteoclastic activity and fibrosis beneath the growth plate. Uremia itself, interferes with cartilage formation. Rapid growth and remodeling of the bones in children renders them more susceptible to the biochemical and hormonal disturbances which occur with progressive renal insufficiency (146).

There is good evidence that the profound acidosis resulting from bicarbonate wasting in children with renal tubular acidosis (RTA) is a cause of growth failure, (143, 144, 147) although the effect on growth may not be the acidosis itself but the loss of electrolytes such as sodium, potassium, and calcium (144). Correction of the acidosis in RTA with bicarbonate results in impressive catch-up growth (147). Chronic hyperchloremic metabolic acidosis itself may also impair growth, however, the contribution of the less severe acidosis seen in chronic renal insufficiency to growth failure is not as certain (147).

Growth hormone levels are normal in children with renal failure (143). Somatomedins have been reported to be low, normal, or high (148). It is not clear whether somatomedin levels are influenced in a specific way by renal insufficiency; whether there may be circulating somatomedin inhibitors, or whether there may be lack of end organ response in uremia (148), but low levels of somatomedin have been noted in end-stage renal disease with normalization of levels after kidney transplantation (148).

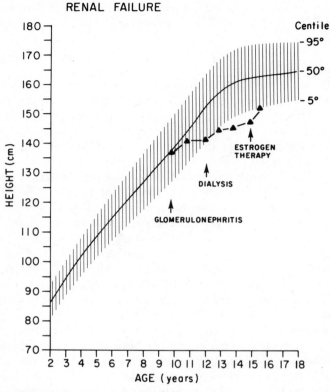

**Figure 9-9.**    Effect of renal disease on growth is shown in the growth chart of girl with renal failure from chronic glomerulonephritis. Growth acceleration was short-lived with dialysis, but noticeable growth spurt did occur when she was given estrogens to stimulate sexual development at age 15. (Courtesy of Dr. Richard Siegler.)

Azotemia per se seems not to be correlated directly with growth deficiency (143). Decreased caloric intake and protein loss during chronic dialysis appear to be correlated with growth deficiency (143), however, although food supplementation seems to exert a salutary effect on the state of nutrition in renal failure, it fails to reverse the growth retardation (144). The use of steroids in children with nephrosis or glomerulonephritis and children with transplanted kidneys in dosages which will achieve the desired therapeutic effect will usually interfere with growth (149). Alternate day therapy causes less growth suppression than does daily therapy, but steroid therapy, even when restricted to alternate days may inhibit growth and cause bone demineralization in children with kidney disease (149). Catch-up growth is generally seen after cessation of steroid therapy, although it may be incomplete when therapy has been prolonged (149).

Transplantation or dialysis, though improving renal status, does not guarantee catch-up growth because the use of steroids is necessary to maintain viability of the transplant and steroids interfere with growth (Figure 9-9). Both with chronic peritoneal dialysis and with hemodialysis, decreased growth velocity is the rule, though there is a wide variation in individual childen (144, 150). If renal osteodystrophy is responsible for the growth deficiency some relief may be expected from treatment with Vitamin D or parathyroidectomy. There are many reasons why growth may be stunted in renal insufficiency but very few measures which can bring relief. It is seldom possible to assure a child with renal failure the prospect of normal growth (143, 144).

### Anemia

In an early report on *congenital hypoplastic anemia*, Hughes named growth deficiency as the most common associated physical anomaly but noted urinary tract, skeletal, and anterior abdominal wall muscle anomalies as well, suggesting that hypoplastic anemia and growth deficiency may be manifestations of a congenital syndrome of multiple defects (151). In a later review of growth retardation with congenital hypoplastic anemia, Diamond et al. considered intermittent anemia and hemosiderosis, especially of endocrine organs, as likely causes of the growth retardation (152). On occasion intrauterine growth retardation occurs with hypoplastic anemia, however, growth failure more commonly becomes noticeable in early childhood. Delayed skeletal maturation is usual, as is delayed or "suspended" pubertal development (153). Growth hormone deficiency, reported in some children with Fanconi's anemia, represents a potentially correctable growth deficiency; however, variable response to human growth hormone has been reported. Norden et al. recently reported a noticeable growth spurt with combined growth hormone and anabolic steroid therapy (154).

Growth deficiency is also seen in children with sickle cell anemia and thalassemia major. Children with *sickle cell anemia* have decreased height and weight, but have normal skinfold thickness; puberty is delayed but normal (155). The factors responsible for the growth failure in children with sickle cell anemia are not known. There is no relationship of the growth failure to degree of anemia, frequency of sickling crises, or frequency of respiratory infections. Although tissue anoxia has been suggested, it has not been proven (156). In *thalassemia major*, stunting of growth is almost invariable after the first decade of life. It has been ascribed to chronic tissue hypoxia due to the severe anemia. Improvement in growth has been noted with vigorous transfusion treatment; however, damage to the endocrine system (especially pancreas and adrenals) by iron deposition within the organs may also contribute to the growth failure (157).

### Chronic infections

Chronic or recurrent infections by themselves may affect weight gain in children but have a lesser effect on linear growth. Growth failure has not usually been demonstrable unless specific organ function is also affected; for example, the kidney in pyelonephritis or the lung in bronchiectasis. In most instances, it is difficult to separate the effect of the infection from that of organ dysfunction. When the infection is cleared, weight is rapidly regained.

### Hepatic Insufficiency

Severe growth deficiency can accompany liver failure with hepatic cirrhosis. Anorexia and malnutrition often complicate the growth failure in chronic liver disease. Recovery from severe liver damage is often not possible and growth failure becomes a moot question. Reduced serum somatomedin activity has been noted in liver failure. Whether this is because of the liver failure or the accompanying malnutrition is not known (158).

### Collagen Vascular Disease

Growth deficiency is a frequent complaint in juvenile rheumatoid arthritis especially in the severe, generalized form. It is also fairly common in children with dermatomyositis or systemic lupus erythematosus (SLE). Most of these disorders respond to treatment with corticosteroids and though the manifestations of the disease can often be controlled with corticosteroids, growth may be curtailed because of the growth suppressing effects of the medication (159) (Figure 9-14).

## Endocrine Disorders

### Hypothyroidism

Hypothyroidism is one of the most common endocrine disorders in childhood. In the neonatal period, hypothyroidism is usually caused by congenital absence or hypoplasia of the thyroid, although chronic lymphocytic thyroiditis accounts for most of the hypothyroidism occurring in childhood and adolescence (160). In addition to thyroiditis, primary hypothyroidism may be seen in children with ectopic (lingual) thyroids, thyroxine synthesis defects (goitrous hypothyroidism), thyroidectomy for tumor or Graves' disease, and in disorders in which the thyroid tissue is replaced by invading tumor tissue (histiocytosis, lymphoma, etc). Hypothyroidism, secondary to hypothalamic or pituitary deficiency, accounts for about 15% of hypothyroidism in children. Table 9-5 displays the relative frequency of childhood hypothyroidism by cause seen at the University of Oregon from 1975 to 1978 (160) and at the University of Utah from 1976 to 1981.

Congenital hypothyroidism occurs with the frequency of 1 in 4000 births. No such figures of incidence are available for acquired hypothyroidism, since many are not reported. Among children seen in referral

Table 9-5. **Frequency of Childhood Hypothyroidism
by Cause**

| Cause of Hypothyroidism | University of Oregon 1975–1978[a] | University of Utah 1976–1981 |
|---|---|---|
| *Primary* | | |
| Lymphocytic thyroiditis | 28 | 72 |
| Thyroxine synthesis defect | 3 | 7 |
| Ectopic thyroid glands | 2 | 2 |
| Miscellaneous | 3 | 2 |
| Total | 36 | 83 |
| *Secondary* | | |
| Pituitary tumor | 4 | 8 |
| Pituitary trauma | 1 | 2 |
| Idiopathic pituitary deficiency | 1 | 6 |
| Total | 6 | 16 |

[a] Taken by permission from LaFranchi. *Pediatr Clin North Am* **26:**33, 1979.

clinics, acquired hypothyroidism appears to be about twice as common as congenital hypothyroidism (160). Since most acquired hypothyroidism is the result of chronic lymphocytic thyroiditis, some idea of its frequency may be derived from the frequency of chronic lymphocytic thyroiditis in childhood. We discovered 62 cases of lymphocytic thyroditis in a survey of 5179 school age children (prevalence of 1.2%) (161). Of these 62 cases of lymphocytic thyroiditis, 10% were hypothyroid (162). We assume that some of the remaining cases will eventually become hypothyroid (163), although spontaneous recovery to normal occurred in approximately half of the 62 with lymphocytic thyroiditis (162). Autoimmune thyroiditis is seen with increased frequency in Down's, Turner's, and Klinefelter's syndromes and in association with diabetes mellitus, Addison's disease, congenital rubella, and toxoplasmosis (160).

Hypothyroidism in childhood or adolescence may be insidious in onset. The most common presenting complaints are growth failure and enlarged thyroid, although anemia or slipped capital femoral epiphyses have provided the clue to hypothyroidism in several children presenting with growth failure to our clinics. Common clinical features of hypothyroidism in childhood are presented in Table 9-6. The child is frequently short and has a stocky appearance. Measurements of body proportion will often show a disproportionately short lower segment (legs). While standing, the child may have a protuberant abdomen and exaggerated lordosis. Weight may be heavy for height due to myxedema, although obesity is not common. Skin may be dry, thick and cool and the child may have a "sallow appearance" (carotenemia, anemia, and intercellular fluid accu-

### Table 9-6. Clinical Features of Hypothyroidism in Children

#### Symptoms

| | |
|---|---|
| Slow growth | Puffiness of face |
| Pallor | Lethargy |
| Poor school performance | Cold intolerance |
| Metrorrhagia or galactorrhea | Fullness of neck |

#### Signs

| | |
|---|---|
| Dry, coarse hair | Short stature |
| Puffiness of eyelids (face) | Decreased growth velocity |
| Low hoarse voice | Stocky appearance |
| Bradycardia | Short lower segment for age |
| Decreased pulse pressure | Dull, placid expression |
| Flabby musculature | Pale, thick, cool skin |
| Delayed deep tendon reflex return | Sallow appearance |

mulation tend to give the skin a pale, yellowish hue). The face has a full or puffy appearance. The hair may be coarse and dry and the muscles flabby, although in some instances myxedematous infiltrate may give the muscles a firm or hypertrophied appearance. Deep tendon reflexes relax slowly. In lymphocytic thyroiditis the thyroid gland is enlarged and of firm consistency with a granular or pebbly surface often with palpable lymph nodes near the gland.

The insidious changes of myxedema in the facial features can be appreciated in photographs of a girl observed in our clinic for acquired hypothyroidism due to lymphocytic thyroiditis (Figure 9-10). Her presenting complaint was growth deficiency. She displayed puffiness of the face, dry skin, delayed skeletal maturation, low serum thyroxine, and elevated TSH. The contribution of hypothyroidism to her appearance is shown dramatically by changes occurring after therapy with thyroxine was instituted. The insidious facial changes of hypothyroidism can be seen beginning at about age 6; after institution of therapy at age 10, there was a rapid return to normal (Figure 9-10).

On occasion, acquired hypothyroidism may be associated with precocious puberty. In girls, premature breast development, galactorrhea, and even vaginal spotting may be seen, and in boys, testicular enlargement, which regresses after treatment with thyroid medication. These phenomenona may result from elevation of gonadotropins and prolactin, accompanying the elevation of TSH caused by the hypothyroidism (hormonal overlap) (164), or from a decreased clearance rate of sex steroids. Hypothyroidism due to hypothalamic–pituitary deficiency is usually mild and commonly presents simply as growth deficiency. These children seldom present with signs or symptoms of hypothyroidism, although an associated deficiency of ACTH and human growth hormone may cause hypoglycemia (165). If a tumor of the hypothalamus or pituitary is the cause of the

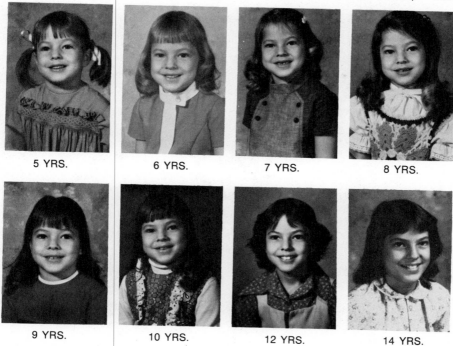

**Figure 9-10.** Serial photos of girl with acquired hypothyroidism (thyroiditis) showing facial changes of hypothyroidism beginning as early as 6 years accompanied by slowdown in growth. Diagnosis made at age 10. Dramatic changes in facial features are seen after beginning thyroid therapy.

pituitary–thyroid deficiency neurologic signs may provide the clue to the cause of the hypothyroidism.

In children with acquired hypothyroidism, the bone-age will be delayed, if the hypothyroidism is of sufficient duration, and epiphyseal dysgenesis may be seen. If hypothyroidism is of long duration, there will be extreme delay in skeletal maturation and possibly loss of potential height. Anemia may be present and is usually normocytic with bone marrow hypoplasia. Cholesterol may be elevated as may also serum carotene. In the EKG, low voltage and prolonged PR interval may be seen with flat or inverted T waves. Thyroxine ($T_4$) will be low in all children with hypothyroidism and $T_3RU$ will generally be low as well. TSH will be elevated in primary hypothyroid disorders, but will be low or normal with pituitary-hypothalamic disorders. If pituitary deficiency is the cause of hypothyroidism, there will be deficient response of TSH to TRH administration (see Chapter 7). In lymphocytic thyroiditis there will generally be elevation of antithyroid antibodies (162, 166). In thyroxine synthesis defects TSH will be elevated and radioiodine uptake will be characteristically elevated.

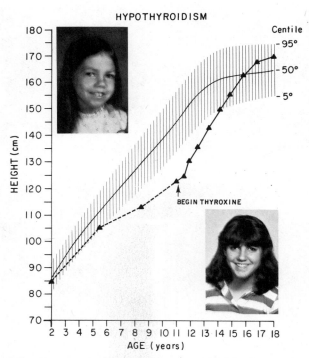

**Figure 9-11.** Growth record in a girl with acquired hypothyroidism (thyroiditis). Slowing down of growth is seen after age 6. Appearance at age 11 when diagnosis of hypothyroidism was made shows delayed maturity, fullness of face, and puffiness of eyes (mild myxedema). Catch-up growth after beginning thyroxine therapy was rapid and consistent throughout adolescence reaching a final height above the 50th percentile. Maturity of facial features is shown in photo at age 18.

Treatment of acquired hypothyroidism requires daily thyroxine therapy. The average dosage of l-thyroxine during the second year of life is 5–6 μg/kg of body weight with a decrease to 4–5 μg/kg/day during early childhood and 3–4 μg/kg/day in later childhood and adolescence (167). Adequate therapy should produce reversal of all symptoms, loss of myxedematous puffiness, and catch-up growth (Figure 9-11). If the period of hypothyroidism extends into the adolescent period, rapid pubertal development is usually seen, however, complete catch-up growth is sometimes not achieved before epiphyses are closed and some potential growth is lost.

Brain development is not affected by acquired hypothyroidism, at least after age 2, but lethargy and poor school performance may be complaints of school age children with acquired hypothyroidism. Recovery of activity level will usually result in better school performance. We have also seen the opposite effect of treatment in school age children. Although slow in school, many hypothyroid children receive good grades because they are persistent and patient in performing assigned tasks (if speed is not demanded or expected). With treatment, such children become more active, with a decrease in attention span resulting in poor school performance, in many cases from good to failing grades. Hyperactive behavior at home may likewise become intolerable when compared to the complacent, compliant hypothyroid state, and it may be necessary to begin with suboptimal thyroid dosage and work up gradually to full replacement dosage allowing child, school, and home to adapt to the return to "normal" status.

### Hypopituitarism

In hypopituitarism, linear growth is retarded so that the velocity of growth is below normal. Growth deficiency is not evident at birth but may be present as early as 3–6 months of age (6). Smith reports that about one-third of growth hormone deficient infants show deceleration of linear growth by 1 year and 75% by 4 years (168). Deceleration in growth beginning in later childhood is usually associated with specific lesions of the pituitary or hypothalamus. Height achievement falls progressively further behind expected levels so there is progressive deviation away from normal range on a growth chart.

Body proportions remain normal, although the general appearance of the child is younger than his/her chronologic age. The face is immature with a short nose and anteverted nostrils, a small mandible, and shallow malar eminences (168). Patients tend to be overweight for their height, with the excess fat deposition concentrated over the trunk (6). The overall appearance has been described as "doll-like" or "cherubic" (Figure 9-12). Although usually of normal intelligence, unless central nervous system damage is responsible for the hypopituitarism, children with hypopituitarism tend to be emotionally infantile exhibiting characteristics of dependency and withdrawal. Most youngsters have a high pitched voice, narrow shoulders, and are relatively weak. The penis is small in males and cryptorchidism occurs in about 20% (17). Micropenis together with hypoglycemia may direct attention to congenital hypopituitarism (see Chapter 8). Deficiency of TSH rarely produces obvious symptoms of hypothyroidism, although low thyroxine levels may be found by testing. ACTH deficiency may contribute to hypoglycemia and poor tolerance of physical stress or illness although adrenal crises with hypovolemia and shock are rare (169).

Growth hormone deficiency is an uncommon cause of growth deficiency. From a survey of children in Newcastle-upon-Tyne, Parkin estimates the incidence of growth hormone deficiency to be about 1 in 30,000 births (1). Growth hormone deficiency may result from disorders of the hypothalamus or pituitary as well as by peripheral insensitivity or soma-

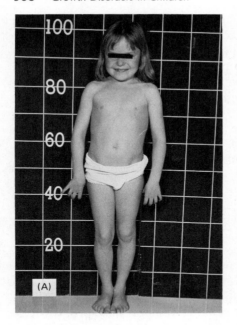

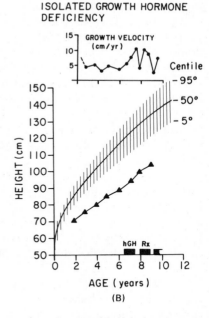

**Figure 9-12.** Isolated human growth deficiency in a 9-year-old girl showing (A) short stature, "cherubic" facial appearance, normal body proportions, and tendency to fat accumulation on torso. (B) Increase in growth velocity after treatment with growth hormone.

tomedin deficiency as listed in Table 9-7. Craniopharyngioma, although a growth of embryonic tissue, is listed among acquired hypothalamic lesions because of the later onset of symptoms and growth failure. Somatomedin deficiencies, responsible for most of the peripheral insensitivity to human growth hormone, will be discussed separately. Idiopathic growth hormone deficiency, which may be due to an abnormality at the level of the hypothalamus or pituitary, is more common than deficiency due to a specific lesion such as craniopharyngioma. In Tanner's series, 18 of 56 subjects with growth hormone deficiency had craniopharyngiomas and 38 had idiopathic growth hormone deficiency (46). Root et al. reported 21 subjects with idiopathic hypopituitarism and 7 with intracranial neoplasia (170). Overall, idiopathic hypopituitarism seems to occur about 2 to 3 times as often as hypopituitarism due to a specific lesion of the pituitary or hypothalamus. Cranial irradiation for CNS tumor or leukemia may produce a growth hormone deficiency and decreased growth velocity (171). It is felt by some that a functional deficiency of GH secretion is caused by the irradiation, curtailing growth while still allowing release of hGH to pharmacologic stimuli (172). Lesions of the hypothalamus or pituitary are likely to produce multiple pituitary deficiencies. Craniophar-

## Table 9-7. Causes of Hypopituitarism

A. *Disorders of the Hypothalamus*
   1. Congenital
      - (a) Absence of growth-hormone releasing factor
      - (b) Syndrome of midline defects, (cleft lip and palate, anosmia, diabetes insipidus)
      - (c) Anencephaly
   2. Acquired
      - (a) Craniopharyngioma
      - (b) Infections (encephalitis, meningitis)
      - (c) Trauma (birth injury, intracranial hemorrhage, hypoxia)
      - (d) Neoplasia (meningioma, ependymoma, metastatic carcinoma)
      - (e) Granuloma (histiocytosis, sarcoidosis, tuberculosis)
      - (f) Emotional deprivation
   3. Idiopathic
B. *Disorders of the Pituitary*
   1. Congenital
      - (a) Congenital absence of pituitary
      - (b) Congenital insensitivity to GHRF
   2. Acquired
      - (a) Vascular Insufficiency
         - (1) Trauma (birth injury or head injury with transection of pituitary stalk)
         - (2) Postpartum hypotension
         - (3) Arteriosclerosis
      - (b) Neoplasia
         - (1) Adenoma, carcinoma (primary or metastatic)
         - (2) Multiple myelomatous infiltration
      - (c) Allergic Hypophysitis
      - (d) Granuloma (histiocytosis, sarcoidosis, tuberculosis)
      - (e) Aneurysm of internal carotid artery
      - (f) Iatrogenic
         - (1) Irradiation
         - (2) Hypophysectomy
   3. Idiopathic
C. *Peripheral Insensitivity to Human Growth Hormone*
   1. Growth hormone receptor deficiency (?)
      (Laron dwarf)
   2. Somatomedin Inhibitors
      (Malnutrition, renal disease, psychosocial deprivation)
   3. End organ resistance
      (pigmy, Turner's syndrome)

Reproduced by permission, Adapted from Root AW, Bongiovanni AM, Eberlein WR: Diagnosis and management of growth retardation with special reference to the problem of hypopituitarism. *J Pediatr* **78**:737, 1971.

yngioma, the most common acquired lesion of the hypothalamus, generally causes panhypopituitarism, while histiocytosis may produce spotty deficiencies (173). Congenital midline defects such as septo-optic dysplasia also commonly result in multiple pituitary deficiencies (growth retardation, hypogylcemia, micropenis).

### Isolated Growth Hormone Deficiency

This is the most common deficiency pattern observed. Idiopathic hypopituitarism and isolated hGH deficiency are assumed to represent functional defects in the hypothalamus or pituitary, but they can seldom be demonstrated. Using growth hormone releasing factor, Grossman et al. have recently demonstrated a hypothalamic defect in growth hormone release, accounting for growth failure in some subjects with idiopathic growth hormone deficiency (174). Goodman et al. reported sixteen cases of isolated growth hormone deficiency in thirty-five subjects with idiopathic pituitary deficiency. Of the remainder, eight displayed full anterior pituitary deficiency and 11 combinations of growth hormone and TSH or growth hormone and ACTH deficiency (175). Tanner found an even higher proportion of children with isolated growth hormone deficiency. Thirty-five out of thirty-eight children with idiopathic hypopituitarism were said to have isolated growth hormone deficiency (46). The frequency of isolated human growth hormone deficiency is of some interest because of their unique growth and maturation pattern (Figure 9-12). Contrary to the subject with total anterior pituitary deficiency who will remain sexually infantile indefinitely, subjects with isolated growth hormone deficiency grow slowly throughout childhood and the usual adolescent period, but sometime in the third decade of life undergo pubertal changes with a modest growth spurt and attain a short adult height with normal appearing sexual development and normal procreative capability (171).

*Diagnosis.* Basal growth hormone levels normally range from 0 to 10 ng/mL. The diagnosis of growth hormone deficiency can ony be made by demonstrating suboptimal release of growth hormone after physiologic or pharmacologic stimulation. Exercise, sleep, estrogen, L-dopa, or clonidine have been used to screen slow-growing youngsters for growth hormone deficiency. Failure to obtain growth hormone levels of 7 ng/mL or more by these stimuli suggests the need for definitive stimulation with L-dopa, arginine, glucagon, clonidine, or insulin. Details of the tests for human growth hormone release are found in Chapter 7. Since none of the tests produce 100% positive results in normal children, it is customary to perform at least two definitive tests of human growth hormone release to assure an accurate and reliable diagnosis of growth hormone deficiency. Suboptimal responses of growth hormone release are commonly seen in primary hypothyroidism, Cushing's disease, obesity, deprivation syndrome, chronic malnutrition, and constitutional delayed growth. Caution should be exercised in making the diagnosis of growth hormone deficiency until each of these states has been taken into consideration or corrected (168).

If growth hormone levels are found to be deficient, testing of the remainder of the anterior and posterior pituitary hormones should be pursued. Thyroid function may be assessed by measurement of $T_4$ and TSH levels and by the TSH response to TRH. Adrenal function may be assessed by measurement of cortisol after hypoglycemia or by measuring 11-deoxycortisol, cortisol, and ACTH after metyrapone. Tests of adrenal function are particularly important if there is a history of hypoglycemia. Gonadotrophin levels (serum or urine FSH and LH) may be measured, but will be of little diagnostic value until the usual age of puberty. Simultaneous urine and serum osmolalities, response of urine volume and urine and serum osmolality to water deprivation, or response to vasopression may be necessary to evaluate posterior pituitary involvement (see Chapter 7).

With no normonal supplements, subjects with growth hormone deficiency grow slowly throughout childhood, deviating progressively from expected growth channels. Bone maturation follows a similar delay so that height age usually equals bone age and both are delayed to about half the expected growth velocity. There is no spontaneous sexual development and the child becomes a young-looking adult but with changes in skin and face suggesting aging—a "young–old" appearance (Figure 9-13).

*Treatment.*    For intracranial lesions, such as craniopharyngioma and other neoplasia, surgical removal must be undertaken. Some investigators have reported accelerated linear growth rates in patients following removal of a craniopharyngioma despite undetectable or low human growth hormone levels (176, 177). Excessive growth after craniopharyngioma is thought by Bucher et al. to be caused by excess insulin associated with hyperphagia and obesity due to the hypothalamic lesion (178). In patients with normal rates of growth after operation, they found elevated prolactin and normal IGF (somatomedin) levels and postulated that the normal growth rate was a result of normal IGF (somatomedin) stimulated by prolactin (178). Most of the other intracranial lesions, such as trauma, or encephalitis, are static and not correctable.

For most growth hormone deficiency states, treatment consists of hormone replacement. Growth hormone may be administrated intramuscularly two to three times per week in dosages of 0.06–0.1 units per kilogram per dose (6, 171). Higher dosages have been used by Tanner (20–40 units/week), who claims some enhanced effectiveness with higher dosages (46). To allow access to hormone for as many youngsters as possible, the lowest effective dose is usually preferred (6, 179). A combination of hGH and oxandrolone has also been tried, but has met with only modest success. The anabolic steroid may diminish the "waning"

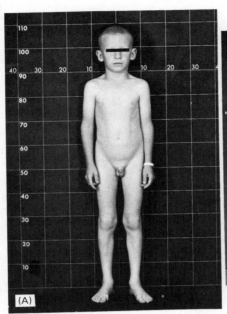
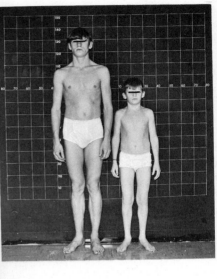

## IDIOPATHIC PITUITARY DEFICIENCY

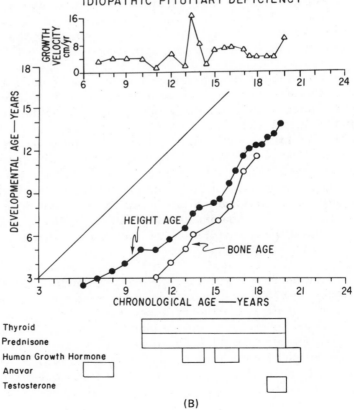

(B)

effect often seen with hGH therapy after the initial growth spurt. Acceleration in skeletal maturation prompted the authors to advise caution in the use of oxandrolone as an adjunct to treatment with hGH (180).

There is some decrease in subcutaneous fat initially, with an increase in lean body mass (46). An initial growth acceleration of two to three times the pretreatment level (from 3 to 6–9 cm/yr on the average) can be expected (46, 171). The increased growth rate is reflected in increases in GH-induced increments in somatomedin levels (181). In subsequent years velocity of growth falls (waning), although generally remains above the pretreatment level until catch-up growth has been accomplished. Some authors have suggested periodic "drug holidays" to counter the deterioration in treatment response (180). Cessation of treatment results in a near cessation of growth; therefore, treatment, once started, should continue till the end of childhood (46).

When the bone-age approaches the usual age of adolescence, a pubertal growth spurt may be enhanced by simultaneous administration of gonadal steroids (estrogen or testosterone) with human growth hormone. Testosterone enanthate 50–200 mg intramuscularly every 3–4 weeks may be used for boys and conjugated estrogen (0.3–1.25 mg/day) or ethinyl-estradiol (50–80 µg/day) may be used as estrogens for girls with medroxy-progesterone, 10 mg/day for 6 days, added at monthly intervals to produce menstrual cycles. For control of diabetes insipidus, pitressin-tannate in oil 0.25–0.5 mL intramuscularly every 48–72 hours or nasal DDAVP in a dosage of 0.025–0.1 mL every 8–12 hours are effective.

Many patients treated with human growth hormone have developed antibodies against the preparation and on occasion inhibition of growth is seen (171, 179). Suboptimal response to human growth hormone is seen in hypothyroid subjects. Plasma somatomedin C concentrations are diminished in hypothyroidism as a result of diminished growth hormone secretion or of decreased somatomedin production due to the hypothyroidism (182). Thyroid status must be determined before treatment with human growth hormone, and if hypothyroidism is found, it should be corrected before beginning human growth hormone therapy. Thyroid may be administered as a therapeutic trial to patients with suboptimal linear growth response to human growth hormone (171). Corticosteroids inhibit growth hormone action and when used in treatment of pituitary deficiency should be given

←

**Figure 9-13.** Idiopathic pituitary deficiency in one of identical twins. In the left panel (A) at age 14 before beginning growth hormone therapy we see short stature, immature facial features, sexual infantilism, and normal body proportions. In right panel (A) the subject is shown with his normal twin at age 16. Response to treatment with hGH and other pituitary replacement therapy is shown in chart (B) displaying developmental achievement (height-age and bone-age) versus chronologic-age. Some acceleration of growth and skeletal maturation is seen with growth hormone and at age 19 with added testosterone.

only in physiologic dosage (12–15 mg/M$^2$/day of hydrocortisone). For mineralocorticoid effect 9-alpha-fluorohydrocortisone 0.05–0.2 mg/day may be used.

There are very few side effects from administration of human growth hormone. Local tenderness or urticaria is occasionally noted at the injection sites, and on occasion, we have noted some general irritability. Increased seizure activity was seen in one subject with craniopharyngioma, although we have not been certain of the cause.

Recently three deaths were reported in subjects receiving hGH injections. The subjects died of a progressive CNS deterioration (Creutzfeldt-Jakob disease) caused by a slow-acting virus, thought to be introduced via the hGH injections. Current preparations of growth hormone from human pituitaries are being scrupulously examined to remove all viral contamination. Use of synthetic hGH will, of course, obviate contamination by CNS viruses.

Human growth hormone is of proven efficacy in treatment of growth hormone deficiency states, but is of variable or uncertain value in other syndromes of short stature. Growth hormone is ineffective in youngsters with genetic short stature, including familial short stature and most dysmorphic syndromes (6, 46). Tanner reported minimal effect in children with intrauterine growth retardation and Turner's syndrome (33), but more recent trials have demonstrated some effect in chidren with both Turner's syndrome and intrauterine growth retardation, provided that large doses of human growth hormone are used (47, 48, 90). When human growth hormone is readily available from recombinant DNA synthesis, it may be possible to offer high dose treatment to girls with Turner's syndrome and to selected children with intrauterine growth retardation who fail to show any spontaneous catch-up growth (14, 91). Children with constitutional delayed growth and deprivational dwarfism, treated by Tanner, failed to achieve useful height acceleration with human growth hormone (33), however, recent reports (16–19) suggest that in some youngsters with "short stature normal variant", who grow at a low rate (less than 4 cm/yr), there may be subtle abnormalties of hGH secretion or action or perhaps a biologically inactive growth hormone (14, 183). Such youngsters may show some improvement in growth rates with growth hormone therapy (91).

### Somatomedin Deficiency (Laron Dwarfism)

In 1966, Laron et al. described a syndrome of familial dwarfism, resembling isolated growth hormone deficiency, but associated with high plasma immunoreactive growth hormone (184). Since then, a number of other investigators have reported similar clinical and biochemical features in children with short stature resembling hypopituitarism (185–187). Children with Laron dwarfism exhibit severe growth retardation, "pinched facies," high pitched voice, and small genitalia, if male. They often have

### Table 9-8. Growth Hormone, Somatomedins and Growth Problems

| Clinical Condition | Human Growth Hormone[c] | Somatomedin Activity[d] |
|---|---|---|
| Hypopituitary dwarf | Low | Decreased |
| Laron dwarf[a] | High | Decreased |
| Malnutrition[e] | Normal or high | Decreased |
| Kwashiorkor | High | Decreased |
| Psychosocial deprivation | Variable | Decreased |
| Renal failure[e] | Normal | Decreased |
| Cushing's syndrome[b,e] | Normal | Normal |
| Turner's syndrome[b] | High | Normal |
| Pigmy[f] | High | Decreased |

Reproduced by permission from Van Wyk JJ and Underwood LE: Growth hormone, somatomedins and growth failure. *Hosp Pract* **13**(August): 57–67, 1978.

Reproduced by permission from Phillips LS and Vassilopoulou-Sellin R: Somatomedins (Med Progress). *New Engl J Med* **302**:371–380 and 438–446, 1980.

[a] hGH receptor deficiency.          [d] Serum SmC levels.

[b] End organ resistance.             [e] Inhibition of Sm activity.

[c] Serum hGH levels.                 [f] Impaired synthesis of Sm.

spontaneous hypoglycemic episodes in infancy. Secretion of ACTH, TSH, gonadotrophins, and ADH is normal, although insulin secretion in response to glucose is suboptimal. Random plasma growth hormone levels are normal to well above normal. Plasma somatomedin levels are low and do not respond to administered human growth hormone. The growth failure in Laron dwarfism has been attributed to a growth hormone receptor abnormality in the liver with a failure of somatomedin production (188). In addition to the growth failure, considered to be due to somatomedin deficiency, a lack of response to the metabolic effects of growth hormone has been reported as well (186–189). This suggests a rather general growth hormone receptor deficiency, resulting not only in deficient somatomedin generation but also in a generalized impaired responsiveness to human growth hormone (188, 189).

Somatomedins may be decreased in a number of conditions other than growth hormone deficiency and Laron dwarfism (104). A number of these conditions have been mentioned earlier in this chapter and include malnutrition, renal failure, and psychosocial deprivation. Table 9-8 presents a number of growth deficiency syndromes in which somatomedins have been measured. Inhibitors of somatomedin activity may be responsible for somatomedin deficiency in malnutrition and renal failure. High corticosteroid levels appear to depress both somatomedin activity and production. In Turner's syndrome and in the African pygmy, growth deficiency is considered to represent an end organ failure of response to somatomedins (104, 188).

### Cushing's Syndrome (Excess Cortisol Production)

Cushing's syndrome is a rare cause of growth failure in childhood. Most of the growth failure associated with excess corticosteroids is a result of the use of corticosteroids in treatment of other disorders, discussed in the section on iatrogenic (drug) growth disorders. Cushing's syndrome is caused by abnormally high levels of cortisol (and other corticosteroids). Excess secretion of corticosteroids may be the result of a tumor of the adrenal cortex, of hypersecretion of ACTH from a pituitary adenoma, or a functional hypothalamic defect. Rarely may ACTH be produced by tumors unrelated to the adrenal or pituitary. Hypothalamic or pituitary disorders tend to cause primarily overproduction of cortisol, whereas tumors of the adrenal cortex often produce excesses of androgens, estrogens, and aldosterone as well.

Excess cortisol produces a deceleration of both linear growth and skeletal maturation and an accumulation of adipose tissue over the trunk, neck, and cheeks. The face is rounded, the cheeks prominent and flushed (moon face), and there is accumulation of fat over the dorsum of the upper thorax (buffalo hump) and in the supraclavicular regions. In young children, generalized obesity is common though there remains a tendency for truncal accumulation of adiposity (Figure 9-14). Hypertension is common and may lead to heart failure in the young subject with Cushing's syndrome. Wide, deep purple striae appear in the skin of the arms, abdomen, and thighs, and the fragile skin may bruise and tear with minimal injury. Weakness and increased susceptibility to infection are common. Virilization may occur if excess adrenal androgens are produced. There may be hair over the face, trunk, and pubes, acne, deepening of the voice, and, in girls, enlargement of the clitoris.

In older children, gradual onset of obesity and deceleration of growth may be the earliest manifestations of Cushing's syndrome. Pubertal development may be delayed or, in a girl with menses established, amenorrhea may occur. Weakness, emotional lability, and deterioration in school work may be prominent complaints. Growth impairment by glucocorticoids involves direct inhibition of growing cartilage, decreased release of human growth hormone, and blunting of growth stimulation by growth hormone (190). The antagonism of growth hormone action appears to involve a decrease in both somatomedin action and somatomedin production (104). The usual physiologic increases in cortisol which occur with stress and illness do not appear to inhibit somatomedin effect on cartilage (104).

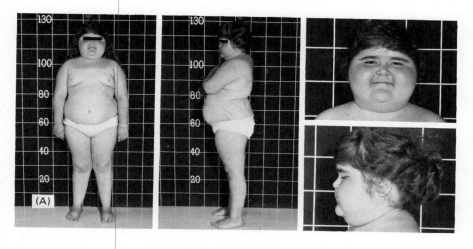

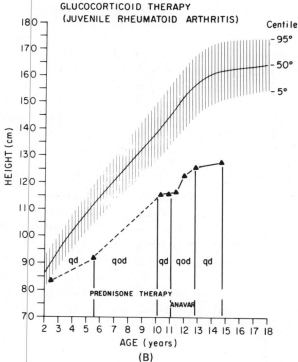

**Figure 9-14.** Cushing's syndrome in a girl treated with prednisone for juvenile rheumatoid arthritis. Photos (A) show pronounced fat accumulation in face, supraclavicular area, and on the trunk. Stiae are present over lower abdomen, flanks, and thighs. Growth slows noticeably (B) during periods of daily prednisone therapy (qd). Resumption of normal growth rate (catch-up growth) occurs with alternate day prednisone therapy (qod) and anavar supplementation.

Cushing's syndrome should be considered as a cause of growth failure if deceleration or cessation of linear growth is seen in a child who is becoming obese and shows other clinical signs of corticosteroid excess. Cortisol levels are usually high in the serum (over 24 $\mu$g/dL in the early morning) and fail to show the usual diurnal rhythm (high in the a.m., low in the p.m.). Free cortisol excretion in a 24-hour urine collection is elevated. High levels of serum androgens, particularly dehydroepiandrosterone (DHEA) and dehydroepiandrosterone sulfate (DHEAS), or urinary 17-ketosteroids are frequently found in children with adrenal tumors. Elevated corticosteroid levels fail to decrease when the child is given dexamethasone. In a normal individual, a single dose of 1 mg of dexamethasone at midnight will suppress the morning serum cortisol level to less than 6 $\mu$g/dL, but the 8 a.m. cortisol level in all forms of Cushing's syndrome will remain elevated. To distinguish adrenal tumors from hypothalamic–pituitary disorders, dexamethasone is administered every 6 hours for 2 days in a dosage 0.5 mg/dose for adults (5 $\mu$g/kg every 6 hours for children) (191) and on the second day urinary free cortisol, urinary 17-OH corticosteroids, or plasma cortisol (other steroids as indicated) are measured. This is followed by 2 days of high dose dexamethasone; 2 mg (20 $\mu$g/kg for children) every 6 hours. Plasma corticoid levels or urinary corticoid excretion in normal individuals will be suppressed by the low dosage. In patients with hypothalamic–pituitary Cushing's syndrome, elevated levels will be suppressed by the high dosage; in adrenal cortical tumors, no suppression occurs even with the high dosage.

Removal of an adrenal cortical tumor by surgery results in cure of Cushing's syndrome, but carcinomas frequently metastasize and careful follow-up is essential. There is no ideal treatment of Cushing's disease (pituitary) in children. Bilateral adrenalectomy has been the most employed treatment, but the appearance of Nelson's syndrome (pituitary tumor with hyperpigmentation) (192) is not unusual. Drugs that inhibit steroidogenesis (mitotane, aminoglutethimide) or that act on neurotransmitters (cyproheptadine) have been used in a few children. Irradiation of the pituitary may be effective in some but carries the risk of damage to other pituitary structures. In the hands of an experienced neurosurgeon, transphenoidal microsurgery has been very successful and deserves careful trial in children (193). Following correction of the endocrine excess, catch-up growth can be expected to occur.

### Metabolic Disorders

A number of metabolic disorders or inborn errors of metabolism may affect growth by a variety of mechanisms. In this section we will discuss disorders associated with diabetes mellitus, hypophosphatemic rickets, hypercalcemia, and hypokalemia (galactosemia and glycogen storage diseases are discussed in Chapter 8).

## Diabetes Mellitus

Though most children with diabetes mellitus enjoy normal growth and adolescence, there are a number who experience some delay in both growth and puberty and a few who exhibit marked deceleration in growth accompanied by truncal obesity, round facies, and hepatomegaly. The syndrome of extreme poor growth in diabetes, first described by Mauriac in 1930, generally develops in poorly controlled juvenile diabetes (194). The hepatomegaly is attributed to fatty infiltration and excess glycogen deposition in the liver, secondary to poor diabetic control. The similarities in appearance of children with Mauriac syndrome and Cushing's syndrome has led some to suggest that chronic cortisol excess may serve as the mechanism for the appearance of the child with Mauriac syndrome (195). Although superficially similar, the data do not confirm cortisol excess in Mauriac syndrome. Most of the manifestations disappear when adequate control of the diabetes is achieved.

Diabetics described as in "fair or good" control exhibit normal growth patterns (196), while those in "poor" control may suffer some impairment of growth (197), suggesting that the level of control of diabetes may influence factors determining growth in diabetic children. Insulin affects somatomedin regulation and a deficiency of insulin might be expected to interfere with somatomedin production or activity. Winter et al. reported a relationship between levels of diabetic control (levels of glycohemoglobin) and somatomedin activity suggesting that slowing of linear growth that occurs in children with poorly controlled diabetes may be related to decreased somatomedin activity (198). This relationship has been examined by others with somewhat tentative conclusions. Rudolf et al. noted acceleration of growth velocity in children who achieved near normal glucose control with pump therapy (and an increase in insulin delivery), but did not measure somatomedin activity (199). In an examination of effects on somatomedin levels of puberty and blood glucose control, Blithen et al. noted deterioration of control of diabetes in adolescence with lack of adolescent rise in somatomedin, which is usually seen with onset of puberty (200). In poorly controlled diabetes Lanes et al. showed blunted somatomedin response to GH administration (201).

Though the studies are not yet conclusive, it appears that control of diabetes does influence somatomedin activity. Deterioration of diabetic control, especially at adolescence, could result in blunting of the adolescent growth spurt and lead to a decrease in ultimate height (200). The key to reversal of the growth deficiency seems to lie in obtaining better control of the diabetes.

## Hypophosphatemic Rickets

Hypophosphatemia and rickets are seen in a wide variety of disorders, most of which are also associated with growth retardation (202).

At one time an almost universal complaint among children living in sunless industrial cities, *Vitamin D deficiency*, is rather uncommon today. Rickets can still be seen in children with decreased dietary intake of Vitamin D or in children denied access to sunshine, however, with the use of cow's milk fortified with Vitamin D and infant formulas containing irradiated ergosterol, dietary deficiency of Vitamin D has been virtually eliminated (203). Very premature infants are still at risk; they seldom receive sufficient Vitamin D from "fortified" formulas and need supplemental Vitamin D. Vitamin D deficiency may also be seen in breast-fed infants whose mothers are strict vegetarians and are themselves deficient in vitamin D (203). Anticonvulsants, particularly phenytoin, phenobarbital, and primidone, are thought to increase the rate of microsomal conversion of 25-hydroxy-Vitamin D to an inactive form (202). Today, rickets is more likely to be seen in children with intestinal malabsorption, liver disease, or in those receiving anticonvulsant therapy (203, 204). Hepatocellular damage can impair 25-hydroxylation of Vitamin D, diminishing production of 1,25-dihydroxycholecalciferol, the active form of Vitamin D, (202). Malabsorption dimishes access to both Vitamin D and calcium. In the nephrotic syndrome, rickets may result from leakage of 25-OH D$_3$ into the urine (205).

Vitamin D deficiency is characterized clinically by hypophosphatemia, hypocalcemia (decreased absorption of calcium from the gut), elevated alkaline-phosphatase, rickets, irritability, muscular weakness, and growth deficiency. Aminoaciduria and phosphaturia are usually present (Table 9-9). Clinically, rickets may be seen in the widening of the metaphyses of long bones, most prominently at the wrists, knees, and ankles; prominence of costochondral rib junctions, an impression at the costal attachment of the diaphragm (Harrison's groove); bowing deformities of long bones, especially those used for weight bearing; bowing of the tibia because of asymmetric muscle pull (saber shin); and frontal bossing of the skull or bulging of the anterior fontanelle (206). Recovery from rickets is rapid with administration of vitamin D$_2$ in dosages of 1000–2000 IU/day and catch-up growth occurs rapidly.

Familial hypophosphatemic rickets takes two forms. *Vitamin D resistant rickets* is an X-linked dominant disorder affecting males more severely than females. The disorder has its onset in infancy, but the rickets may not be discovered until the child begins to learn to walk. The child then displays muscle weakness and bowing of weight-bearing long bones characteristic of rickets (Figure 9-15). In infancy, growth failure, late dentition, deformities of the skull and legs, and disproportionate dwarfism affecting primarily the legs may occur (202). Serum phosphorus is decreased and serum alkaline-phosphatase increased, but serum calcium is normal. Fraser speaks of this as the "phosphopenic" form of Vitamin D refractory rickets (207).

**Table 9-9. Characteristics of Hypophosphatemic Rickets**

|  | *Vitamin D Deficiency Rickets* | *Vitamin D Dependency Rickets* | *Vitamin D Resistant Rickets* |
|---|---|---|---|
| Inheritance pattern | None | Autosomal recessive | X-Linked autosomal dominant |
| **Presentation** |  |  |  |
| Growth retardation | Present | Present | Present |
| Rickets/ weakness | Present | Present | Present |
| **Laboratory findings** |  |  |  |
| Serum Ca | Decreased | Decreased | Normal |
| Serum PO$_4$ | Decreased | Decreased | Decreased |
| Alkaline phosphatase | Elevated | Elevated | Elevated |
| Aminoaciduria | Present | Present | None |
| Urinary PO$_4$ | Increased | Increased | Increased |
| Primary defect | Nutritional deficiency, lack of sun, intestinal malabsorption, 25-OH enzyme deficiency | Deficiency of 1-OH enzyme in liver | Backleak of phosphate from renal tubule |
| Treatment | Cholecalciferol 400–2000 IU/ day or 1,25(OH)$_2$D$_3$ 0.5 μg/day + Good nutrition | Cholecalciferol 10,000–50,000 IU/day or 1 alpha (OH)D$_3$ 1 μg/day or 1,25 (OH)$_2$D$_3$ 1 μg/day | Cholecalciferol 25,000–50,000 IU/day + phosphate supplement 1–2 g/day + high phosphate diet |

Reproduced by permission from Henry D, Elders MJ: Growth retardation syndromes associated with hypophosphatemia. *J Arkansas Med Soc* **74:**481, 1978.

Mild to severe rachitic changes may be seen on x-rays (206). (Figure 9-15) There is widening of the growth plate, under-mineralization, and "fraying" of the trabecular bone in the metaphyseal region. In advanced rickets, there is widening and cupping of the metaphysis. There is a transport defect of phosphate anion, leading to heavy phosphate loss in the urine and severe hypophosphatemia. Serum levels of 25-hydroxy-vitamin D and parathyroid hormone are normal (207). Therapy requires high phosphate supplements to overcome the urinary phosphate losses and to raise serum phosphate levels sufficiently to allow bone mineralization and growth. Foods high in phosphate, such as milk, cheese, eggs,

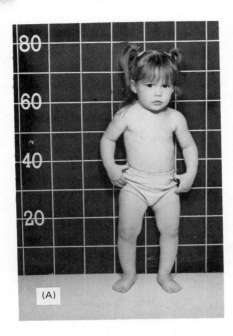

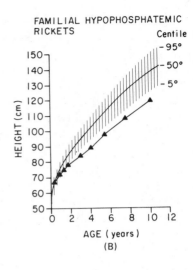

FAMILIAL HYPOPHOSPHATEMIC RICKETS

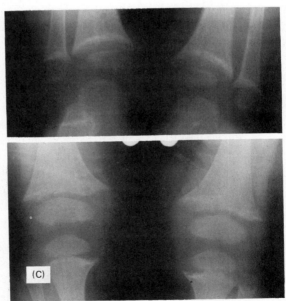

**Figure 9-15.** Child with familial hypophosphatemic rickets at age 2½ (A) showing bowing of lower extremities and swelling of wrists and ankles from metaphyseal flaring. Growth (B) falls below 5th percentile by age 3 and remains below but roughly parallel to 5th percentile through childhood despite treatment with Vitamin D and phosphate supplements. X-rays (C) show poor ossification of growth plates at knee and ankle.

lean meat, beans, and nuts should be encouraged, in addition to which an oral phosphate supplement may be prescribed containing combinations of mono and dibasic sodium and potassium phosphate (Table 9-9).

*Vitamin D dependent rickets* is an autosomal recessive disorder resembling Vitamin D deficiency that occurs despite normal intake of Vitamin D and adequate exposure to sunlight. This disorder has its onset in early infancy with hypotonia (muscular weakness), motor retardation, irritability, seizures or tetany, hypocalcemia, rickets, and enamel hypoplasia of teeth formed postnatally. Males and females are equally affected (202, 207). Laboratory findings are similar to those of Vitamin D deficiency with hypophosphatemia, hypocalcemia, and elevated serum alkaline-phosphatase. Serum PTH levels are elevated and the x-ray findings are characteristic of hyperparathyroidism. There is some increased excretion of urinary phosphate and amino acids. Fraser suggests the name "calciopenic" for this form of familial rickets to distinguish it from the "phosphopenic" Vitamin-D-resistant form (207).

The defect in Vitamin D dependent rickets is a deficient 1-alpha-hydroxylation of vitamin D. Physiologic doses of Vitamin D or 25-hydroxy-vitamin D have no effect, however, complete healing of the rickets occurs with 10,000–50,000 units of vitamin D daily or 1µg of 1,25(OH)$_2$D3 (calcitriol) per day. Once healing has begun there is generally a catch-up growth spurt (Table 9-9).

Hypophosphatemia and rickets may also occur with Fanconi's syndrome in any of its several forms. *Cystinosis* is the most common form of Fanconi's syndrome seen in childhood. In the nephropathic form of this disorder, growth retardation may be seen during the latter part of infancy and radiographic and clinical evidence of rickets are usually present by 2 years of age. Abnormal deposition of cystine crystals in the cornea, conjunctivae, bone marrow, lymph nodes, leukocytes, and internal organs lends to the disorder some of its characteristic findings. Photophobia is usually present; refractive crystalline deposits may be seen in the cornea and conjunctivae. Retinal depigmentation may contribute to the photophobia. Renal tubular loss of bicarbonate leads to metabolic acidosis further compromising growth, which is generally severely affected. Although some relief of the renal tubular acidosis can be achieved with bicarbonate solutions, progressive renal damage usually leads to death by 10 years of age (202, 208). An intermediate variety of cystinosis, beginning in adolescence, has slower progress toward renal insufficiency. Growth through childhood may be delayed or normal (208).

Management of cystinosis or other forms of Fanconi's syndrome with renal tubular acidosis should include correction of the metabolic acidosis and hypokalemia with a sodium/potassium alkalinizing solution such as Shohl's solution which provides 1 mEq of sodium and 1 mEq of potassium per milliliter as a citrate salt. The daily requirement of this solution is 3–10 mEq/kg given in four divided doses. Vitamin D, in dosage of

10,000–25,000 units/day, will lead to healing of rickets. Phosphate salts with calcium supplement may be used either in place of or in combination with reduced Vitamin D dosage. Phosphates must be used cautiously in combination with alkalinizing solutions for fear of triggering tetany (202).

Osteomalacia or rickets may occur in *renal tubular acidosis* (RTA), interfering with normal growth. The pathogenesis of rickets in RTA is usually attributed to hypophosphatamia and acidosis. The acidosis promotes increased release of calcium from bones and loss of calcium in the urine. Hypocalcemia leads to elevated levels of PTH which increasesa the renal excretion of phosphate. Hypophosphatamia ensues, leading to decreased bone mineralization and rickets. Serum phosphate levels return to normal if the acidosis is corrected. The rickets respond either to alkali therapy alone or in combination with small doses of Vitamin D, 2000–5000 units/day (202).

*Hypercalcemia* gives rise to slow growth, together with weakness, hypotonia, anorexia, constipation, and impaired renal function. In our experience, hypercalcemia is most likely to occur in a child being treated with excessive amounts of Vitamin D for rickets or hypoparathyroidism. In such circumstances, adjusting the vitamin D dose is usually sufficient to correct the hypercalcemia and restore normal growth. In other rare disorders, such as hypophosphatasia, William's syndrome or sarcoidosis, use of steroids or other substances to reduce calcium absorption from the gut may be useful. In primary hyperparathyroidism, removal of the hyperfunctioning parathyroid tissue results in correction of the hypercalcemia.

*Hypokalemia* may cause retarded growth, weakness, and impaired renal function. Most hypokalemia is of a transient nature and does not materially affect growth, although the hypokalemia of Bartter's syndrome, renal tubular disease, Cushing's disease, or thyrotoxicosis may be of sufficient severity and duration to interfere with growth. Correction of the underlying disorder will reverse the growth failure due to hypokalemia.

### Iatrogenic Disorders

There are a number of hormones or drugs which, when used for therapy of specific illnesses or disorders, may affect growth. Foremost among the agents currently in use which profoundly affect growth are the steroid hormones; corticosteroids, estrogens, and androgens. Stimulant medications used in the treatment of hyperkinetic children have also been reported to suppress growth. Virtually any agent which must be used for a prolonged period in growing children may have the capacity to influence some aspect of growth, however, we will restrict our discussion to those named above.

*Corticosteroids* are used in pharmacologic dosage for control or treatment of a variety of disorders in children including nephrosis, glomerulonephritis, collagen-vascular diseases, asthma, eczema and a variety of other skin disorders, hypoplastic anemia, and for immunosuppression following kidney or other organ transplants. When used for long term therapy, corticosteroids are capable of retarding growth. The amount of growth retardation encountered with the use of corticosteroids depends upon the type and amount of corticosteroid used, the duration and mode of therapy, and the nature of the underlying disorder.

Dosages of cortisol in excess of 45 mg/m.$^2$/day, prednisone in dosage greater than 4–6 mg/m.$^2$/day, or betamethasone in a dosage greater than 0.6 mg/m$^2$/day have been reported to cause noticeable growth suppression in children (138, 159, 209). Cushing's syndrome, however, has been reported to occur from long term use of dexamethasone administered by nasal spray (210) or from percutaneous absorption of triamcinolone cream (211). In hypopituitary subjects, dosages of cortisone greater than 20 mg/m.$^2$/day may cause growth suppression (209).

Any corticosteroid preparation can cause suppression of normal adrenal function, and if continued on a daily basis for a period of 7 days or longer can produce prolonged hypothalamic–pituitary suppression, resulting in adrenal insufficiency during periods of stress (212). Growth retardation is noticeable within a few weeks (209). The severity of growth retardation and delay in skeletal maturation is related to the duration of therapy (Figure 9-14). Sobel suggests that even small excesses of cortisol production in depressed children may contribute to some measurable growth failure (213).

The effect of corticosteroids on growth can be diminished and in some cases reversed by the use of alternate day therapy. A single dose of steroids may exert a therapeutic affect long beyond its effect on adrenal suppression. In disorders that can be controlled by alternate day therapy, adrenal and growth suppression is minimal (214–216). Growth of children with asthma has been reported to be normal on alternate day steroid therapy (140, 217), but growth retardation is not always spared in renal disease even with alternate day therapy (149).

When therapy with corticosteroids is stopped, growth resumes, and in most children who do not have an underlying condition, which by itself may affect growth, there is a catch-up growth spurt. If the corticosteroid therapy is prolonged, catch-up growth may be incomplete (Figure 9-14). Children with hypopituitarism fail to show any catch-up growth (209). In asthmatic children receiving corticosteroids, skeletal maturation tends to be retarded more than height during steroid treatment; time of pubertal onset seems not to be influenced much by corticosteroid therapy even though skeletal maturation is delayed (217). Catch-up growth after discontinuation of corticosteroid therapy is quite slow in asthmatic children and in those with renal disease and may result in permanent growth deficiency (140, 149).

In addition to the effects on growth, corticosteroid therapy may lead to a decrease in bone mineralization, leading to compression fractures, peptic ulcer disease, suppression of the immune system, and overwhelming infections. Corticosteroid therapy also suppresses endogenous adrenal secretion and hypothalamic–pituitary regulation of the adrenal. It is important to remember that in the period after discontinuation of corticosteroids (when awaiting a catch-up growth spurt), there may be adrenal failure or crisis with illness or with stress occurring within 3–9 months after the steroid has been discontinued (212). "Protective therapy" with hydrocortisone must be supplied during such stressful periods. A dosage of 100–200 mg/m.$^2$/24 hr of hydrocortisone IV or IM should be provided during periods of stress, serious illness, or surgery.

Corticosteroid therapy of *adrenogenital syndrome* (congenital virilizing adrenal hyperplasia—CAH) poses a special problem in growth regulation. Untreated CAH results in adrenal production of excess amounts of androgen, resulting in a growth spurt and acceleration of bone and sexual maturation (Figure 9-17). Administration of hydrocortisone in a dosage of 25 mg/m.$^2$/day blocks the overproduction of androgens, but an excess of hydrocortisone (usually more than 45 mg/m.$^2$/day) suppresses linear growth. Even in moderate doses, too little to cause obvious signs of cortisol overdosage or Cushing's syndrome, there may be growth suppression (213). Careful titration between dosages of hydrocortisone which control virilization and those which produce growth suppression is necessary.

The manner in which corticosteroids suppress growth appears to be complex. Growth hormone release is blunted by corticosteroids (218), however, growth hormone does not reverse the growth deficiency (159, 216, 219). Serum somatomedin activity is diminished by glucocorticoid administration; less effect is seen with alternate day therapy (216). Corticosteroids also suppress growth by direct action on cell metabolism. Steroid therapy suppresses calcium absorption, promotes phosphate excretion, and decreases serum Vitamin D concentrations that interfere with bone mineralization (149). On a cellular level the actions of steroids are not known, however, corticosteroids appear to inhibit DNA synthesis and block cell proliferation (159). Baxter thinks there might be steroid induced synthesis of inhibitory proteins or blocking of RNA synthesis by receptor–steroid complexes (220).

If administrated over long periods of time, *anabolic steroids* may be responsible for reduced stature (221). Anabolic steroids are all chemically altered derivatives of testosterone and share with testosterone growth accelerating actions. Such steroids will cause an increase in growth rate and are used frequently for this purpose but will also increase the rate of skeletal maturation and may produce signs of virilization as well (12). Although some anabolic steroids may have less androgenic activity than testosterone, all of them will cause acceleration of skeletal maturation if used in dosages capable of stimulating acceleration of linear growth (5). Acceleration of epiphyseal closure will eventually lead to loss of growth potential and short stature.

*Estrogens* inhibit growth despite normal or increased secretion of growth hormone. The metabolism and growth promoting effects of growth hormone are blunted by administration of estrogens and epiphyseal closure is accelerated. Somatomedin production is decreased by estrogen (104). These actions form the basis for the use of estrogen pharmacologically to prevent excessive height in girls.

*Stimulant medications* used in treatment of children with hyperkinetic behavior may have a growth suppressant effect (222, 223). The drugs produce a temporary retardation in rate of weight gain and rate of linear growth, but there is no evidence that ultimate height or weight are materially affected (223). Catch-up growth tends to occur during "holidays" from the drugs. Effects on growth with long-term continuous therapy will need to be carefully documented. The cause of the growth suppression by stimulant drugs is not known. Variable effects on growth hormone release have been reported but no consistent effect has been demonstrated (223).

## DISORDERS OF EXCESSIVE GROWTH IN CHILDHOOD

Excessive growth from pathologic conditions presents less frequently as a growth disorder than does growth deficiency. Although natural growth excess such as familial tall stature or accelerated growth occurs with about the same frequency as familial short stature or delayed growth patterns, excessive or accelerated growth is not viewed as a problem as often as growth deficiency. Normal variants of growth excess are discussed in an earlier section of this Chapter and growth excess disorders with onset in infancy are discussed in Chapter 8. In this section we will discuss chromosomal, genetic, or dysmorphic syndromes characterized by excessive growth in childhood and endocrine or hormonal disorders which cause excess growth in children (Table 9-10). Disorders of accelerated or delayed puberty which affect growth are discussed in Chapter 10.

### Intrinsic Disorders

Some of the intrinsic disorders of growth which exhibit growth acceleration in infancy (see Chapter 8) also have a marked effect on growth later in childhood, producing characteristic childhood patterns of excess growth which merit emphasis.

### Chromosomal Disorders

There are only a few chromosomal disorders which are apt to produce excessive growth in childhood. *Klinefelter's syndrome* (XXY) is a common cause of hypogonadism and infertility (224), occurring in about 1 in 500 males. Beginning in childhood, there is a tendency toward tall, slim stature with long limbs and low upper segment/lower segment ratio. In childhood the penis and testes are relatively small (225). At adolescence the testes

**Table 9-10. Growth Excess Disorders
in Childhood**

A.   *Intrinsic growth excess disorders*
  1.   Chromosomal disorders
       (a)   Klinefelter's syndrome
       (b)   XYY syndrome
  2.   Genetic disorders
       (a)   Marfan's syndrome
       (b)   Homocystinuria syndrome
  3.   Congenital malformation syndromes
       (a)   Cerebral gigantism
       (b)   Weaver's syndrome
B.   *Extrinsic growth excess disorders*
  1.   Endocrine growth excess disorders
       (a)   Pituitary gigantism (acromegaly)
       (b)   Hyperthyroidism
       (c)   Excess sex steroids
  2.   Iatrogenic–endocrine disorders
  3.   Nonendocrine disorders

remain small, although testosterone is generally adequate to provide virilization (225). Gynecomastia is found in most subjects. Seminiferous tubules become hyalinized and fibrotic, and infertility is the rule (226). There is a tendency toward mental dullness with 15–20% of patients having an IQ below 80. There are frequently behavior problems associated with emotional immaturity, insecurity, shyness, poor judgment, and unrealistic boastful activity (36).

The diagnosis is often not suspected in childhood unless the dull mentality and behavioral problems prompt medical attention. The incomplete virilization and gynecomastia, together with poor body image, draw attention to the syndrome, which then can be recognized by the growth pattern, body habitus, and pubertal deficiencies. Diagnosis is confirmed by the XXY chromosomal karyotype pattern.

Testosterone replacement therapy may be considered if virilization is noticeably deficient. Some judicious waiting to see how much spontaneous puberty will occur is reasonable, but the social and psychological needs of the young man must be met and supplemental testosterone supplied if spontaneous development lags appreciably behind expected sexual development (36, 226). Low dose depo-testosterone may be started by 12–13 years of age (25–50 mg every 3–4 wk) with gradual increases up to 200–300 mg/every 2 weeks by 16–17 years of age. When full development has occurred, low dosage every 4–6 weeks may be sufficient to maintain virilization (36).

*XYY syndrome* occurs in 1 in 840 newborn males, but the syndrome is seldom recognized during childhood and only fortuitously in adulthood. Although occasionally long at birth, the tendency toward tall stature usually does not become evident until 5–6 years of age. Youngsters are not strong or well coordinated and a fine intention tremor may be present (36). There is a tendency toward mental dullness and explosive antisocial behavior. Temper tantrums and aggressive or defiant behavior start in early childhood. Psychosexual problems appear to be common. The incidence of XYY karyotype among institutionalized male juvenile delinquents may be as high as 1 in 35; 24 times as frequent as XYY karotype among newborn males (227, 228).

### Genetic Disorders

In a few genetic disorders growth excess is an expected characteristic. *Marfan's syndrome* is characterized by tall stature with long, slim limbs, muscular hypotonia, and diminished subcutaneous fat (Figure 9-16). Features of the syndrome include arachnodactyly with hyperextensibility of the joints, a tendency toward scoliosis (60%) and kyphosis, breast bone deformity (either pectus excavatum or carinatum), narrow face and narrow palate, upward lens subluxation, myopia, bluish sclerae, inguinal and femoral herniae, and dilatation of the ascending aorta with or without dissecting aneurysm of the aorta (229, 230). The disorder is transmitted as an autosomal dominant trait with variable expression; it appears to be a basic defect in connective tissue, but the defect has not been defined (231). Cultured fibroblasts from individuals with Marfan syndrome show metachromatic cytoplasmic inclusions (230).

During childhood and adolescence, measures to prevent scoliosis should be attempted. We have tried speeding up the epiphyseal closure in two preadolescent girls with Marfan's syndrome by administration of estrogen, but have not been very successful in either preventing excessive height or in preventing progression of the scoliosis (Figure 9-16). Glaucoma may occur, especially if the lens dislocates into the anterior chamber of the eye. Dissecting aneurysm or other vascular complications may occur at any age and such complications are the major cause of death (232). Mean survival age is 43–46 years (36).

*Homocystinuria syndrome* is an inborn error of aminoacid metabolism associated with defective development of connective tissue and blood vessels resembling Marfan's syndrome (233). Normal to tall stature is the usual growth pattern, although failure to thrive has also occurred. There is a resemblance to Marfan's syndrome in the slim skeletal build, pectus excavatum or carinatum, and kyphoscoliosis. Downward subluxation of the lens occurs by late childhood and most children are myopic. Medial degeneration of the aorta and intimal hyperplasia leads to pads and ridges within the vessels frequently leading to arterial and venous thrombosis (36). In contrast to Marfan's syndrome, in which intelligence is normal,

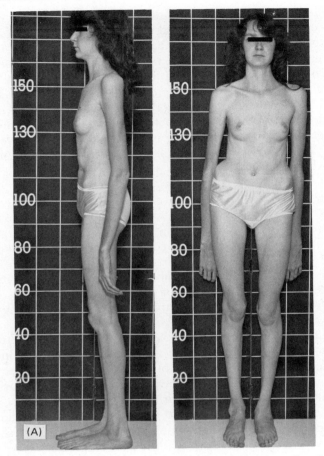

**Figure 9-16.** Marfan's syndrome in a 14-year-old girl (A) showing excessive height, thin body habitus, and normal pubertal development, (B) thin face, (sublexed lenses), and long, thin (spidery) hands and feet. Scoliosis was treated with body brace. (C) Estrogens given to speed up skeletal maturation and prevent excessive height and worsening of scoliosis.

mental defect occurs in nearly 60% of cases of homocystinuria (233); the EEG is usually abnormal and seizures have occurred frequently. Spasticity, nervousness or even schizophrenic behavior have been noted. Thromboembolic phenomena are a constant danger and are frequently a cause of morbidity and death (36, 233).

### Congenital Malformation Syndromes
A few of the congenital malformation syndromes resulting in excessive growth which were introduced in Chapter 8 have characteristic growth

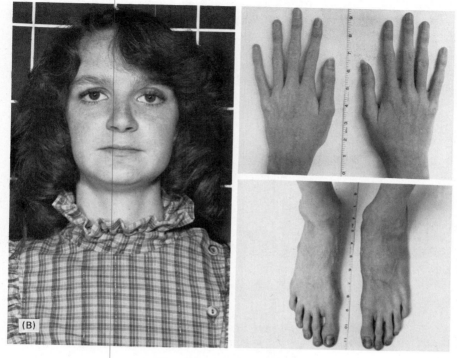

**Figure 9-16.** (Continued)

patterns in childhood. In *cerebral gigantism*, growth is rapid during the first 3–4 years with accelerated osseous maturation commensurate with height. By 10–11 years, the height age is that of a 14–15-year-old (234). In addition to rapid early growth, this syndrome is characterized by macrocephaly and dolicocephaly, large hands and feet, down slanting palpebral fissures, hypertelorism, prognathism, high narrow palate, and coarse looking features (Figure 8-8). There is poor coordination and variable mental deficiency (36). General health in childhood is good, but excessive size, mental dullness, and poor coordination may lead to behavioral problems (234, 235). *Weaver's syndrome* is characterized by accelerated growth and maturation of prenatal onset. Children with this syndrome have camptodactyly and unusual facies, consisting of large bi-frontal diameter of the skull with flat occiput, ocular hypertelorism, large ears, long philtrum, and micrognathia (236). Rapid skeletal maturation in infancy would be expected to be associated with large size as an infant and child with short stature as an adolescent and adult, although, so far, the natural history of growth, beyond infancy, is not known (36).

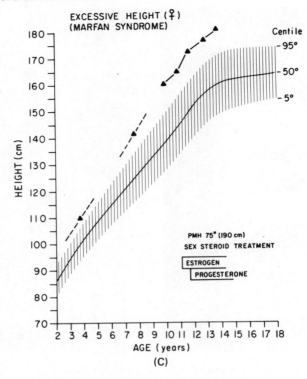

**Figure 9-16.** (Continued)

## Extrinsic Disorders

The growth excess disorders, which are extrinsic in origin, involve excesses of hormones which stimulate either accelerated or excess growth.

### *Endocrine Disorders*

*Pituitary gigantism* (acromegaly) is the prototype for all giant syndromes and perhaps the only disorder which has the capacity to truly produce gigantism—that is, growth in excess of intended genetic potential. There are pituitary giants who have grown to a height of 7–9 feet and whose feats have become legendary, such as Goliath, whose armored figure in the ranks of the Philistines struck terror into the hearts of opposing troops until David laid him low with a sling shot. There is also the legendary "Irish giant" who enjoyed notoriety in the early 19th century because of his size and physical prowess (237). He died, however, in early adulthood, weakened by progressive pituitary deficiency, as did, also, the more recently described Alton giant whose life was followed at Barnes Hospital in St. Louis early in this century (238, 239).

Despite the notoriety earned by a few pituitary giants, excessive growth in childhood from a growth-hormone-producing pituitary tumor is an exceedingly rare event. If the excessive growth hormone is produced in childhood, rapid growth of all tissues ensues and "gigantism" is the result. Pituitary tumors occurring in adolescence are associated with signs of acromegaly in addition to gigantism (240–243). In most reported cases of pituitary gigantism, excessive acceleration of growth is noted shortly before or during puberty (169), however, the excessive growth rate of the Alton giant was noted within the first year of life, when the child grew 45 cm, and growth was most pronounced during the first 4 years of life (239).

The first indication of a pituitary, growth-hormone-producing tumor is usually a period of rapid growth not associated with accelerated skeletal maturation. Growth is proportionate in childhood, but as the child enters puberty, hands and feet become very large, the jaw becomes prominent, bones of the skull become thickened, and bones of the face, especially the supraorbital bones, become overgrown, giving the individual a coarse facial appearance (169). The extreme to which this coarseness of facial features may occur is reflected in the appearance of an acromegalic professional wrestler, whose professional name was "The Angel", but whose distinction was his ability to frighten opponents with his grotesque facial features during wrestling bouts.

Generalized visceromegaly occurs and subcutaneous tissue becomes thickened. Excessive sweating and seborrhea may occur; basal metabolism is slightly increased, although thyroid function is normal (170). Degenerative changes may develop in joints, leading to joint discomfort and deformities. Daughaday draws attention to the occurrence of severe peripheral neuropathy and neuropathic arthropathy in several pituitary giants (239). The pituitary tumor or skull thickening may give rise to headaches, visual impairment, and paresthesias. Persistent long-term elevation of human growth hormone gives rise to abnormal glucose tolerance which may lead to permanent diabetes mellitus.

Pubertal development is frequently suboptimal due to disturbances in gonadotrophin secretion. As a result, it is possible for the pituitary giant to continue a "eunuchoid" type of growth into young adulthood. This kind of growth was well documented in the Alton giant who was still growing at the time of his death at age 24. By that time, he had achieved a height of 272 cm (nearly 9 feet) (239). Untreated patients usually die during the second or third decade of life with clinical symptoms of deficiencies of all pituitary hormones except growth hormone (170). The Alton giant, the tallest human being for whom verifiable records exist, died at age 24 from a cellulitis of the ankle caused by braces which he needed for ambulation because of progressive neuropathy (239).

Most pituitary gigantism is a result of growth-hormone-producing pituitary tumors, although a case of hypothalamic tumor producing gigantism, without any evidence of pituitary defect, has also been reported

(243). Classically, growth-hormone-producing tumors are eosinophilic adenomas, however, many of the adenomas are "chromophobic" to standard stains, although they have the characteristics of somatotrophs with electron microscope or immunostaining. The diagnosis of growth hormone excess is established by demonstrating an elevated level of somatomedin C or of growth hormone that is not suppressed by raising the blood sugar. Hyperglycemia is induced by administering glucose 1.75 g/kg (up to 75 g) orally. Blood samples for growth hormone are obtained at 0, 60, 90, and 120 minutes. In normal persons, the level of growth hormone in the blood should fall to 5 ng/mL or less within 60 to 120 minutes after ingestion of the glucose. Careful radiographic evaluation of the sella turcica should be made to determine the location and size of the tumor to aid in directing therapy (6).

Treatment is aimed at interrupting the production of human growth hormone while preserving as much normal pituitary function as possible. This may be accomplished by surgical removal of the tumor, cryo-ablation, or tumor irradiation. The last of these appears to be least effective, although is acceptable when neurologic signs are not present. If signs of intracranial neurologic involvement are found, surgery offers the only reliable relief. Transsphenoidal microsurgery offers the best possibility of removal of tumor and preservattion of pituitary function (6). There is frequently need for substitution therapy of cortisol, thyroid, sex hormone, and vasopressin because of deficiencies of other pituitary hormones.

*Hyperthyroidism* in infancy results in a striking acceleration of skeletal maturation together with modest acceleration of linear growth and premature closure of cranial sutures (see Chapter 8). In childhood and adolescence, there is a moderate acceleration of both linear growth and skeletal maturation (244). Coupled with the accelerated increase in linear growth is a lack of weight gain or even weight loss as a consequence of the hypermetabolic state. There are also typical signs and symptoms of hyperthyroidism which overshadow the growth spurt. Such children tend to exhibit emotional lability, excessive activity, restlessness, and weakness. The eyes become prominent and may protrude (exophthalmos). There is usually a stare with lid lag and sometimes weakness of the eye muscles. The thyroid is diffusely enlarged, the skin is warm and moist, the pulse rate rapid, and the pulse pressure increased.

The diagnosis of hyperthyroidism is confirmed by elevation of serum thyroxine, $T_3$ RIA, or rapid, high uptake of radioiodine by the thyroid. Hyperthyroidism is usually treated by medical suppression with propylthiouracil or methimazole, or by partial surgical removal of the thyroid. The latter therapy often renders the individual hypothyroid eventually and thyroid replacement therapy should be started after surgery. Successful therapy of the hyperthyroid state allows return to a normal rate of growth (168).

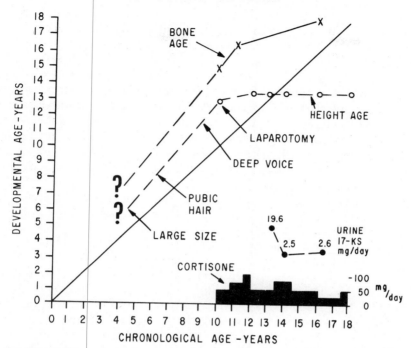

**Figure 9-17.** Growth chart of subject with congenital virilizing adrenal hyperplasia showing rapid early growth, early virilization, and ultimate short stature. Growth was virtually complete by the time cortisol therapy was instituted, showing effects on growth and skeletal maturation of unchecked adrenal androgens.

Linear growth and skeletal maturation may be remarkably affected in individuals with isosexual precocious puberty, tumors which produce excess amounts of estrogens or androgens, or *congenital virilizing adrenal hyperplasia* in which adrenal androgens are produced in excessive amounts. The sex hormones, especially androgens, have the capacity to imitate the pubertal growth spurt and accelerate both linear growth and skeletal maturation (Figure 9-17). Accelerated growth in childhood leads to excessive size and may produce peculiar psychological problems. Because of the rapid acceleration of skeletal maturation produced by these hormones, closure of the epiphyses occurs at a much earlier than average age; the result is a short teenager and adult.

## Iatrogenic–Endocrine Disorders

The use of estrogens to "limit" excessive height in tall girls or the use of androgens to "enhance" the strength and competitive fervor of young male or female athletes may produce undesirable side effects on growth and/or pubertal development. The natural effect of sex hormones on growth and pubertal development has been reviewed in Chapter 5. Acceleration of linear growth and of skeletal maturation in "experiments of nature" in which enzyme deficiencies or tumors cause secretion of excess sex steroids has been mentioned in the preceeding section. The same effect on growth and skeletal development can be achieved by administration of estrogen or androgen to prepubertal children.

In the treatment of prepubertal girls for excessive height with estrogens, some initial acceleration of linear growth is usually seen. This is accompanied by rapid weight gain and appearance of sexual characteristics. Blockage of growth hormone effect and acceleration of skeletal maturation usually combine to eventually reduce female height achievement below that expected from normal puberty (22).

The use of androgens in prepubertal male or female athletes would have the same effect. Linear growth and skeletal maturation would be accelerated, the skeletal acceleration usually exceeding the linear growth (5). In addition, virilization would occur, perhaps not unwelcome in a boy if he is near the age of puberty, but clearly undesirable in a girl (245). The use of such agents in prepubertal children is clearly contraindicated (246). Even in adolescents or young adults, the administration of sex steroids for "increased strength" or "competition" in sports is of questionable value and carries with it potential for harm (245–249).

Although growth in young adults would likely be unaffected by the use of sex steroids, normal function of the reproductive system could suffer damage—irreparable if of sufficient duration (245, 247). Estrogens in a female or androgens in a male suppress the normal hypothalamic–pituitary mechanism by which the reproductive organs and gonads are controlled (247). Excessive use of sex steroids may result in loss of cyclicity of menses in a female, resulting in functional sterility. Excess testosterone in a male results in depression of testicular function and azoospermia and may eventually cause hyalinization and fibrosis of tubules within the testes and loss of function (246). Cholestasis occurs in most subjects who take anabolic agents in large dosage—hepatitis and malignant liver tumors, although rare, may also occur (245, 247). Although serious side effects are seldom seen, sex hormones should not be prescribed unless precautions are taken to minimize side effects and there is some assurance that the hormones will achieve the desired result (245–249).

### Nonendocrine Disorders

In addition to familial or genetic tall stature, one of the few nonendocrine disorders which is associated with excessive or accelerated growth is *obesity*. In many obese children, height, as well as weight, is above average and skeletal maturation is modestly accelerated as well. The acceleration of height and bone maturation is usually overshadowed by the weight gain and is seldom of such a degree that it prompts concern. Attention is rightly directed to the excess weight gain. The cause of modest increase in linear growth and skeletal maturation in obesity is not known. Reduction in the rate of weight gain is usually accompanied by a return to normal growth rate.

## REFERENCES

1. Lacey KA, Parkin JM: The normal short child, community study of children in Newcastle-upon-Tyne. *Arch Dis Child* **49:**417, 1974.
2. Horner JM, Thorsson AV, Hintz RL: Growth deceleration patterns in children with constitutional short stature: An aid to diagnosis. *Pediatrics* **62:**529, 1978.
3. Garn SM: Determinants of size and growth during the first 3 years, *Mod Prob Paediatr* **7:**50, 1962.
4. Marti-Henneberg C, Nirrianen AK, Rappaport R: Oxandrolone treatment of constitutional short stature in boys during adolescence. *J. Pediatr* **86:**783, 1975.
5. Jackson ST, Rallison ML, Buntin WH, et al: Use of oxandrolone for growth stimulation in children. *Am J Dis Child* **126:**481, 1973.
6. Frasier SD: Growth disorders in children. *Pediatr Clin North Am* **26**(February):1, 1979.
7. Smith DW, Truog W, Rogers JE, et al: Shifting linear growth during infancy: Illustration of genetic factors in growth from fetal life through infancy, *J Pediatr* **89:**225, 1976.
8. Illig R, Prader A: Effect of testosterone on growth hormone secretion in patients with anorchia and delayed puberty. *J Clin Endocrinol Metab* **30:**615, 1970.
9. Blethen SL, Gaines S, Weldon V: Comparison of predicted and adult heights in short boys: Effect of androgen therapy. *Pediatr Res* **18:**467, 1984.
10. Kaplan JG, Moshang T Jr, Bernstein R, et al: Constitutional delay of growth and development: Effects of treatment with androgens. *J Pediatr* **82:**38, 1973.
11. Bettmann HK, Goldman HS, Abramowics M, et al: Oxandrolone treatment of short stature: Effect on predicted mature height. *J Pediatr* **79:**1018, 1971.
12. Moore, DC, Tattoni DS, Limbeck GA, et al: Studies of anabolic steroids: Effect of prolonged oxandrolone administration on growth in children and adolescence with uncomplicated short stature. *Pediatrics* **58:**412, 1976.
13. Rosenfeld RG, Northcraft GB, Hintz RL: A prospective, randomized study of testosterone treatment of constitutional delay of growth and development in male adolescents. *Pediatrics* **69:**681, 1982.
14. Ad hoc committee on growth hormone usage: Growth hormone in the treatment of children with short stature. *Pediatrics* **72:**891, 1983.
15. Kowarski AA, Schneider J, Ben-Galim E, et al: Growth failure with normal serum RIA-GH and low somatomedin activity: Somatomedin restoration and growth acceleration after exogenous GH. *J Clin Endocrinol Metab* **47:**461, 1978.
16. Rudman D, Kutner MH, Goldsmith MA, et al: Further observations on four subgroups of normal variant short stature. *J Clin Endocrinol Metab* **51:**1378, 1980.
17. Frazer T, Gavin JR, Daughaday, et al: Growth hormone-dependent growth failure. *J. Pediatr* **101:**12, 1982.
18. Van Vliet G, Styne DM, Kaplan SL, et al: Growth hormone treatment for short stature, *N Engl J Med* **309:**1016, 1983.
19. Grant JA, Howard CP, Daughaday WH: Comparison of growth and somatomedin C responses following growth hormone treatment in children with small-for-date short stature, significant idiopathic short stature and hypopituitarism, *Acta Endocrinol* **106:**168, 1984.

20. Underwood LE: Growth hormone treatment for short children. *J Pediatr* **104:**237, 1984.

21. Gertner JM, Genel M, Gianfredi SP, et al: Propsective clinical trial of human growth hormone in short children without growth hormone deficiency. *J Pediatr* **104:**172, 1984.

22. Rallison ML, Wood CM, Lester PD: Use of estrogenic preparations in limiting excessive linear growth in girls. (Unpublished Observations).

23. Wettenhall, NB, Cahill C, Roche AF: Tall girls: A survey of 15 years of management and treatment. *J Pediatr* **86:**602, 1975.

24. Greenblatt RB, McDonough PG, Mahesh VB: Estrogen therapy inhibition of growth. *J Clin Endocrinol Metab* **26:**1185, 1966.

25. Schoen EJ, Solomon IL, Warren O, et al: Estrogen treatment of tall girls. *Am J Dis Child* **125:**71, 1973.

26. Frasier SD, Smith FG, Jr: Effect of estrogens on mature height in tall girls: A controlled study. *J Clin Endocrinol Metab* **28:**416, 1968.

27. Zachmann M, Ferrandez A, Muerset G, et al: Treatment of excessively tall stature in girls. *Helv Paediatr Acta* **30:**11, 1975.

28. Anderson H, Jacobsen BB, Kastrup KW, et al: Treatment of girls with excessive height prediction. *Acta Paediatr Scand* **69:**293, 1980.

29. CDC: Long-term oral contraceptive use and the risk of breast cancer. *JAMA* **249:**1591, 1983.

30. Vessey MP, Lawless M, McPherson K: Neoplasia of the cervix uteri and contraception: A possible adverse effect of the pill. *Lancet* **2:**930, 1983.

31. Schaffner F: The effect of oral contraceptives on the liver. *JAMA* **198:**155, 1966.

32. Prader A: Behandlung des Grosswuchses. *Monatsschr. Kinderheilkd,* **123:**328, 1975.

33. Zachmann M, Ferrandez A, Muerset G, et al: Testosterone treatment of excessively tall boys. *J Pediatr* **88:**116, 1976.

34. Van den Bosch JSG, Smals AGH, Pieters GFFM, et al: Instant growth inhibition by low dose oestrogens in excessively tall boys. *Acta Endocrinol* **100:**327, 1982.

35. Tolksdorf M, et al: Clinical aspects of Down's syndrome from infancy to adult life. *Hum Genetics* **2**(Suppl):3, 1981.

36. Smith DW: *Recognizable Patterns of Hfuman Malformation,* ed 3. Philadelphia, WB Saunders Co, 1982.

37. Turner HH: A syndrome of infantilism, congenital webbed neck and cubitus valgus. *Endocrinology* **23:**566, 1938.

38. Polani PE, Hunter WF, Lennox B: Chromosomal sex in Turner's syndrome with coarctation of the aorta. *Lancet* **2:**120, 1954.

39. Ford CE, Jones KW, Polani PE, et al: A sex-chromosome anomaly in a case of gonadal dysgenesis (Turner's syndrome). *Lancet* **1:**711, 1959.

40. Haddad HM, Wilkins L: Congenital anomalies associated with gonadal aplasia—review of 55 cases. *Pediatrics* **23:**885, 1959.

41. Matthies F, MacDiarmid WD, Rallison ML, et al: Renal anomalies in Turner's syndrome. *Clin Pediatr* **10:**561, 1971.

42. Lindsten J: The nature and origin of X chromosome aberrations in Turner's syndrome. A cytogenetical and clinical study of 57 patients. Stockholm, Almquist and Wiksell, 1963.

43. Smith DW: Growth deficiency dysmorphic syndromes. *Postgrad Med J* **54**(Suppl 2):147, 1978.

44. Park E, Bailey JD, Cowell CA: Growth and maturation of patients with Turner's syndrome. *Pediatr Res* **17:**1, 1983.

45. Pelz L, Timm D, Eyermann E, et al: Body height in Turner's syndrome. *Clin Genet* **22**:62, 1982.

46. Tanner JM, Whitehouse RH, Hughes PCR, et al: Effect of human growth hormone treatment for 1 to 7 years on growth of 100 children, with growth hormone deficiency, low birthweight, inherited smallness, Turner's syndrome, and other complaints. *Arch Dis Child* **46**:745, 1971.

47. Butenandt O: Growth hormone deficiency and growth hormone therapy in Ulrich–Turner syndrome. *Klin Wochenschr* **58**:99, 1980.

48. Lenko HL, Leisti S, Perheentupa J: The efficacy of growth hormone in different types of growth failure. *Eur J Pediatr* **138**:241, 1982.

49. Johanson AJ, Brasel JA, Blizzard RM: Growth in patients with gondal dysgensis receiving fluoxymesterone. *J Pediatr* **75**:1015, 1969.

50. Ross JL, Cassorla FG, Skerda MC, et al: A preliminary study of the effect of estrogen dose on growth in Turner's syndrome. *N Engl J Med* **309**:1104, 1983.

51. Spranger JW: Metaphyseal chrondrodysplasia. *Postgrad Med J* **53**:480, 1977.

52. Bongiovanni AM, Album MM, Root AW, et al: Studies in hypophosphatosia and response to high phosphate intake. *Am J Med Sci* **255**:163, 1968.

53. Jansen M: Ueber atypische Chondrodystrophie (Achondroplasia) und über eine noch nicht beschriebene angeborene Wachstumstörung des Knochensystems: Metaphysäre Dysostosis. *Ztschr. f. Orthop Chir* **61**:253, 1934.

54. Schmid F: Beitrag zur Dysostosis Enchondralis Metaphysaria. *Monatsschr. Kinderheilkd* **97**:393, 1949.

55. Schwachman H, Diamond LK, Oski F, et al: The syndrome of pancreatic insufficiency and bone marrow dysfunction. *J Pediatr* **65**:645, 1964.

56. McLennan TW, Steinbach HL: Schwachman's syndrome: The broad spectrum of bony abnormalities. *Radiology* **112**:167, 1974.

57. Siggers DC, Burke JB, Morris B, et al: Cartilage–hair hypoplasia. *Postgrad Med J* **53**:473, 1977.

58. Bailey JA: Multiple epiplyseal dysplasias, in *Disproportionate Short Stature, Diagnosis and Treatment*. Philadelphia, WB Saunders Co, 1973, pp 380–437.

59. Wolcott CD, Rallison ML: Infancy-onset diabetes mellitus and multiple epiphyseal dysplasia. *J Pediatr* **80**:292, 1972.

60. Leri A, Weill J: Une affection congenitale et symetrique du developpement osseus: la dyschondrostose. *Bull Mem Soc Med Hosp (Paris)* **45**:1491, 1929.

61. Langer LO: Mesomelic dwarfism of the hypoplastic ulna, fibula, mandible type. *Radiology* **89**:654, 1967.

62. Maroteaux P, Lamy M: La pycnodysostose. *Presse Med* **70**:999, 1962.

63. Forland M: Cleidocranial dysostosis. A review of the syndrome and report of a sporadic case with hereditary transmission. *Am J of Med* **33**:792, 1962.

64. Albright F, Burnett CH, Smith PH, et al: Pseudohypoparathyroidism—an example of "Seabright-Bantam Syndrome". Report of three cases. *Endocrinol* **30**:922, 1942.

65. Mann JB, Alterman S, Hills G: Albright's hereditary osteodystrophy comprising pseudohypoparathyroidism and pseudopseudohypoparathyroidism. With a report of two cases representing the complete syndrome occurring in successive generations. *Ann Int Med* **56**:315, 1962.

66. Fitch N: Albright's hereditary osteodystrophy: A review. *Am J Med Genet* **11**:11, 1982.

67. Spranger JW: Catabolic disorders of complex carbohydrates. *Postgrad Med J* **53**:441, 1977.

68. Hurler G: Ueber einen Typ multipler Abartungen, vorwiegend am Skelettsystem. *Zeitschrift Kinderheilkd* **24**:220, 1919.

69. Scheie HG, Hambrick GW, Jr, Barness LA: A newly recognized forme fruste of Hurler's disease (Gargoylism). *Am J Ophthalmol* **53:**753, 1962.

70. Hunter C: A rare disease in two brothers. *Proc R Soc Med* **10:**104, 1917.

71. Sanfilippo SJ, Podosin R, Langer LO Jr, et al: Mental retardation associated with acid mucopolysacchariduria (heparitin sulfate type), *J Pediatr* **63:**837, 1963.

72. Robbins MM, Stevens HF, Linker A: Morquio's disease: An abnormality of mucopolysaccharide metabolism. *J Pediatr* **62:**881, 1963.

73. Maroteaux P, Lamy M: Hurler's disease, Morquio's disease and related mucopolysaccharidoses. *J Pediatr* **67:**312, 1965.

74. Sly WS, Quinton BA, McAlister WH, et al: Beta glucuronidase deficiency: Report of clinical, radiologic and biochemical features of a new mucopolysaccharidosis. *J Pediatr* **82:**249, 1973.

75. Tanner JM, Lejarraga H, Cameron N: The natural history of the Silver–Russell syndrome: A longitudinal study of thirty-nine cases. *Pediatr Res* **9:**611, 1975.

76. Hutchinson J: Congenital absence of hair and mammary glands with atrophic condition of the skin and its appendages in a boy whose mother had been almost totally bald from alopecia areata from the age of six. *Trans Med Chir Soc Endinburgh* **69:**473, 1886.

77. Gilford H: Progeria: A form of senilism. *Pract* **73:**188, 1904.

78. DeBusk FL: The Hutchinson–Gilford progeria syndrome. *J Pediatr* **80:**697, 1972.

79. MacDonald WB, Fitch KD, Lewis IC: Cockayne's syndrome. An heredo-familial disorder of growth and development. *Pediatrics* **25:**997, 1960.

80. Fujimoto WY, Greene ML, Seegmiller JE: Cockayne's syndrome: Report of a case with hyperlipoproteinemia, hyperinsulinemia, renal disease, and normal growth hormone. *J Pediatr* **75:**881, 1969.

81. Cockayne EA: Dwarfism with retinal atrophy and deafness. *Arch Dis Child* **21:**52, 1946.

82. Cunningham M, Godfrey S, Moffat WMV: Cockayne's syndrome and emphysema. *Arch Dis Child* **53:**722, 1978.

83. Noonan JA, Ehmke DA: Associated non-cardiac malformations in children with congenital heart disease. *J Pediatr* **63:**468, 1963.

84. Collins E, Turner G: The Noonan syndrome. *J Pediatr* **83:**941, 1973.

85. Theintz G, Savage MO: Growth and pubertal development in five boys with Noonan's syndrome. *Arch Dis Child* **57:**13, 1982.

86. Aarskog D: A familial syndrome of short stature associated with facial dysplasia and genital anomalies. *J Pediatr* **77:**856, 1970.

87. Sugarman GI, Rimoin DL, Lackman RS: The facial–digital–genital (Aarskog) syndrome. *Am J Dis Child* **126:**248, 1973.

88. Miller HC, Merritt TA: *Fetal Growth in Humans*. Chicago, Year Book Medical Publishers, Inc, 1979.

89. Walther FJ, Ramaekers LHJ: Growth in early childhood of newborns affected by disproportionate intrauterine growth retardation. *Acta Paediatr Scand* **71:**651, 1982.

90. Lanes R, Plotnick LP, Lee PA: Sustained effect of human growth hormone therapy on children with intrauterine growth retardation. *Pediatrics* **83:**731, 1979.

91. Schaff-Blass E, Burstein S, Rosenfeld RL: Advances in diagnosis and treatment of short stature, with special reference to the role of growth hormone. *J Pediatr* **104:**801, 1984.

92. Winick M, Rosso P: The effect of severe early malnutrition on cellular growth of human brain. *Pediatr Res* **3:**181, 1969.

93. Stock MB, Smythe PM: A 15 year developmental study of effects of severe undernutrition during infancy on subsequent physical growth and intellectual functioning, *Arch Dis Child* **51:**327, 1976.

94. Garrow JS, Pike MC: The long-term prognosis of severe infantile malnutrition. *Lancet* 1:1, 1967.

95. Briers PJ, Hoorweg J, Standfield JP: The long-term effects of protein energy malnutrition in early childhood on bone age, bone cortical thickness and height. *Acta Paediatr Scan* 64:853, 1975.

96. Widdowson EM, McCance RA: The effect of finite periods of undernutrition at different ages on the composition and subsequent development of the rat. *Proc R Soc Edinburgh Biol Sci* 158:329, 1963.

97. Krueger RH: Some long-term effects of severe malnutrition in early life. *Lancet* 2:514, 1969.

98. McWilliam KM, Dean RFA: The growth of malnourished children after hospital treatment. *East Afr Med J* 42:297, 1965.

99. Davis DR, Apley J, Fill G, et al: Diet and retarded growth. *British Med J* 1:539, 1978.

100. Naeye RL, Diener MM, Hareke HT Jr, et al: Relation of poverty and race to birth weight and organ and cell structure in the newborn. *Pediatr Res* 5:17, 1971.

101. Powell GF, Brasel JA, Raiti S, et al: Emotional deprivation and growth retardation simulating idiopathic hypopituitarism. *New Engl J Med* 276:1279, 1967.

102. Monckeberg F, Donoso G, Oxman S, et al: Human growth hormone in infant malnutrition. *Pediatrics* 31:58, 1963.

103. Parra A, Garza C, Garza Y, et al: Changes in growth hormone, insulin, thyroxine values, and in energy metabolism of marasmic infants. *J Pediatr* 82:133, 1973.

104. Phillips LS, Vassilopoulu-Sellin R: Somatomedins. *New Engl J Med* 302:371, 438, 1980.

105. Vest M, Talbot NB, Crawford JD: Hypocaloric dwarfism and hydronephrosis in diabetes insipidus. *Am J Dis Child* 105:175, 1963.

106. Prasad AS: Zinc deficiency in man. *Am J Dis Child* 130:359, 1976.

107. Halsted JA, Smith JC Jr, Irwin MI: A conspectus of research on zinc requirement of man. *J Nutr* 104:345, 1974.

108. Prasad AS, Schoomaker EB, Ortega J, et al: Zinc deficiency in sickle cell disease. *Clin Chem* 21:582, 1975.

109. Solomens NW, Rosenfield RL, Jacob RA, et al: Growth retardation and zinc nutrition. *Pediatr Res* 10:923, 1976.

110. Collipp PJ, Castro-Magana M, Petrovic M, et al: Zinc deficiency: Improvement in growth and growth hormone levels with oral zinc therapy. *Ann Nutr Metab* 26:247, 1982.

111. Butrimovitz GP, Purdy COC: Zinc nutrition and growth in a childhood population. *Am J Clin Nutr* 31:1409, 1978.

112. Sobel EH, Silverman FN, Lee CM Jr: Chronic regional enteritis and growth retardation. *Am J Dis Child* 103:569, 1962.

113. Prader A, Tanner JM, von Harnack GA: Catch-up growth following illness or starvation. *J Pediatr* 62:646, 1963.

114. Cacciari E, Salardi S, Lazzari R, et al: Short stature and celiac disease: A relationship to consider even in patients with no gastrointestinal symptoms. *J Pediatr* 103:708, 1983.

115. Kirschner BS, Voinchet O, Rosenberg IH: Growth retardation in inflammatory bowel disease. *Gastroenterology* 75:504, 1978.

116. Motil KL, Grand RJ, Maletskos CJ, et al: The effect of disease, drug, and diet on whole body protein metabolism in adolescents with Crohn's disease and growth failure. *J Pediatr* 101:354, 1982.

117. McCaffery TD, Nasr K and Lawrence AM, et al: Effect of administered human growth hormone on growth retardation in inflammatory bowel disease. *Am J Digestive Dis* 19:411, 1974.

118. Sadeghy-Nejad A, Senior B: The treatment of ulcerative colitis in children with alternate-day corticosteroids. *Pediatrics* **43:**840, 1968.

119. Kirschner BS, Klich JR, Kalman SS, et al: Reversal of growth retardation in Crohn's disease with therapy emphasizing oral nutritional supplementation. *Gastroenterology* **80:**10, 1981.

120. Driscoll RH, Rosenberg IH: Total parenteral nutrition in inflammatory bowel disease. *Med Clin of North Am* **62:**185, 1978.

121. Mosier HD, Grossman HJ, Dingman HF: Physical growth in mental defectives. *Pediatrics* **36:**465, 1965.

122. O'Connell EJ, Feldt RH, Stickler GB: Head circumference, mental retardation and growth failure. *Pediatrics* **36:**62, 1965.

123. Mosier HD Jr, Jansons RA: Stunted growth in rats following X-irradiation of the head. *Growth* **31:**139, 1967.

124. Castells S, Voeller KK, Vinas C, et al: Cerebral dwarfism: Association of brain dysfunction with growth retardation. *J Pediatr* **85:**36, 1974.

125. Addy DP, Hudson FP: Diencephalic syndrome of infantile emaciation. *Arch Dis Child* **47:**338, 1972.

126. Silver HK, Finkelstein M: Deprivation dwarfism. *J Pediatr* **70:**317, 1967.

127. Whitten CF, Pettit MG, Fischoff J: Evidence that growth failure from maternal deprivation is secondary to undereating. *JAMA* **209:**1675, 1969.

128. Guilhaume A, Benoit O, Gourmelen M, et al: Relationship between sleep stage IV deficit and reversible hGH deficiency in psychosocial dwarfism. *Pediatr Res* **16:**299, 1982.

129. Frasier SD, Rallison ML: Growth retardation and emotional deprivation: Relative resistance to treatment with human growth hormone. *J Pediatr* **80:**603, 1972.

130. Money J: The syndrome of abuse dwarfism (psychosocial dwarfism or reversible hyposomatotropism). *Am J Dis Child* **131:**508, 1977.

131. Suoninen P: Physical growth of children with congenital heart disease. Pre- and post-operative study of 355 cases. *Acta Paediatr Scand* **225:**1, 1971.

132. Mehrizi A, Drash A: Growth disturbance in congenital heart disease. *J Pediatr* **61:**418, 1962.

133. Adams FH, Lund GW, Disenhouse RB: Observations on the physique and growth of children with congenital heart disease. *J Pediatr* **44:**674, 1954.

134. Levy RJ, Rosenthal A, Miettinen OS, et al: Determinants of growth in patients with ventricular septal defect. *Circulation* **57:**793, 1978.

135. Umansky R, Hauch AJ: Factors in growth of children with patent ductus arteriosus. *Pediatrics* **30:**540, 1962.

136. Richards MR: Pre- and post-operative growth patterns in congenital heart disease as shown by the Wetzel Grid. *Pediatrics* **9:**77, 1952.

137. Bate TWP, Price DA, Holme CA, et al: Short stature caused by obstructive apnoea during sleep. *Arch Dis Child* **59:**78, 1984.

138. Falliers CJ, Tan LS, Szentivanyi J, et al: Childhood asthma and steroid therapy as influences on growth. *Am J Dis Child* **105:**127, 1963.

139. Ferguson AC, Murray AB, Tze W-J: Short stature and delayed skeletal maturation in children with allergic disease. *J Allergy Clin Immunol* **69:**461, 1982.

140. Chang KC, Miklich DR, Barwise G, et al: Linear growth of chronic asthmatic children: The effects of the disease and various forms of steroid therapy. *Clin Allergy* **12:**369, 1982.

141. Hauspie R, Susanne C, Alexander F: A mixed longitudinal study of the growth in height and weight in asthmatic children. *Hum Biol* **48:**271, 1976.

142. Worthen HG: Growth failure due to diseases of the proximal tubule. *J Pediatr* **57**:14, 1960.

143. Potter DE, Greifer I: Statural growth of children with renal disease. *Kidney Int* **14**:334, 1978.

144. Broyer M: Growth in children with renal insufficiency. *Pediatr Clin No Am* **29**:991, 1982.

145. Hodsen EM, Shaw PF, Evans RA, et al: Growth retardation and renal osteodystrophy in children with chronic renal failure. *J Pediatr* **103**:735, 1983.

146. Avioli LV: Childhood renal osteodystrophy. *Kidney Int* **14**:355, 1978.

147. McSherry E: Acidosis and growth in nonuremic renal disease. *Kidney Int* **14**:349, 1978.

148. Lewy JE, Van Wyk JJ: Somatomedin and growth retardation in children with chronic renal insufficiency. *Kidney Int* **14**:261, 1978.

149. Travis LB, Chesney R, McEnery P, et al: Growth and glucocorticoids in children with kidney disease. *Kidney Int* **14**:365, 1978.

150. Stefanidis CJ, Hewitt IK, Balfe JW: Growth in children receiving continuous ambulatory peritoneal dialysis. *J Pediatr* **102**:681, 1983.

151. Hughes DWO: Hypoplastic anemia in infancy and childhood. *Arch Dis Child* **36**:349, 1961.

152. Diamond LK, Allen DM, Magill FB: Congenital hypoplastic anemia. *Am J Dis Child* **102**:403, 1961.

153. Clarke WL, Weldon VV: Growth hormone deficiency and Fanconi anemia. *J Pediatr* **86**:814, 1975.

154. Norden UZ, Humbert JR, MacGillivray MH, et al: Fanconi's anemia with growth hormone deficiency. *Am J Dis Child* **133**:291, 1979.

155. Luban NLC, Leikin SL, August GH: Growth and development in sickle cell anemia. *Am J Pediatr Hemat/Oncol* **4**:61, 1982.

156. Whitten CF: Growth status of children with sickle cell anemia. *Am J Dis Child* **102**:355, 1961.

157. McIntosh N: Endocrinopathy in thalassaemia major. *Arch Dis Child* **51**:195, 1976.

158. Wu A, Grant DB, Hambley J, et al: Reduced serum somatomedin activity in patients with chronic liver disease. *Clin Sci* **47**:359, 1974.

159. Loeb JN: Corticosteroids and growth. *New Engl J Med* **295**:547, 1976.

160. La Franchi SH: Hypothyroidism. *Ped Clin North Am* **26**:33, 1979.

161. Rallison ML, Dobyns BM, Keating FR Jr, et al: Thyroid disease in children: A survey of subjects potentially exposed to fallout radiation. *Am J Med* **56**:457, 1974.

162. Rallison ML, Dobyns BM, Keating FR Jr, et al: Occurrence and natural history of chronic lymphocytic thyroiditis in childhood. *J Pediatr* **86**:675, 1975.

163. Winter J, Eberlein WR, Bongiovanni AM: The relationship of juvenile hypothyroidism to chronic lympocytic thyroiditis. *J Pediatr* **69**:709, 1966.

164. Costin G, Kershnar AK, Kogut MD, et al: Prolactin activity in juvenile hypothyroidism and precocious puberty. *Pediatrics* **50**:881, 1972.

165. Raiti S, Trias E, Maclaren NK: Primary hypothyroidism, differentiation from primary hypopituitarism. *Am J Dis Child* **129**:1397, 1975.

166. Fisher DA, Oddie TH, Johnson DE, et al: The diagnosis of Hashimoto's thyroiditis. *J Clin Endocrinol Metab* **40**:795, 1975.

167. Rezvani I, DiGeorge AM: Reassessment of the daily dose of oral thyroxine for replacement therapy in hypothyroid children. *J Pediatr* **90**:291, 1977.

168. Smith DW: *Growth and Its Disorders.* Philadelphia, WB Saunders Co, 1977.

169. Labhart A, Zachmann M: Clinical physiology of pituitary tumors. *Prog in Neurological Surgery* **6**:1, 1975.

170. Root AW, Bongiovanni AM and Eberlein WR: Diagnosis and management of growth retardation with special reference to the problem of hypopituitarism. *J Pediatr* **78:**737, 1971.

171. Preece MA: Diagnosis and treatment of children with growth hormone deficiency. *Clin Endocrinol Metab* **11**(Mar):1, 1982.

172. Romshe CA, Zipf WB, Miser A, et al: Evaluation of growth hormone release and human growth hormone treatment in children with cranial irradiation-associated short stature. *J Pediatr* **104:**177, 1984.

173. Latorre H, Kenny FM, Lahey ME, et al: Short stature and growth hormone deficiency in histiocytosis X. *J Pediatr* **85:**813, 1974.

174. Grossman A, Savage MO, Wass JH, et al: Growth-hormone-releasing factor in growth hormone deficiency: Demonstration of a hypothalamic defect in growth hormone release. *Lancet* **2**(8342):137, 1983.

175. Goodman HG, Grumbach MM, Kaplan SL: Growth and growth hormone: II. A comparison of isolated growth hormone deficiency and multiple pituitary hormone deficiencies in 35 patients with idiopathic hypopituitary dwarfism. *New Engl J Med* **278:**57, 1968.

176. Kenny FM, Iturzaeta MF, Mintz D, et al: Iatrogenic hypopituitarism in craniopharyngioma: Unexplained catch-up growth in three children. *J Pediatr* **72:**766, 1968.

177. Frasier SD, Smith FG Jr: Return of normal growth following removal of a craniopharyngioma. *Am J Dis Child* **116:**311, 1968.

178. Bucher H, Zapf J, Torresoni T, et al: Insulin-like growth factors I and II, prolactin, and insulin in 19 growth hormone-deficient children with excessive, normal, or decreased longitudinal growth after operation for craniopharyngioma. *N Engl J Med* **309:**1142, 1983.

179. Prader A, Zachmann M, Poley JR, et al: Long-term treatment with human growth hormone in small doses: Evaluation of 18 hypopituitary patients. *Helv Paediatr Acta* **22:**423, 1967.

180. Howard CP, Takahashi H, Hayles AB: Children with growth hormone deficiency, Intermittant treatment with somatotropin and oxandrolone. *Am J Dis Child* **135:**326, 1981.

181. Shalch DS, Tollefson SE, Klingensmith GJ, et al: Effects of human growth hormone administration on serum somatomedins, somatomedin carrier proteins, and growth rates in children with growth hormone deficiency. *J Clin Endocrinol Metab* **55:**49, 1982.

182. Chernausek SD, Underwood LE, Utiger RD, et al: Growth hormone secretion and plasma somatomedin-C in primary hypothyroidism. *Clin Endocrinol* **19:**337, 1983.

183. Spiliotis BE, August GP, Hung W, et al: Growth hormone neurosecretary dysfunction: A treatable cause of short stature. *JAMA* **251:**2223, 1984.

184. Laron Z, Pertzelan A, Mannheimer S; Genetic pituitary dwarfism with high serum concentration of growth hormone. A new inborn error of metabolism? *Israeli J Med Sc* **2:**152, 1966.

185. Najjar SS, Khachadurian AK, Ilbawi MN, et al: Dwarfism with elevated levels of plasma growth hormone. *New Engl J Med* **284:**809, 1971.

186. New MI, Schwartz E, Parks GA, et al: Pseudohypopituitary dwarfism with normal plasma growth hormone and low serum sulfation factor. *J Pediatr* **80:**620, 1972.

187. Van den Brande JL, DuCaju MVL, Visser HKA, et al: Primary somatomedin deficiency. *Arch Dis Child* **49:**297, 1974.

188. Macaron C, Fumuyiwa O: Receptor dysfunction and hormone resistance in human diseases—a review. *Am J Med Sci* **275:**149, 1978.

189. Clemens RD, Costin G, Kogut MD: Laron dwarfism: Growth and immunoreactive insulin following treatment with human growth hormone. *J Pediatr* **88:**427, 1976.

190. Strickland AL, Underwood LE, Voina SJ, et al: Growth retardation in Cushing's syndrome. *Am J Dis Child* **123:**207, 1972.

191. Frasier SD: Laboratory evaluation of endocrine function, in *Pediatric Endocrinology*, New York, Grune and Stratton, 1980, pp 23–53.

192. Nelson DH, Meakin JW, Thorn GW: ACTH producing pituitary tumors following adrenalectomy for Cushing's syndrome. *Ann Int Med* **52:**560, 1960.

193. Bergstrand CG, Nilsson KO: Treatment of Cushing's disease in children. *Acta Paediatr Scand* **71:**1, 1982.

194. Guest CM: The Mauriac syndrome: Dwarfism, hepatomegaly, and obesity with juvenile diabetes mellitus. *Diabetes* **2:**415, 1953.

195. Najjar S, Ayash MA: The Mauriac syndrome. *Clin Peds* **13:**723, 1974.

196. Jackson RL, Holland E, Chatman ID, et al: Growth and maturation of children with insulin-dependent diabetes mellitus. *Diabetes Care* **1:**96, 1978.

197. Jackson RL: Growth and maturation of children with insulin-dependent diabetes mellitus. *Pediatr Clin No Am* **31**(Jun):545, 1984.

198. Winter RJ, Phillips LS, Klein MN, et al: Somatomedin activity and diabetic control in children with insulin-dependent diabetes. *Diabetes* **28:**952, 1979.

199. Rudolf MCJ, Sherwin RS, Markowitz R, et al: Effect of intensive insulin treatment on linear growth in the young diabetic patient. *J Pediatr* **101:**333, 1982.

200. Blethen SL, Sargeant DT, Whitlow MG, et al: Effect of pubertal stage and recent blood glucose control on plasma somatomedin C in children with insulin-dependent diabetes mellitus. *Diabetes* **30:**868, 1981.

201. Lanes R, Recker B, Fort P, et al: Impaired somatomedin generation test in poorly controlled insulin dependent diabetes mellitus. *Pediatr Res* **18**(Apr):169A, 1984.

202. Henry D, Elders MJ: Growth retardation syndromes associated with hypophosphatemia. *J Arkansas Med Soc* **74:**481, 1978.

203. Bachrach S: Vitamin D deficiency rickets in American children. *Comprehensive Therapy* **7:**29, 1981.

204. Tolman KG, Jubiz W, Sannella JJ, et al: Osteomalacia associated with anticonvulsant drug therapy in mentally retarded children. *Pediatrics* **56:**45, 1975.

205. Felsenfeld A, Llach F: Vitamin D and metabolic bone disease: A clinicopathologic overview. *Path Ann* **17**(1):383, 1982.

206. Pitt MJ: Rachitic and osteomalacic syndromes. *Radiol Clin No Am* **19:**581, 1981.

207. Fraser D, Scriver CR: Familial forms of vitamin D-resistant rickets revisited. X-linked hypophosphatemia and autosomal resessive vitamin D dependency. *Am J Clin Nutri* **29:**1315, 1976.

208. Schulman JD, Schneider JA: Cystinosis and the Fanconi syndrome. *Pediatr Clin North Am* **23:**779, 1976.

209. Blodgett FM, Burgin L, Iezzoni D, et al: Effects of prolonged cortisone therapy on the statural growth, skeletal maturation and metabolic status of children. *New Engl J Med* **254:**636, 1956.

210. Champion PK: Cushing syndrome secondary to abuse of dexamethasone nasal spray. *Arch Inter Med* **134:**750, 1974.

211. May P, Stein EJ, Ryter RJ, et al: Cushing Syndrome from percutaneous absorption of triamcinolone cream. *Arch Inter med* **136:**612, 1976.

212. Graber AL, Ney RL, Liddle GW, et al: Natural history of pituitary-adrenal recovery following long-term suppression with corticosteroids. *J Clin Endocrinol Metab* **25:**11, 1965.

213. Sobel EH: Abnormal growth patterns in infancy and childhood, in *Endocrine and Genetic Disease of Childhood and Adolescence.* Gardner LI (ed), Philadelphia, WB Saunders Co, 1975, pp 74–84.

214. Sadeghi-Nejad A, Senior B: Adrenal function, growth and insulin response in patients treated with corticoids on alternate days. *Pediatr* **43:**277, 1967.

215. Soyka LF: Treatment of the nephrotic syndrome in childhood. Use of an alternate day prednisone regimen. *Am J Dis Child* **113:**693, 1967.

216. Elders MJ, Wingfield BS, McNatt ML, et al: Glucocorticoid therapy in children, effect on somatomedin secretion. *Am J Dis Child* **129:**1393, 1975.

217. Kerrebijn KF, DeKroon JPM: Effect on height of corticosteroid therapy in asthmatic children. *Arch Dis Child* **43:**556, 1968.

218. Frantz AG, Rabkin MT: Human growth hormone, clinical measurement, response to hypoglycemia and suppression by corticosteroids. *New Engl J Med* **271:**1375, 1964.

219. Morris HG, Jorgensen JR, Elrick H, et al: Metabolic effects of human growth hormone in corticosteroid treated children. *J Clin Invest* **47:**436, 1968.

220. Baxter JD: Mechanisms of glucocorticoid inhibition of growth. *Kidney Int* **14:**330, 1978.

221. Van der Werf ten Bosch JJ, Haak A: *Somatic Growth of the Child,* Springfield, Charles C. Thomas, 1966.

222. Safer D, Allen R, Barr E: Depression of growth in hyperactive children on stimulant drugs. *New Engl J Med* **287:**217, 1972.

223. Roche AF, Lipman RS, Overall JE, et al: The Effects of stimulant medication on the growth of hyperkinetic children. *Pediatrics* **63:**847, 1979.

224. Klinefelter HF Jr, Reifenstein EC Jr, Albright F: Syndrome characterised by gynecomastia, aspermatogenesis without aleydigism, and increased secretion of follicle-stimulating hormone. *J Clin Endocrol Metab* **2:**615, 1942.

225. Ratcliffe SG: The sexual development of boys with the chromosome constitution 47, XXY (Klinefelter's syndrome). *J Clin Endocrinol Metab* **11:**703, 1982.

226. Caldwell PD, Smith DW: The XXY syndrome in childhood. Detection and treatment. *J Pediatr* **80:**250, 1972.

227. Vallentine GH, McClelland MA, Sergovich FR: The growth and development of four XYY infants. *Pediatrics* **48:**583, 1971.

228. Nielson J, Friedrich U, Zeuthen E: Stature and weight in boys with the XYY syndrome. *Humangentik* **14:**66, 1971.

229. Marfan AB: Un cas de deformation congenitale des quatre membres plus prononcee aux extremites characterisee par e'allongement des os avec un certain degre d'amincissement. *Bull Mem Soc Med Hosp (Paris)* **13:**220, 1896.

230. Pyeritz RE, McKusick VA: The Marfan syndrome. Diagnosis and management. *N Engl J Med* **300:**772, 1979.

231. Boucek RJ, Noble NL, Gunja-Smith Z, et al: The Marfan syndrome: A deficiency in chemically stable collagen cross-links. *N Engl J Med* **305:**988, 1981.

232. Roberts WC, Honig HS: The spectrum of cardiovascual disease in the Marfan syndrome: A clinico-morphologic study of 18 necropsy patients and comparison to 151 previously reported necropsy patients. *Am Heart J* **104:**115, 1982.

233. Carson NAJ, Cusworth DC, Dent CE, et al: Homocystinuria: A new inborn error of metabolism associated with mental deficiency. *Arch Dis Child* **38:**425, 1963.

234. Sotos JF, Dodge PR, Muirhead D, et al: Cerebral gigantism in childhood. A syndrome of excessively rapid growth with acromegalic features and a non-progressive neurologic disorder. *New Engl J Med* **271:**109, 1964.

235. Jaecken J, Vanderschueren-Lodeweyckx M, Eeckels R: Cerebral gigantism syndrome. *Zeitschr Kinderheilkd* **112:**332, 1972.

236. Weaver DD, Graham CB, Thomas IT, et al: A new overgrowth syndrome with accelerated skeletal maturation, unusual facies and camptodactyly. *J Pediatr* **84:**547, 1974.

237. Sinclair D: *Human Growth After Birth*, ed 3. London Oxford University Press, p 43, 1978.

238. Behrens LH, Barr DP: Hyperpituitarism beginning in infancy: The Alton giant, *Endocrinol* **16:**120, 1932.

239. Daughaday WH: Extreme gigantism: Analysis of growth velocity and occurrence of severe peripheral neuropathy and neuropathic arthropathy. *New Engl J Med* **297:**1267, 1977.

240. Frasier SD, Kogut MD: Adolescent acromegaly: Studies of growth hormone and insulin metabolism. *J Pediatr* **71:**832, 1967.

241. Saxena KM, Crawford JD: Acromegalic gigantism in an adolescent girl. *J Pediatr* **62:**660, 1963.

242. Spence HJ, Trias EP, Raiti S: Acromegaly in a 9½ year old boy. *Am J Dis Child* **123:**504, 1972.

243. Costin G, Fefferman RA, Kogut, MD: Hypothalamic gigantism. *J Pediatr* **83:**419, 1973.

244. Schlesinger S, MacGillivray MH, Munschauer RW: Acceleration of growth and bone maturation in childhood thyrotoxicosis. *J Pediatr* **83:**233, 1973.

245. Lamb DR: Anabolic steroids in athletics: How well do they work and how dangerous are they? *Am J Sports Med* **12:**31, 1984.

246. Frasier SD: Androgens and athletes. *Am J Dis Child* **125:**479, 1973.

247. Ryan AJ: Anabolic steroids are fools gold. *Fed Proc* **40:**2682, 1981.

248. Wright JE: Anabolic steroids and athletics. *Exercis Sports Scien Rev* **8:**149, 1980.

249. Brooks R: Olympic up-date: Anabolic steroids and athletes. *The Physician and Sports Medicine* **8:**161, 1980.

# 10
# Growth Disorders
## of Adolescence

Growth throughout adolescence and ultimate adult height are closely related to events of sexual maturation (puberty). In Chapter 5 we discussed the normal relationships between growth and pubertal events, and in this chapter we will direct attention to abnormalities of growth accompanying pubertal disorders (see Table 10-1). Some disorders, such as familial short stature, skeletal dysplasias, congenital dysmorphic syndromes, and intrauterine growth retardation are associated with short stature in childhood and adolescence, but pubertal development and the pubertal growth spurt occur at about the usual time and in a normal sequence. Such children will receive only casual attention in this section. Disorders of puberty, which have little or no effect on growth (such as testicular feminization syndrome, Kallmann's syndrome, and many disorders producing amenorrhea), will be listed in tables for completeness but will not be discussed in detail.

## NORMAL PHYSIOLOGIC VARIANTS OF ADOLESCENCE

Physiologic delay or acceleration of sexual maturation (puberty) represent the extremes of normal variation in tempo of growth and sexual maturation and are the adolescent counterparts of constitutional delayed or accelerated growth patterns of childhood (Chapter 9). They are not strictly disorders of either growth or of puberty, but since they deviate strikingly from the average tempo of growth and development, they frequently excite concern.

### Constitutional Delay of Adolescence

Constitutional delay appears to be the result of a delayed maturation of the hypothalamic mechanism which regulates the endocrinologic phenomena of puberty (1). It is not an endocrine disorder but rather an extreme

348

**Table 10-1.**

1. *Normal Physiologic Variants*
   Constitutional delayed adolescence
   Constitutional accelerated adolescence
2. *Delayed Adolescence (Puberty)*
   Hypothalamic disorders
   Pituitary disorders
   Gonadal disorders
   Endocrine disorders
   Systemic disease
3. *Precocious Puberty*
   Hypothalamic (pituitary) precocity
   Gonadotropin-producing tumors
   Sex hormone excess from tumor or hyperplasia
   Exogenous hormone administration

of a normal phenomenon. In Prader's longitudinal study of normal children in Zurich, over 97% of boys showed initial testicular enlargement by 14 years and first pubic hair by 15 years (2). Similarly, over 97% of girls could expect breast budding and first pubic hair by 13–13½ years (2). Although these limits are often used to define the "normal" range beyond which careful evaluation for organic delay in puberty should be sought, Prader rightly points out that 2.5% of *normal* adolescents will be delayed in their pubertal onset beyond these limits (2).

Constitutional delay of puberty is the most common problem in adolescents who seek medical counsel because of pubertal delay (1). It occurs with equal frequency in males and females, although far more males seek medical relief because ". . . in our society they are more likely to be openly ridiculed, abused, bullied by their peers . . . or excluded from social and athletic activities because of inappropriate size and development for their chronologic age" (1).

## Clinical Characteristics and Natural History

Typically the youngster with delayed adolescence is a boy age 14–17 (or a girl age 13–16) who looks younger than his (her) stated age. These youngsters are short for age, but in good health. Generally, they are short throughout childhood, but become acutely aware of their small size and lack of sexual development and may begin to wonder whether something is wrong when their peers begin their pubertal development and growth spurt (2) (Figure 9-1).

In about 60% of families, there is a history of late maturation in other family members (1). In order to elicit this information, it may be necessary to specifically ask the age of menarche in adult female family members and ask how much male members grew after leaving high school or after enlisting in armed forces.

The children are generally of normal length and weight at birth but have a growth deceleration during the first few years of life accompanied by a delay in skeletal maturation (3). They are frequently at or below the 3rd percentile. Linear growth proceeds through childhood more or less parallel to the 3rd percentile at a normal rate of about 5 cm/yr, however, actual measurements are not often available (1). At about the time that a pubertal growth spurt might be expected, the growth rate of the child with delayed puberty is slowing down (Figure 9-1). This serves merely to exaggerate the differences between the slow-maturer and his or her peers and excites anxiety about growth.

Physical examination of the child is usually normal. Precise measurements of height, weight, and body proportion are needed to be sure that the child is progressing normally, and particular note should be made of nutritional status. Genitalia are normal. Sometimes evidence of early puberty is present, although it is not always appreciated by the child. Testicular size may already be approaching early pubertal levels in boys (2) and changes in vaginal mucosa and labial hairs or even very early breast budding may be present in the girl. Skeletal maturation is delayed (usually 1–3 years) by about the same proportion as are height and weight (1).

Laboratory testing, including endocrinologic investigation, is normal. Hemogram, erythrocyte sedimentation rate, urinalysis, serum thyroxine, and skull x-rays are all normal and help separate constitutional delayed puberty from systemic diseases and hypothyroidism, which might present with delay in puberty (1). The levels of gonadotropins and their response to GnRH are low for chronologic age but appropriate for physiologic stage (bone age) (4–6). The response of plasma growth hormone to stimulation tests is normal or low (2), but normal levels are found after administration of small amounts of sex hormones (7).

If untreated, the child with constitutional delay of puberty will grow and develop about as expected for a child the age of his or her bone age. Skeletal maturation seems to represent the physiologic status with considerable accuracy (2). Testicular volume will start to increase in the boy at a bone age of about 12 and pubic hair will appear at a bone age of about 13. The pubertal growth spurt will begin soon thereafter, and peak height velocity will be reached at a bone age of about 14 (2). Similar predictions of timing of events of puberty for the late-maturing girl can be made with expectation of breast budding and growth spurt when the bone age is between 11 and 12, and menarche when the bone age reaches about 13 years. Growth rate is very low just before the pubertal growth spurt, giving the impression of cessation of growth. Late in starting, the growth spurt tends to be less noticeable than average, but continues well past the age when growth has usually ceased and the ultimate height attained is usually within the range expected, based on mid-parent height (2).

Since constitutional delay of puberty is a normal state and not a disease, the diagnosis is one of exclusion of other causes of delayed puberty. However, a positive diagnosis can be made, in most instances, if one finds growth retardation and modestly delayed skeletal maturation in a healthy boy or girl who has grown at a normal rate through childhood and has a family history of delayed puberty (2). One may add a negative review for systemic disease, appropriate nutrition, good eating habits and normal screening lab tests (1). Patients who fail to show the typical characteristics, described above, for constitutional delayed puberty or who fail to progress through puberty at a satisfactory rate (approximately 4–5 years from beginning to culmination) should be studied further (1).

The differential diagnosis for delayed puberty is long, but there are a few disorders which closely simulate constitutional delay of puberty. These include chronic diseases such as renal tubular acidosis or inflammatory bowel disease, dysmorphic syndromes such as Silver–Russell syndrome, chromosomal syndromes such as Turner's or Klinefelter's syndrome, gonadotropin deficiencies (hypopituitarism), and primary gonadal failure (1, 2). These entities are discussed in the section on delayed puberty in this chapter.

The GnRH (LHRH) stimulation test may be useful in determining the normal status of the hypothalamic–pituitary–gonadal axis in the subject with delayed puberty. The intravenous injection of GnRH produces an age-dependent peak of plasma LH and FSH (4–6). In primary gonadal failure and in Turner's syndrome, the response is enhanced; in hypo-thalamic and pituitary failure, the levels are low. In constitutional delay of puberty the values are normal for the child's bone-age (2, 5). A decreased response to LHRH is seen in children with constitutional delay of puberty if the LHRH test is repeated on consecutive days (7). Decreased responsiveness of the gonad to gonadotropin and of the pituitary to clomiphene stimulation (8) seem to point to delayed maturation or delayed sensitivity of the hypothalmic–pituitary–gonadal axis in constitutional delay of puberty.

### Treatment of Constitutional Delay of Puberty

A normal but delayed physiologic state needs no therapy because puberty will eventually occur spontaneously. The treatment of choice, therefore, is to provide counsel, assuring the youngster that he or she is normal and that with time full normal growth and maturation will occur. A growth chart depicting the rate of growth, a description of the events of puberty as they relate to bone-age, and a prediction of ultimate adult height may help the youngster to see his or her pattern in perspective. Evidence of normal laboratory tests may also be reassuring, including a response to GnRH if deemed desirable. If reassurance is accepted by the young person and by his or her parents, he/she should be followed at intervals of about 6–12 months in order to document progress toward spontaneous puberty and to reassure both patient and parent of the physician's concern but conviction that all is normal (1).

For some boys and most girls, such reassurance is sufficient, but for some young men, the psychosocial pressures of sexual immaturity and small size seem insurmountable and of extreme urgency. Short stature and sexual immaturity set the adolescent apart from his or her peers, distort his/her self-image, and create anxiety. They may feel rejected by peers and avoid physical education classes or fail to shower because of taunting and bullying in the shower room by their peers, or in other ways withdraw from peer contact or act out in antisocial ways to show their extreme discomfort. Patience in waiting out the time-table of nature is difficult for a teenager, and sometimes the burden of feeling different or deprived of natural sexual development leaves long-standing psychological scars. The extent of their feelings may not be evident during the initial examination and time may need to be provided for an open discussion without social pressures.

If psychosocial pressures seem to warrant medical intervention, it is possible to provide hormonal therapy over a short period of time to stimulate appearance of sex characteristics. Both the expected benefits and the possible undesirable side effects of a short course of gonadal hormones should be outlined to the patient and the parents so they can intelligently participate in the decision to use such therapy or await the natural occurrence of puberty.

For a boy, treatment with a long-acting injectable preparation of testosterone is preferred. Suggested dosage varies from 50 mg of testosterone enanthate at monthly intervals for 3–4 months to 200 mg monthly for 4–6 months (1, 9). Prader suggests 100 mg at first, followed by 250 mg monthly (2). We have used an adaptation of these regimens, beginning with 50 mg of testosterone enanthate intramuscularly and at 3 week intervals increasing the dosage by 50 mg progressively up to 200 mg and thereafter, administering 200 mg every 3 weeks for the remainder of a 6 month period. This dosage schedule has been well accepted and within the 6 month period, noticeable acceleration of growth and appearance of sex characteristics are usually seen. Some continued growth and development occurs for several months after the medication is stopped, so examination for changes in size, sexual maturation, and for estimation of skeletal maturation (and predicted mature height) should be continued for at least 6 months after therapy before additional treatment is considered. The desired acceleration of growth and sexual development is more likely to occur if treatment can be deferred until the bone-age is approaching the usual age for onset of puberty; that is, 12–13 years. If insufficient growth and development has occurred, a second course of therapy may be initiated, but it must be understood by the patient and parent that prolonged therapy with testosterone can reduce ultimate height achievement, produce some tubular damage, and possible infertility can result (10–11). Brief courses of androgen, as described here, have not been shown to adversely affect ultimate height (12).

Accelerated growth and sexual development have also been achieved by use of oral testosterone derivatives such as methyl testosterone in dosages of 10–20 mg/day or fluoxymesterone 5–10 mg/day for 4–6 months or the use of human chorionic gonadotropin (hCG) 1500–2000 units intramuscularly weekly for 3–4 months (13). The latter therapy, though having some theoretical advantage in stimulating activity of the subject's own testes, is inconvenient because of the frequency of injections required. There is also some fear that permanent tubular damage may occur with prolonged administration of hCG (14). The propensity of methyltestosterone to cause cholestatic jaundice, the relative costs of medication, and less effective stimulation of sexual development with testosterone derivatives have led us to prefer testosterone injections to other forms of therapy. The dosage used to stimulate accelerated puberty must be the least amount which will accomplish the aim of therapy. Larger amounts of androgens over longer periods of time will compromise eventual height and are more likely to be accompanied by gynecomastia and tubular damage in the testes (1, 11).

Though girls require therapy less often than boys, initiation of pubertal development can be accomplished by treatment with ethinyl estradiol 50–80 µg/day for 90 days (9) or with conjugated estrogen 0.3 to 0.625 mg/day, adding medroxyprogesterone for 6 days each month to allow menstrual periods (1). We have found the use of conjugated estrogens either continuously or interrupted with medroxyprogesterone for a 3–6 month period to be quite satisfactory in initiating puberty in girls with a skeletal maturation near the usual time for puberty (11–12 yrs). Estrogens accelerate epiphyseal fusion and may compromise predicted adult height, although for brief periods of 3–6 months the effect on ultimate height is undetectable. If growth acceleration is desired, together with promotion of sexual maturation, it may be desirable to combine estrogen therapy with an anabolic steroid such as oxandrolone (0.1–0.25 mg/kg/day). The use of combined hormones increases the likelihood of unwanted acceleration of skeletal maturation, depending on dosage and length of treatment. The treatment should, for these reasons, be reserved for "the adolescent female who has severe psychological and social disability resulting from her maturational delay" (1).

Children with *familial short stature* will also be short as adolescents, but their pubertal development can be expected to appear at the usual time and they will progress normally through puberty, achieving their full mature height and development appropriate for their genetic endowment. Bone age tends to be approximately equal to the chronologic age and the height of the adolescent is within the range expected from the mid-parent height. No endocrine abnormalities are present and no treatment will increase the ultimate height achievement.

## Constitutional Accelerated Puberty

Some children who are tall for age have tall parents and normal rate of skeletal maturation. They enter puberty at the usual time and ultimately achieve a tall adult height (familial tall stature). Other children who are tall for age have accelerated skeletal maturation. The bone age is one or more years advanced when compared to their chronologic age. These children are large throughout childhood, enter puberty earlier than the average, and complete their full growth at an early age, achieving an ultimate height lower than expected from their childhood growth pattern but consistent with their mid-parent height.

For a boy the average age for appearance of pubic hair is 12–13 years. Enlargement of the testes begins by about age $11\frac{1}{2}$ and marks the true beginning of puberty in the boy, however, testicular enlargement is not noticeable, except by careful examination. Boys with constitutional accelerated puberty exhibit noticeable signs of puberty as early as $9$–$9\frac{1}{2}$ years. The sequence of pubertal events is normal though accelerated, and the children achieve full sexual development and adult height at an early age. The choice of 9 or $9\frac{1}{2}$ years (2–2.5 standard deviations early) as a definition of normal accelerated puberty is arbitrary (18). There may be normal adolescents who begin puberty earlier and some with pathologic pubertal development beginning later.

For a girl, breast development is usually the first noticeable sign of puberty, beginning on the average at $11$–$11\frac{1}{2}$ years (15). Girls with constitutional accelerated adolescence may be expected to exhibit breast development as early as $8\frac{1}{2}$–9 years (2–2.5 standard deviations early). As with early maturing boys, the sequence of events of puberty is normal, though generally proceeding at a slightly more rapid than normal rate, and full height and sexual maturity are achieved as early as 12–13 years. The dividing line between constitutional accelerated puberty and idiopathic precocious puberty is arbitrary, because idiopathic precocious puberty is indistinguishable in all respects from normal puberty except by timing.

The only treatment needed is reassurance to the patient and parents that the phenomenon is normal. Prediction of mature height can be offered from Greulich–Pyle height prediction charts if it is felt that short stature may occur and may present problems with psychological acceptance. In such cases, some reassurance or counseling may be of help. Counseling should also direct attention to the possible effects of early full sexual maturation, the possibility of sexual aggressiveness in boys or of shyness and withdrawal in girls. If the danger of conception is viewed as real in girls, contraception may be considered seriously as girls achieve an age of possible fertility 1–2 years after menses.

Table 10-2. Definitions of Delayed Adolescence

|  | Boy | Girl |
|---|---|---|
| Marshall/Tanner (16, 17) (1969, 1970) | Less than stage G2 by 13.6 years | Less than stage B2 by 13.4 years |
|  | or | or |
|  | excessive delay in passing from G2 to G5 | failure to pass from stage B2 to menarche within 5 years |
| Prader (2) (1975) | Testes less than 4–6 mL by 13.9 years | No breast development by 13.4 years |
| Root (18) (1973) | No testicular enlargement by 13.5 years | No Breast development by 13 years |
|  | or | or |
|  | more than 5 years to achieve full maturity | greater than 5 years from earliest breast development to menarche |

## DELAYED ADOLESCENCE

The point at which puberty is considered to be unnaturally delayed is somewhat arbitrary, but if it is assumed that most children will begin puberty within two standard deviations of the mean time for first noticeable signs of puberty, the age at which puberty may be said to be delayed may be defined as suggested in Table 10-2. The definitions, all of which are arbitrary, are sufficiently uniform that we may accept the definition of delayed puberty for boys as failure to exhibit testicular enlargement (Tanner stage G2) by age 13.5 to 14 years and for girls as failure to show breast development (Tanner stage B2) by 13 to 13.5 years (16–18).

### Causes of Delayed Adolescence

The most common cause of delayed adolescence is constitutional delay which has been defined and described in the preceeding section. The remainder of the causes can be considered as hypothalamic, pituitary, or gonadal disorders, or as involving other endocrine or systemic disorders (19) as outlined in Table 10-3. We have chosen to consider delayed puberty as a function of the hypothalamic–pituitary–gonadal axis, although it may be useful from a diagnostic viewpoint to consider the causes of *hypogonadism* (Turner's syndrome XO and its variants versus ovarian failure in a 46XX female—radiation, infection, etc.), *hypogonadotropism* (physiologic delay, endocrine disorders, systemic diseases, congenital deficiency disorders, or anatomic lesions of the pituitary–hypothalamus), or *eugonadism* (absence of the uterus, polycystic ovaries, or androgen insensitivity) as suggested by Reindollar and McDonough (20).

## Table 10-3. Causes of Delayed Adolescence (Puberty)

A. *Hypothalamic Disorders*
1. Congenital deficiency of GnRH
   (a) Familial or sporadic
   (b) Kallmann's syndrome
   (c) Lawrence–Moon–Biedl syndrome
   (d) Prader–Willi syndrome
2. Acquired deficiency of GnRH
   (a) Infections
   (b) Neoplasms
   (c) Trauma

B. *Pituitary Disorders*
1. Congenital gonadotrophin deficiency
   (a) Idiopathic hypopituitariam
   (b) Isolated LH or FSH deficiency
   (c) Midline brain defects
2. Acquired gonadotrophin deficiency
   (a) Neoplasms
       (1) Craniopharyngioma, histiocytosis
       (2) Pituitary adenomas
   (b) Infections (meningitis, etc)
   (c) Trauma
   (d) Radiation Damage

C. *Gonadal disorders*
1. Congenital gonadal deficiency
   (a) Turner's syndrome (45 XO + mosaics)
   (b) Klinefelter's syndrome
   (c) Gonadal agenesis or dysgenesis
   (d) Familial testicular deficiency syndromes
   (e) Myotonia dystrophica
2. Acquired gonadal deficiency
   (a) Infections (gonorrhea, orchitis, etc)
   (b) Mechanical, post-operative, irradiation
       (1) Torsion of ovary or testes
       (2) Oophrectomy/orchiectomy
       (3) Post-orchiopexy atrophy
       (4) Post-irradiation necrosis
   (c) Post-Traumatic
       (1) Spinal cord damage
       (2) Testicular injury/atrophy

D. *Endocrine Disorders*
1. Hypothyroidism/hyperthyroidism
2. Cushing's syndrome/adrenogenital syndrome
3. Diabetic mellitus
4. Androgen insensitivity

Table 10-3. (Continued)

E.  Systemic (Major Organ) Disease
    1.  Socioeconomic malnutrition
    2.  Regional enteritis/ulcerative colitis
    3.  Renal failure/Renal tubular acidosis
    4.  Cyanotic heart disease
    5.  Asthma
    6.  Anemia/leukemia
    7.  Juvenile rheumatoid arthritis/SLE
    8.  Anorexia nervosa

Reproduced by permission and adapted from Shenker IR, et al, *Pediatric Annals* **7**(9): 605, Sept 1978 and Barnes VD, *Med Clin North Am* **59**:1337, 1975.

## Hypothalamic/Pituitary Disorders

The initiation of puberty depends upon the maturation of the hypothalamic–pituitary–gonadal axis. Puberty will fail to occur naturally if there is a deficiency of the hypothalamic gonadotropin releasing hormone (GnRH).

In some people there is familial or sporadic absence of GnRH; in others the deficiency of GnRH is associated with characteristic features. *Kallmann's syndrome* is characterized by hypogonadotropic hypogonadism and anosmia. Children with this syndrome fail to develop sexually but are usually of normal size with increased arm span, long legs, and relative shortening of the trunk. Both FSH and LH remain at prepubertal levels; however, elevations occur after test administration of GnRH (21). Inability to smell, due to agenesis of the olfactory lobes, is present from early childhood, although often not a complaint, unless specifically sought. In some patients, gynecomastia, cryptorchidism, deafness, cleft lip or palate, and renal anomalies may occur (19). Familial occurrence suggests an autosomal dominant or recessive mode of inheritance with variable expression and penetrance (22). In the *Prader–Willi syndrome*, delayed puberty and cryptorchidism due to hypothalamic dysfunction is associated with infantile hypotonia, massive obesity, short stature, mental deficiency, characteristic facial appearance with almond-shaped eyes, small broad hands and feet, and carbohydrate intolerance (23). The *Lawrence–Moon–Biedl syndrome* is an autosomal recessive condition characterized by hypogonadotropic hypogonadism (deficiency of hypothalamic GnRH) or primary gonadal failure and polydactyly, obesity, mental retardation, and retinitis pigmentosa (24).

Deficiency of GnRH can also occur from acquired lesions of the hypothalamus. Infections involving the hypothalamus, such as encephalitis, sarcoidosis, or tuberculosis; trauma or hypothalamic neoplasms such as craniopharyngiomas, gliomas, astrocytomas, and pinealomas; or histiocytosis may interfere with release of GnRH and lead to hypogonadotropic delay in puberty. Neoplasms are often small and occult, causing no neurologic symptoms and the delay in puberty may be considered to be a constitutional delay for some time or until more definitive symptoms suggest an intracranial lesion.

Many of the disorders that affect releasing factors from the hypothalamus affect the pituitary gland as well. It is common to see multihormonal pituitary defects from involvement of pituitary and hypothalamic tissue by the disease process. Tumors of the pituitary may be intrasellar (pituitary adenomas) or may originate in extrasellar tissues but invade the sella and destroy pituitary function (histiocytosis).

In *idiopathic hypopituitarism*, congenital hypothalamic dysfunction results in deficiency of gonadotropins and other pituitary hormones. Growth hormone deficiency from early childhood results in a low rate of growth and progressive deviation from expected growth achievement. A variety of combinations of pituitary hormone deficiencies are seen, ranging from isolated growth hormone deficiency to complete pituitary deficiency. If gonadotropin production is deficient, pubertal development will not take place and sexual infantilism will persist. Partial GnRH deficiency in the male produces the "fertile eunuch" syndrome with lack of LH stimulated sexual development but normal spermatogenesis (18). *Midline malformations of the brain* may be associated with deficiencies of hypothalamic–pituitary function. In infancy this may be manifest by micropenis in the male, hypoglycemia or optic hypoplasia (see Chapter 8). At adolescence there will be pituitary deficiency of gonadotropins resulting in pubertal delay (21).

*Craniopharyngioma*, arising from the remnants of Rathke's pouch, is the most common of the hypothalamic–pituitary tumors in children, accounting for the majority of the brain lesions producing pubertal delay (25). Growth failure, increased intracranial pressure, and loss of vision beginning in mid to late childhood form the typical triad of signs of the tumor. Decreased visual acuity, bitemporal field deficits or even blindness emphasize the central location of the tumor. Hydrocephalus, headache, vomiting, or other signs of increased intracranial pressure may obscure the endocrine abnormalities. Multiple endocrine abnormalities may occur because of destruction or compression of the pituitary and hypothalamus, including short stature (growth hormone deficiency), lack or arrest of sexual development, diabetes insipidus, and less frequently, hypothyroidism and hypoadrenalism (25).

*Histiocytosis* X (Hand–Schüller–Christian disease) is a chronic, disseminating reticuloendotheliosis characterized by infiltration of histiocytes into skin, viscera and bone. Diabetes insipidus from infiltration of the hypothalamus is the most common endocrine deficiency, although growth hormone deficiency and lack of sexual development have also been observed (21, 26). *Pituitary adenomas* are uncommon in children. Pituitary deficiency is produced by compression of the normal pituitary tissue by the intrasellar tumor, or from impairment of the hypophyseal–portal circulation. Extrasellar expansion of the tumor may produce pressure on the optic chiasm, optic nerve, or hypothalamus. Pituitary deficiency is recognized by decreased linear growth and delayed sexual development. Hypothyroidism and deficiency of adrenocortical hormones may be detected later (25). Prolactin producing tumors or isolated hyperprolactinemia may also produce a delay in puberty (27). *Basilar meningitis*, most commonly due to meningeal tuberculosis, may lead to scarring and impaired hypothalamic–pituitary function. *Head trauma* may result in transsection of the pituitary stalk, resulting in deficient pituitary function. Children who receive *radiation therapy* for intracranial tumors may develop complete or partial gonadotropin deficiency, usually associated with human growth hormone deficiency (28). Similarly, children treated for leukemia with *radiation* and *chemotherapeutic agents* may have growth failure and pubertal delay from pituitary or hypothalamic failure.

### Gonadal Disorders

Gonadal deficiency may arise from congenital disorders such as Turner's or Klinefelter's syndromes, or from acquired disorders including infection, trauma, or physical factors.

*Klinefelter's syndrome* represents a chromosomal excess disorder (XXY) in males with an abnormality of the seminiferous tubules. In childhood, the individual with Klinefelter's syndrome has a relatively small penis and testes, and in adolescence and adulthood, the testes remain small. The seminiferous tubules become hyalinized and fibrotic and infertility is usual. Testosterone production and virilization are diminished in some patients, but most have adequate testosterone production to produce normal virilization (29). Gynecomastia occurs in most cases. FSH levels are characteristically high because of deficient inhibin formation by the Sertoli cells from the abnormal testes. Elevation of gonadotropins has been seen as early as age 10–11 (30). Individuals with Klinefelter's syndrome tend to be tall and slim with long limbs. Mental dullness or behavioral problems are common (31), but in many the variations from normal in growth, intelligence tests scores, and psychosexual development are of small degree (29).

In previous chapters we have emphasized the appearance and growth characteristics of individuals with *Turner's syndrome* in infancy (Chapter 8) and childhood (Chapter 9). The most consistent features of Turner's syndrome are short stature and gonadal dysgenesis (32). As the child approaches the age of puberty, lack of sexual development may become the most noticeable feature of the syndrome. Because the characteristic physical features, which allow recognition, may be absent, it is important to consider Turner's syndrome in any girl presenting with short stature and sexual infantilism.

Typically, girls with Turner's syndrome grow slowly during childhood, fail to have a pubertal growth spurt, and achieve a mean final height of about 142 cm (55 inches) depending somewhat on mid-parent height (32, 33). Physical anomalies that may aid in recognition include distinct facial appearance with micrognathia, fish mouth, ptosis, low-set or malformed ears, and high arched palate. The neck is short, with a low hairline and webbing (pterygium colli). The chest is shield-shaped with hypoplastic nipples. The hands may be short (metacarpals) and the nails hypoplastic; and there is an increased carrying angle of the arms (cubitus valgus) (Figure 9-4). In addition, left-sided cardiac anomalies (such as coarctation of the aorta, or aortic stenosis), positional anomalies of the kidney, frequent otitis media with mild deafness, and acquired hypothyroidism (Hashimoto's thyroiditis) may be associated (21, 32).

Dysgenesis of the ovaries prevents sexual development in the girl with Turner's syndrome at the usual time of puberty, though adrenarche may occur because of normal androgen secretion from the adrenal glands. This usually occurs a little later than usual and pubic and body hair are generally somewhat sparse. Because of the ovarian agenesis, serum FSH and LH levels are elevated. Levels are elevated during the first few years of life, then fall to nearly normal levels until the age at which adolescent development is expected to occur when levels rise to characteristically high (menopausal) levels (20, 34).

Some sexual development does occur in individuals with variants of the syndrome, including individuals with mosaic chromosomal patterns and those with isochrome or partial sex chromosome deletion patterns. In individuals with mosaic karyotypes the phenotype may range from typical Turner's syndrome to normal appearing female (20). Functioning ovarian tissue may be present leading to pubertal development, menarche, and rarely even pregnancy (21). Gonadal dysgenesis with a structurally abnormal X chromosome leads to a variety of patterns of growth and sexual development. Loss of one complete chromosome in all tissues results in short stature, gonadal dysgenesis, and somatic anomalies. But loss of either short arm or long arm of one of the X chromosomes leads to partial expression of the syndrome. Deletion of the short arm of the X chromosome as in XXqi or XXp- results in short stature and somatic anomalies, although feminization may occur normally, occasionally even with menses. Loss of the long arms as in XXpi or XXq- results in gonadal dysgenesis and lack of feminization but normal height and variable somatic anomalies (35).

A congenital absence of gonads in either sex, *gonadal agenesis*, will result in lack of sexual development at puberty, but may not affect growth appreciably until the usual time of puberty. In utero an ovary is not necessary for female development to take place, but functioning testes are necessary for male development. It is presumed, therefore, in male "anorchia" that testes were present during intrauterine life but that sometime after formation of male organs the testes underwent total atrophy, leaving the child approaching puberty without any identifiable testicular tissue (36).

Several forms of *familial testicular insufficiency* have been described (37). *Reifenstein's syndrome* is characterized by hypospadius, postpubertal sclerosis of spermatogenic tubules, decreased virilization, and gynecomastia. In *Weinstein's syndrome*, hyalinization of tubules and failure of germ cell development is associated with obesity, blindness, nerve deafness, and hyperuricemia (18). Subjects with *myotonic muscular dystrophy* commonly have postpubertal sclerosis of the spermatic tubules, premature balding, and cataracts (37). Individuals with *familial germinal cell aplasia* are infertile but virilize normally.

Destruction of gonadal tissue by *trauma* or *infections* can lead to hypogonadal function of variable degree. If the destruction is severe enough, both fertility and endocrine function can be diminished or absent. *Orchitis* from mumps or other viral infections, at or after puberty, may produce gonadal atrophy and decreased function, as can tuberculous invasion of the gonads. Severe gonorrheal infection can lead to scarring of either gonads or internal genital duct structures, producing sterility, but only leads to complete gonadal atrophy on rare occasions. Direct *trauma* to the testicle can lead to atrophy, and if both testes are involved, lack of sexual development would follow. Spinal cord damage may lead to infertility and to pubertal delay, but less commonly to total lack of pubertal development. *Torsion of ovary or testes* may lead to infarction and atrophy. Gonads may need to be surgically removed because of tumor or injury. The testes may undergo atrophy after *orchiopexy for cryptorchidism* and ovary or testes may become atrophic after pelvic irradiation. If any of these events occur before puberty and both gonads are involved, puberty will be delayed and require hormonal replacement.

### Endocrine Disorders

A number of endocrine disorders, not directly involved in the hypothalamic–pituitary–gonadal axis, may also cause a delayed or deficient puberty.

*Hypothyroidism* will delay growth, skeletal maturation, and pubertal development. On occasion, especially in girls, precocious pubertal development may occur despite retardation in growth and skeletal maturation. Characteristically, hypothyroidism in childhood is insidious in onset; gradual growth failure and delay in onset or progression of secondary sexual characteristics may be the only signs noted initially. Easy fatigue or lethargy, mild constipation, and dry skin may also be present. Short, stocky appearance with mild puffiness of the face, sallow complexion, slow pulse rate, delayed reflex relaxation, modest-sized goiter, and delay in sexual maturation may be seen on examination (Figure 9-10). Serum thyroxine ($T_4$) will be low and serum thyroid stimulating hormone (TSH) elevated. In thyroiditis, antithyroid antibodies may be elevated. Thyroiditis may be associated on occasion with other autoimmune disorders, including Addison's disease, hypoparathyroidism, and diabetes mellitus. A low $T_4$ with normal or low TSH suggests secondary hypothyroidism due to hypothalamic or pituitary deficiency. Tests of pituitary function should be completed before beginning thyroxine therapy since unrecognized and untreated adrenal (ACTH) deficiency could result in an adrenal crisis (1). Although *hyperthyroidism* generally causes an acceleration of growth and skeletal maturation, there may be modest delay in pubertal development or secondary amenorrhea in a menstruating adolescent.

In *Cushing's syndrome*, linear growth is delayed in the presence of truncal obesity. Pubertal development may be delayed or secondary amenorrhea may occur in girls after menarche. If excess adrenal androgens are produced, hirsutism and other signs of virilization may occur, including acceleration of skeletal maturation and linear growth, at times canceling out the retardation of linear growth caused by the glucocorticoid excess (somatomedin deficiency). In *adrenogenital syndrome* associated with 17-alpha-hydroxylase deficiency, estrogen, androgen, and cortisol synthesis are diminished, resulting in failure of sexual maturation and adrenarche in the female. Amenorrhea and absence of sexual hair are commonly seen in adult females with this disorder. Deoxycorticosterone is produced in large amounts leading to hypokalemic alkalosis and hypertension. Children with familial cytomegalic adrenocortical hypoplasia fail to enter puberty despite treatment with corticosteroids and have been shown to have a gonadotropin deficiency (38).

Normal growth and pubertal development is expected in most juvenile diabetics; however, in *uncontrolled diabetes mellitus* with frequent episodes of ketoacidosis, pubertal development may be delayed. Rising gonadal or adrenal hormones of puberty may increase the need for insulin and increase the glycemic dysequilibrium. Extreme glycemic dysequilibrium and ketoacidosis, in turn, interfere with growth through suppression of somatomedin production or activity. Hormonal events of puberty are also inhibited.

In the *syndrome of gonadal dysgenesis with androgen insensitivity* (testicular feminization), classical female secondary sexual development occurs in a person with an XY karyotype (37). There is sparse or absent pubic and axillary hair and sparse body hair. Administration of androgen fails to stimulate hair growth because of the tissue androgen insensitivity due to deficiency of target cell androgen receptors or to defects in specific binding of androgens to receptors (33). The external genitalia are normal for a female with a short blind vagina. The uterus is absent. Testes are present either intraabdominally or in the inguinal or labial region. The disorder is X-linked with the heterozygous mother often demonstrating some mild androgen insensitivity. After completion of secondary sexual development, the gonads should be removed because of risk of gonadal malignancy. Gonads may be removed earlier for psychosocial reasons and feminization accomplished with estrogen therapy. Replacement estrogen therapy prevents menopausal symptoms and osteoporosis, and preserves the secondary sexual development. At no time should these girls be told of their genetic or gonadal sex. They are totally female in their phenotype and psychosocial behavior.

### Systemic Disorders

Delay in puberty can occur in association with a number of systemic illnesses, especially if associated with *malnutrition*. Socioeconomic deprivation or voluntary decrease in food intake can have the same effect. Weight loss to about 80% of ideal body weight can lead to gonadotropin deficiency with delayed puberty or delay in progression through the stages of puberty (Figure 5-17). With removal of the cause of the malnutrition and return to normal weight, hypothalamic–pituitary–gonadal function will usually resume (21, 39).

The first signs of *inflammatory bowel disease* may be a loss of weight, lack of linear growth, and delay or cessation of pubertal development (40). This may be accompanied by elevated ESR, mild anemia, and hypoalbuminemia. In some subjects, especially those with Crohn's disease, the growth failure and lack of pubertal development may be the only overt sign of inflammatory bowel disease leading one to consider constitutional delay of puberty until a thorough gastrointestinal examination is performed (41).

Acidosis seems to be primarily responsible for growth retardation and delay in pubertal development in *renal disorders*. In renal tubular acidosis growth failure may occur without renal failure. The exact mechanism by which acidosis retards growth is unknown, but it appears to inhibit somatomedin activity. Correction of the acidosis may be followed by resumption of growth and pubertal development, although progressive renal failure requiring dialysis to maintain correction of azatemia and acidosis may continue to interfere with normal pubertal progress (Figure 9-9). Leydig cell function seems to be affected less than spermatogenesis in males (42). *Cyanotic heart disease, asthma, anemia,* and *collagen vascular disease*, when severe enough to affect linear growth, may also contribute to delay in pubertal development. Children with *leukemia* in early childhood, who have experienced long-term remission, may enter puberty at the usual time; however, girls with onset late in childhood may manifest a delay in puberty. Primary ovarian failure may follow use of anti-leukemic medications (21).

*Anorexia nervosa* in adolescent age girls is characterized by voluntary pernicious refusal of food—even when food is accepted, it is frequently regurgitated or vomited. Psychologically, there is distortion of body image so that even a slim figure is viewed as overweight. Functional pituitary deficiency occurs in anorexia nervosa which may be manifest by amenorrhea in a menstruating female or delay or cessation of pubertal development in the prepubertal or developing adolescent (43). Plasma levels of FSH, LH, and estradiol are decreased and there is reversion of the LH response to GnRH to a prepubertal pattern. There are increased levels of plasma growth hormone and cortisol, low levels of DHEA and DHEAS, and decreased plasma $T_3$ (21). The sensitivity of the hypothalamic–pituitary endocrine systems to good nutrition is dramatically demonstrated in anorexia nervosa (43).

## Evaluation and Diagnosis of Delayed Adolescence

Evaluation of the cause for delayed adolescence may be undertaken in any child for whom concern about pubertal delay is expressed by the patient or by his/her parents, bearing in mind the normal ranges of pubertal onset discussed earlier in this chapter and in Chapter 5. Initial efforts should be directed toward discovering those children with constitutional delayed adolescence who make up the majority of children with delayed pubertal development.

Initial evaluation of an individual with delayed puberty should include a careful history, physical examination, and estimate of skeletal maturation. The *history* should include information concerning gestation and neonatal health and nutrition, growth and development during infancy and childhood, exposure to drugs or toxins, nutritional status in childhood, chronic illnesses, significant head trauma, symptoms of central nervous system dysfunction, and growth and development patterns of parents, siblings and close relatives. The psychological impact of the delay in puberty on the individual should be assessed. During the *physical examination*, particular attention should be paid to height, weight, body proportions, and nutritional status; the stage of sexual development, especially testicular size in males and breast budding or labial hair in females; and the neurologic status including examination of the ocular fundus and visual fields. Specific physical features of systemic illness, such as hypothyroidism, Turner's syndrome, or Klinefelter's syndrome should be sought. An estimate of *skeletal maturation* is made from x-rays of the hand and wrist (9, 18).

The child with *constitutional delay of adolescence* usually displays a healthy past which includes a normal birth and infancy and normal nutritional status. Growth after age 2–3 is of normal velocity with height near the lower limits of normal. Physical examination is normal except for immaturity and small size, both of which are consistent with the child's level of skeletal maturation. Unsuspected early signs of puberty are often already present at the time of the initial examination. The youngster with constitutional delayed puberty should be followed to confirm that the anticipated pattern of growth and development ensue. Should the individual not begin sexual maturation when the bone age reaches 12–13 years, further evaluation is necessary.

If the individual with delayed sexual maturation does not fit the criteria for constitutional delay or if clues from the history or physical examination suggest a more complex etiology, further evaluation and testing will be needed. Signs of systemic illness or endocrine disturbance may require gastrointestinal, cardiac, or renal evaluation, or tests of thyroid, adrenal, or pancreatic function as suggested by the historical or physical clues. Other causes of delay in sexual maturation may be divided for convenience into those with gonadal dysfunction versus those with hypothalamic or pituitary dysfunction (20).

In *gonadal deficiency disorders* (hypergonadotropic hypogonadism) an elevation of FSH and LH will be found in either serum or urine in early adolescence. Lack of gonadal steroids leads to elevation of pituitary gonadotropins, even in childhood, because of lack of negative feedback on the hypothalamic or pituitary regulating systems (30). Response of FSH and LH to GnRH administration is variable, although generally exaggerated (44). Klinefelter's and Turner's syndromes may be recognized through their distinctive chromosomal patterns. Since both of these disorders are common causes of pubertal delay, it is recommended that chromosomal karyotype be performed in any male adolescent with delay or deficient puberty who has small testes and in any female who is short and has delayed or deficient pubertal development.

*Hypothalamic–pituitary disorders* (hypogonadotropic hypogonadism) are not as simple to evaluate as the gonadal deficiency disorders. A few of the syndromes of hypothalamic deficiency such as Kallmann's or Prader–Willi syndromes have some specific associated features which may provide appropriate clues. Neoplasms, trauma, and infections may affect the central nervous system characteristically so that specific lesions may be detectable. Skull x-rays or CT scan and visual field examinations may be helpful in detecting and locating CNS tumors or lesions causing pubertal delay. If growth as well as puberty has been affected and pituitary deficiency is suspected, measurements of human growth hormone, TSH, and ACTH with appropriate provocative tests may be helpful.

Isolated deficiency of gonadotropins due to either hypothalamic or pituitary deficiency are not simple to separate from constitutional delayed adolescence. Basal levels of LH and FSH do not permit a distinction. A number of stimulatory and inhibitory tests have been suggested, but in prepubertal individuals anti-estrogens (clomiphene) or anti-androgens (flutamide) are of no value in separating constitutional delay from pathologic hypogonadotropism (30). GnRH may be administered to adolescents with delayed puberty to stimulate release of FSH and LH (44). In subjects with constitutional delayed growth, levels of FSH and LH rise to levels appropriate for their status of sexual development (or skeletal maturation) (44). Sizonenko claims that values of FSH and LH obtained from delayed adolescence overlap with those obtained from hypogonadotropism making this an unreliable test for differentiation of the two entities (30), but others have found the response to GnRH helpful for diagnostic discrimination (45, 46); however, obese, adolescent boys may have delayed sexual maturation and low gonadotropin response to GnRH with later spontaneous normal maturation (47). Because hypersecretion of prolactin induces hypogonadism and galactorrhea in both sexes and may cause delayed puberty (27), Sizonenko suggests measurement of prolactin in cases of delayed puberty (30). Levels of adrenal androgens may provide some diagnostic distinction as well. Cohen et al. report lower levels of DHEA, DHEA sulphate, and androstenedione in subjects with growth hormone deficiency than in those with constitutional delay in adolescence; by contrast, subjects with hypogonadotropic hypogonadism had significantly raised values (48). GnRH given repeatedly over several days may serve to distinguish GnRH deficiency from pituitary gonadotropin deficiency. In the patient with GnRH deficiency, repeated administration of GnRH will cause a rise in basal FSH and LH or gonadal steroids (9). Despite much interest in pubertal endocrinology, it is still very difficult to precisely characterize some hypothalamic or pituitary disorders of delayed puberty.

Sex steroids (testosterone or estradiol) can be measured in a basal state or after stimulation with human chorionic gonadotropin (hCG). Low basal levels would be found in all forms of hypogonadism. In constitutional delayed puberty, sex steroid levels would be in the prepubertal range and indistinguishable from those of hypogonadotropic hypogonadism. Stimulation with hCG in either single or multiple dosage will produce no respone in subjects with anorchia or gonadal deficiency, however, a significant increase in gonadal hormone secretion will occur in individuals with hypogonadotropic hypogonadism who have normal gonads. This test is not often used in girls because of the danger of producing hemorrhagic cysts in the ovary. In cryptorchidism, in which it should be most useful, conflicting results have been obtained. Zachmann reported an increase in urinary testosterone within 4–6 days after a single injection of 5000 units of hCG intramuscularly (49). By contrast, Gendrel et al. found decreased response of the cryptorchid gonads compared to normal (50), while others have reported normal gonadal steroid levels after hCG (30).

## Management of Delayed Adolescence

The management of constitutional delayed adolescence, including consideration of psychological stresses, need for counseling, and the use of hormones to accelerate puberty, is presented in the section of this chapter entitled "Constitutional Delay of Adolescence." Tumors of the hypothalamus or pituitary may be surgically removed, ablated with laser or cryotherapy, or irradiated, although pituitary replacement therapy may be necessary therafter. Systemic disorders require treatment aimed at correcting the lung, heart, gastrointestinal, or immune system disorder.

Girls with Turner's syndrome should receive female hormones at about the usual age of puberty or when the skeletal maturation has achieved a level of 11–12 years. Some consideration can be given to size and social maturity in deciding the best time to begin replacement hormonal therapy. There is some evidence that anabolic steroids such as oxandrolone or fluoxymesterone, given either alone or together with estrogen, may improve height achievement (51, 52). It may be desirable to begin the androgen therapy just before the estrogen and to continue androgen during the female hormone replacement therapy period. We generally being oxandrolone 0.1 mg/kg/day about 1–2 years before we contemplate beginning estrogen replacement therapy and continue the androgen in the same or slightly higher dosage (up to 0.2 mg/kg/day) with the estrogen. At about the time the skeletal maturation reaches the 11–12 year level, we begin low dose conjugated estrogen (Premarin) 0.3 mg/day. This is increased up to 1.25 mg/day and combined with medroxyprogesterone to allow menses about every 6–8 weeks. When secondary sexual development is complete, estrogen may be reduced to 0.625 mg/day continuing to allow menses every 6–8 weeks. Anabolic steroids are discontinued as growth is completed.

Testosterone therapy for the patient with Klinefelter's syndrome who has subnormal plasma testosterone values, may be considered in a schedule similar to that used for hypogonadotropic hypogonadism. Testicular prostheses should be considered for the boy with anorchia. These are available in graduated sizes and can be inserted in childhood and replaced with gradually increasing sized prostheses until adulthood.

In individuals with hypogonadotropic hypogonadism, estrogen or androgen replacement therapy should be started at the appropriate age for puberty. In *girls* conjugated estrogens 0.3–0.625 mg/day or ethinyl estradiol 0.02–0.05 mg/day may be administered with the addition of progesterone after 6–9 months when the higher dosage is achieved, or when estrogen breakthrough bleeding occurs (53). Thereafter, estrogen is administered for 21 days with the addition of medroxyprogesterone 10 mg/day for days 16–21 of each cycle. For the final 6–7 days of each cycle, no medication is given to allow withdrawal menstrual bleeding. This cyclic therapy should be continued until the usual time for menopause. In *males* testosterone enanthate in dosages of 200–400 mg intramusuclarly should be administered with sufficient frequency (every 2–4 weeks) to assure normal testosterone levels and continued throughout life (1, 16). It is best to begin with a low dosage and gradually increase to full adult levels (47).

Infertility is usual in hypogonadotropic states, although it may be possible to stimulate gonadal maturation with hCG or specific gonadotropin preparations (53, 54). GnRH may induce ovulation in subjects with hypothalamic deficiency (55). Subjects with gonadal dysgenesis require removal of dysgenetic gonads (as in testicular feminization) because of the danger of malignancy within the dysgenetic gonad. After removal of the gonad, such subjects will require replacement gonadal steroid therapy. Subjects with 17-alpha-hydroxylase deficiency will require cortisol for prevention of adrenal insufficiency and suppression of excess ACTH and will also need gonadal steroids for sexual development (18).

## PRECOCIOUS PUBERTY

A girl may be considered to be sexually precocious if secondary sexual characteristics appear before 8 years of age (more than 2.5 standard deviations earlier than the mean time of pubertal onset) (18, 21). A boy may be considered sexually precocious if pubertal development begins before 9.5 years of age (18). Some European observers, more restrictive in their definition, suggest that menarche in a girl before the eighth birthday or breast development before age 6 should be considered pathologic (56, 57). For boys, appearance of sexual characteristics before the age of 8 would be considered precocious (56). We have generally accepted the former definition (18) as our guide for distinguishing normal from precocious puberty, although we acknowledge that by doing so, we are knowingly including 2½% of a normal population within our definition. We agree with Bierich (56) that it may be sensible to consider more than 2.5 standard deviations but less than 4 standard deviations early as constitutional accelerated puberty unless obvious pathology is noted on the initial examination.

Sexual precocity may be *isosexual* or *heterosexual*. Isosexual precocity is used to describe sexual development which is appropriate for the phenotype of the child, while heterosexual precocity suggests virilization of the female or feminization of the male child (18). Except for virilizing adrenal hyperplasia, we will be discussing only isosexual precocious puberty in this section. Isosexual precocious puberty may in turn involve the complete hypothalamic–pituitary–gonadal axis and is then called true sexual precocity, or it may arise from hormonal secretions from the gonads or from extragonadal tissues and is then termed pseudoprecocious puberty. In the former, there is premature activation of the normal pubertal control mechanism while in the latter, the hormonal secretions are independent of the normal control mechanism (18).

In isosexual precocious puberty, the sexual development follows the usual pattern of normal puberty. In the girl breast development is seen first, followed by pubic hair as the body takes on feminine proportions. Later the genitalia mature and a leukorrhea appears. In the boy, the first sign of precocious puberty is testicular enlargement, followed by appearance of pubic hair and penile enlargement (19, 56). Variation in the sequence of appearance of sexual characteristics is seen both in normal and precocious children. Vaginal bleeding may even be the first sign of precocious puberty (58). Sudden appearance and rapid progression of pubertal characteristics raises the suspicion of tumor or ectopic source of hormone. Accelerated somatic growth becomes evident early in the course of precocious puberty. This growth spurt is accompanied by rapid acceleration of bone maturation which leads to premature epiphyseal closure and early cessation of growth (Figure 10-1). Most youngsters with precocious puberty are large as children but short as adults (58).

## Incomplete Sexual Precocity

Premature breast development (premature thelarche), early isolated pubic and axillary hair appearance (premature pubarche), or premature isolated vaginal bleeding (premature menarche) without generalized accelerated puberty appear to be benign incomplete signs of puberty. Their etiology is poorly understood (59). In all conditions, serum gonadotropin levels may be within the normal range or slightly elevated (18).

### *Premature Thelarche*

Premature thelarche or isolated breast development may be unilateral or bilateral and may occur any time in childhood but as a rule appears within the first 2 years of life and tends to disappear spontaneously (56). Persistence beyond 2 years is thought to be unusual (19), although Mills et al. reported that over half (57%) of their series of 46 patients with premature thelarche showed palpable breast tissue for at least 3–5 yrs. Most of the patients did not show progressive enlargement (only 11%) (60). When premature thelarche occurs shortly after birth, it may be confused with neonatal breast enlargement which generally subsides within a few weeks after birth. Those cases in which breast tissue is present from the neonatal period are more likely to have progressive breast enlargement (60). Premature thelarche may represent extreme sensitivity of the breast tissue to usual childhood levels of estrogen, although there are subtle estrogen effects also noted on vaginal cells examined by urocytogram (61). Slightly elevated estrogen levels have been seen in some children, although in most, plasma estradiol and gonadotropin levels are normal (62). Intermittent spikes of FSH and LH adequate to stimulate small amounts of estrogen have also been suggested as a pathophysiologic mechanism for premature thelarche (63). In some cases, there may be exposure to unrecognized environmental sources of estrogen (18). Since it is a benign physiologic event, premature thelarche needs no therapy, although there may be some anxiety until observation and absence of other indications of puberty prove the benign nature of the phenomenon.

### *Premature Pubarche*

Premature pubarche or isolated appearance of pubic or axillary hair at about 5–8 years of age is seen more frequently in girls than boys and seems to occur more often in children with brain damage (64). Growth in height and skeletal maturation are usually slightly accelerated (56). Adolescent plasma levels of DHEA, DHEA sulfate, and androstenediol (18) and elevated urine 17-ketosteroids have been found in most children with premature sexual hair (65); this appears to be early activation of androgen

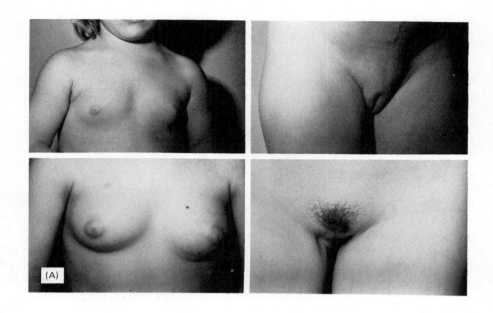

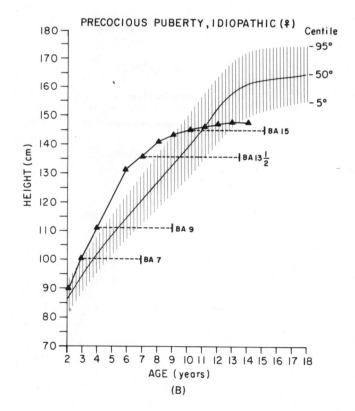

PRECOCIOUS PUBERTY, IDIOPATHIC (♀)

Centile

— 95°

— 50°

— 5°

BA 15

BA 13½

BA 9

BA 7

HEIGHT (cm)

AGE (years)

(A)

(B)

370

secretion from the adrenal gland and is termed premature adrenarche by some (56, 59, 66). Premature adrenarche does not usually lead to early onset of complete sexual development (19), but only intermittant folow-up with androgen/estrogen and gonadotropin levels will ensure that premature pubarche is not the expression of an androgen-producing tumor or the beginning of puberty (19, 59, 67).

## Premature Menarche

Premature menarche represents isolated vaginal bleeding in the absence of other signs of secondary sexual development (breast or pubic hair). The cyclic vaginal bleeding is transient, although it may persist for several years. There is no acceleration of growth nor any effect on ultimate height. Normal pubertal development occurs at the usual time and fertility appears unaffected (68). It is important to consider vaginal neoplasma or foreign body with the initial episode, but if no cause is found, no treatment is necessary since the disorder is self-limiting and has no long-term effect on menstrual pattern or fertility (68).

## Causes of Precocious Puberty

The causes of precocious puberty are shown in Table 10-4. These include hypothalamic–pituitary disorders, gonadotrophin producing tumors, gonadal tumors or adrenal hyperplasia, and exogenous hormone administration.

## Hypothalamic–Pituitary Dysfunction

Abnormalities or lesions or the hypothalamus or pituitary can result in early release of gonadotropins to produce precocious puberty.

*Idiopathic precocious puberty.* From the relative frequencies of causes of precocious puberty (Table 10-5), it may be noted that fully two-thirds of all published cases of sexual precocity are "idiopathic". This form of precocious puberty is more common in girls than in boys, nearly an 8:1 ratio. Idiopathic precocious puberty accounts for over 80% of cases of precocious puberty in girls and only about 40% in boys (69). In some instances a familial pattern of precocious puberty is evident, but most cases are sporadic and the cause is unknown. Abnormal EEG findings in some youngsters with idiopathic precocious puberty (70, 71) has led to the suggestion that the "gonadostat" in the hypothalamus of such individ-

**Figure 10-1.**  Girl with idiopathic sexual precocity (A). At age 2 years (upper panel), breasts were well established, but no pubic hair was evident. Menses began at age 12 months. Progression of breast development and pubic hair by age 6 is shown in the lower panel (A) of the figure despite blocking therapy with medroxyprogesterone. (B) Typical growth pattern showing early accelerated growth and accelerated skeletal maturation with early cessation of growth which has resulted in short stature by early teenage.

### Table 10-4. Causes of Precocious Puberty

A. *Hypothalamic (Pituitary) Disorders*
  1. Incomplete forms
     (a) Premature thelarche
     (b) Premature adrenarche
  2. Idiopathic precocious puberty
  3. McCune–Albright syndrome
  4. Cerebral disorders
     (a) Tumors of hypothalamus, pineal
     (b) Hydrocephalus, encephalitis, trauma
  5. Hormonal overlapping
     (a) Hypothyroidism
     (b) Addison's disease
     (c) Post-steroid or late AGS therapy
  6. Blindness
B. *Gonadotropin-Producing Tumors*
  1. Chorioepitheliomas, teratomas
C. *Sex Hormone Excess From Tumor/Hyperplasia*
  1. Congenital adrenal hyperplasia (AGS)
  2. Ovarian/testicular tumors
D. *Exogenous Hormone Administration*
  1. Anabolic steroids
  2. Estrogens

Reproduced by permission from Bierich JR, *Clin Endocrinol Metabol* **4:**107, March, 1975 and Blunck W, *Pediatr Ann* **3**(July):30–46, 1974.

uals prematurely matures to pubertal sensitivity levels (56, 21). Since the majority of such patients are girls, it may be that the regulatory centers of the diencephalon in girls are particularly susceptible to external disturbances (56).

Idiopathic precocious puberty is characterized by early sexual maturation, accelerated growth, and skeletal maturation (Figure 10-1). Skeletal development is not generally as advanced as sexual development. Menarche in a girl often occurs several years before the bone-age reaches a level of 12–13 years. Growth and height, however, lag behind the skeletal maturation, leading to very short stature when the epiphyses close (56). Girls with idiopathic precocious puberty reach an average height of 145–149 cm (58) (Figure 10-1). Biochemically, precocious puberty is associated with pubertal levels of FSH, LH, gonadal steroids, and 17-ketosteroids. Responsiveness to GnRH is enhanced. Hormonal levels correlate well with the stage of sexual development or with skeletal maturation. The diagnosis of idiopathic precocious puberty is made by exclusion of other causes of isosexual precocity.

**Table 10-5. Relative Frequency of Causes
of Precocious Puberty**[a]

| | |
|---|---|
| Hamartomas of the hypothalamus | 40 cases |
| Other cerebral lesions | over 200 cases |
| Idiopathic precocious puberty | over 600 cases |
| Weil–Albright syndrome | 48 cases |
| Untreated hypothyroidism | 9 cases |

Reproduced by permission from JR Bierich: *Clin Endocrinol Metabol*
**4:**107, 1975.

[a] Number of published cases reported up to 1969.

Intellectual, psychic, and psychosexual development correspond to chronologic age and does not undergo any noticeable acceleration. Youngsters are often treated as older children, leading to excessive expectations and emotional stress (69). Girls who are immature in their sexual attitudes, although mature physically, are easily seduced. The number of pregnancies before the age of 15 years is high. Maturity of psychosexual status does not occur with pregnancy. Most of the children lack any concept of mothering, placing a serious emotional burden upon both the patient and the family.

In *the McCune–Albright syndrome*, (Weil–Albright–McCune–Sternberg syndrome), first described by Weil in 1922 (72), sexual precocity is associated with polyostotic fibrous dysplasia and characteristic cafe-au-lait skin pigmentation. An incomplete form of McCune–Albright syndrome was reported in 3 girls by Grant and Martinez; polyostotic fibrous dysplasia and precocious puberty were present without the typical skin pigmentation (73). Spontaneous fractures occur frequently at points of cystic bone involvement and may be the first sign of the disorder. Fractures become less frequent after full pubertal development. The sexual precocity, which occurs almost exclusively in females, may begin at a very early age but usually progresses slowly (71, 56). Hyperthyroidism, acromegaly, and hyperadrenocorticism have been associated with the McCune–Albright syndrome suggesting a congenital hypothalamic anomaly, resulting in hypersecretion of several hypothalamic releasing factors (74). Some children with *neurofibromatosis* display precocious sexual development which may begin very early and progress rapidly (71). Many subjects do not have noticeable space-occupying cerebral lesions, though hypothalamic gliomas have been assumed to be the proximate cause of the sexual precocity. The *Silver–Russell syndrome* of short stature, intrauterine growth retardation, and somatic asymmetry may be associated with elevated urine and serum gonadotropin levels and sexual precocity (75).

*Intracranial disorders* involving the hypothalamus are a common organic cause of precocious puberty. Precocious puberty has occurred after encephalitis, head trauma, brain abscess, supracellar cysts, sarcoid or tubercular granulomas, and hypothalamic tumors. Sexual precocity due to tumor of the central nervous system is more common in boys than in girls, accounting for one-third to one-half of sexual precocity in boys (19). Optic and hypothalamic gliomas with or without neurofibromatosis, astrocytomas, ependymomas, teratomas, and hamartomas may all produce sexual precocity. They are often found in combination with other CNS anomalies (56). Hamartoma of the tuber cinereum, a rare cause of early sexual development, causes an autonomous proliferation of cells which produce gonadatropin-releasing hormone (71, 56). The pineal gland has a suppressive influence on sexual maturation. If the pineal gland is destroyed by tumor, precocious development may occur. Likewise, a cerebral tumor between the hypothalamus and pineal gland may interrupt the connection between pineal and hypothalamus or destroy the CNS puberty-inhibitory centers and produce sexual precocity (65). Hydrocephalus, especially with widening of the third ventricle, may be complicated by sexual precocity, which may not stop with normalization of the intracranial pressure (71). Inflammatory diseases of the CNS, such as encephalitis or meningitis, may lead to hydrocephalus or by themselves be a cause of sexual precocity. Sexual precocity has even been described in children with septo-optic dysplasia and hypothalamic hypopituitarism (with intact median eminence-anterior pituitary unit) (76). It is not certain how the cerebral centers which control puberty are affected by this wide variety of cerebral lesions, but it is believed that abolition of inhibitory impulses from the posterior parts of the diencephalon may be a common denominator, leading to release of hypothalamic hormones to begin the chain of events which result in early puberty (56–58).

A phenomenon known as *"hormonal overlap"* may be responsible for sexual precocity in *hypothyroidism* and *Addison's disease*. This phenomenon is seen most commonly in primary hypothyroidism, although it is a rare event. Linear and skeletal growth are retarded, while sexual maturation is accelerated. Galactorrhea and enlarged cystic ovaries may also be found (77). TSH, prolactin, and gonadotropins are elevated and the sella turcica may be shown to be enlarged by lateral skull x-ray. It is postulated that increased secretion of TRH is responsible for the elevated concentrations of the pituitary hormones. With adequate thyroid hormone therapy the progression of sexual precocity ceases as does the galactorrhea, and the pituitary size may decrease to normal (21). Although less common, sexual precocity may accompany untreated *Addison's disease*, characterized by elevations of ACTH and gonadotropins (78). It is supposed that increased secretion of corticotropin releasing hormone causes elevation of LH and FSH along with ACTH; regression in sexual precocity is seen with adequate cortisol therapy. A similar phenomenon may be seen in children with *virilizing adrenal hyperplasia* who are treated after virilization and skeletal maturation has already occurred. Premature maturation of the hypothalamic–pituitary axis appears to occur from the effects of the adrenal androgens and sexual development may begin shortly after the cortisol therapy is started (21). Precocious puberty may also be seen after stopping long-term androgen therapy during childhood (71).

True premature sexual development is seen commonly in *blind children*. The cause of the sexual precocity is not known, although it is tempting to speculate on the influence of light perception on the pineal gland and in turn the influence of the pineal gland on sexual precocity.

## Sexual Precocity from Excess Gonadotropins

Gonadotropins administered or produced by tumor bypass the hypothalamic–pituitary axis and lead to sexual precocity by stimulation of the gonads to produce their natural hormones. Prolonged administration of gonadotropin (hCG injections) for cryptorchidism or other perceived medical need will lead to enlarged penis and testes, appearance of pubic hair, and nocturnal emission in a male child. If the medication is stopped, progression of the pubertal signs will cease, however, pubic hair will remain and the penis will remain enlarged. Malignant chorioepitheliomas or teratomas may arise from the gonads, pituitary, or mediastinum and hepatoblastomas from the liver. Human chorionic gonadotropin is produced by trophoblastic tumors (teratomas and chorioepitheliomas), while liver tumors produce a substance with LH activity. So far gonadotropin-producing liver tumors have only been described in males (56).

## Gonadal/Adrenal Tumors or Hyperplasia

*Testicular tumors* are rare in childhood, but reach a peak incidence in adolescence. Leydig cell tumors are usually unilateral, firm, and demarcated from the remaining testicular tissue. As a rule they are benign neoplasms, but if malignant, they tend to secrete excessive amounts of androgens. The rate of virilization is quite variable and may occur either from testosterone or large amounts of androstenedione. Operative removal of the tumor results in arrest or regression in about half of the children, the rest progress on to full sexual maturation despite surgery (56).

*Granulosa or theca-cell tumors* of the ovary are rare in children but still represent one of the more common organic lesions which cause sexual precocity in the female (79, 80). Most of the tumors are palpable by careful bimanual palpation of the abdomen and pelvis. In childhood such tumors are usually benign. Clinically there is rapidly progressing isosexual maturation and irregular menstrual bleeding (withdrawal bleeding). Pubic and axillary hair appear from small amounts of androgen produced by the tumors or from estrogen stimulated adrenarche (56). Urinary estrogen excretion is moderately or greatly increased and in theca-cell tumors there is increase in pregnanediol as well. Gonadotropins are suppressed (19). Removal of the tumor results in arrest or regression of the sexual precocity, although progression to complete maturity may occur if skeletal maturation

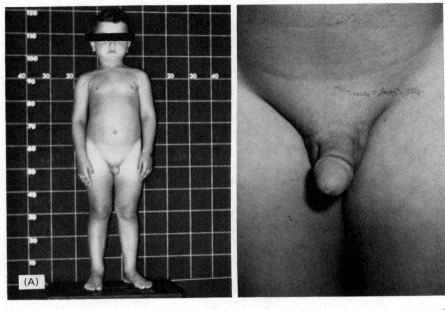

**Figure 10-2.** Boy with congenital virilizing adrenal hyperplasia showing (A) early growth spurt with genital enlargement and pubic hair by age 4 when treatment with hydrocortisone was begun. (B) Growth rate was controlled to some extent by steroid therapy, but early cessation of growth has resulted in low average adult height. Full sexual development was achieved by about age 12 despite hydrocortisone therapy.

is advanced to the usual time of puberty. Ovarian tumors which produce only androgens are very rare.

Small *follicular cysts* are often seen on the ovary of prepubertal girls. Occasionally the cysts are large and actively secrete sufficient estrogen to induce feminization (79, 80). Regression of the cyst may be associated with arrested feminization, but recurrence of cysts may lead to repeated breast development and menstrual bleeding (21).

Excessive amounts of androgens from *tumor or hyperplasia of the adrenal gland* produce incomplete isosexual precocious puberty in the boy or virilization in a girl. Adrenal hyperplasia or tumor accounts for nearly one-third of the cases of sexual precocity in boys. Virilization occurs rapidly, including enlargement of the penis, appearance of pubic hair, rapid somatic growth with a muscular appearance, acceleration of skeletal maturation, and later lowering of the voice and acne if the androgen excess is not interrupted (Figure 10-2). The testes, which are not participants in the production of androgen, remain small, though on occasion aberrant adrenal tissue in the testes enlarges irregularly in response to

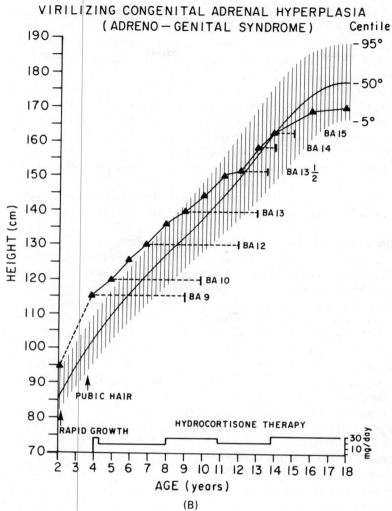

VIRILIZING CONGENITAL ADRENAL HYPERPLASIA
( ADRENO — GENITAL SYNDROME )

**Figure 10-2.** (Continued)

the high ACTH levels. In congenital adrenal hyperplasia (CAH), there is characteristically elevation not only of adrenal androgens measured as urinary 17-ketosteroids, but of cortisol precursors as well. In the most common form of CAH, 17-OH-progesterone is elevated in plasma and its excretory product, pregnanetriol, in the urine. In adrenal tumors there is usually elevation of not only androgens, but glucocorticoids as well. Hypertension from elevation of both glucocorticoids and mineralocorticoids may occur either with tumors (81) or in adrenal hyperplasia associated with 11-hydroxylase deficiency in which excess amounts of DOC are produced.

Removal of an adrenal tumor results in cessation of virilization and some regression of signs, although penile enlargement and pubic hair remain. Recurrence of adrenal tumors is common. Virilization from adrenal hyperplasia may be controlled with replacement dosages of hydrocortisone, 25 mg/m$^2$/day orally, although true puberty may supervene with treatment; prolonged exposure to elevated androgen levels may induce precocious maturation of the hypothalamic pubertal mechanism of LH secretion (82). Hyperplastic *aberrant adrenocortical tissue* may be found in the testes of the untreated male with adrenogenital syndrome or if suppressive corticosteroid therapy is discontinued. Histologically, such tissue cannot be distinguished from Leydig cell adenomas, but the tissue will be responsive to cortisol or dexamethasone suppression (56).

### Administration of Anabolic Steroids or Estrogens

The administration of anabolic steroids, estrogen, or human chorionic gonadatropin (hGC), either intentionally or accidentally will produce either virilization or feminization. Not only will secondary sex characteristics appear under the stimulus of administered hormones, but a growth spurt and skeletal acceleration will also generally be seen. Used over prolonged periods, exogenously administered sex hormones or hCG are capable of inducing precocious development of secondary sex characteristics and closing skeletal epiphyses to reduce height achievement. In certain circumstances, these are precisely the effects desired, but if they are considered undesirable side effects, such medications should be used with caution, and certainly should not be used for frivolous or unnecessary reasons such as weight control or "muscle-building" in children (83).

### Diagnosis of Precocious Puberty

In the *history* of the child with sexual precocity, particular attention should be directed to symptoms suggesting central nervous system involvement, such as headache, vomiting, ataxia, and visual changes and to the possibility of environmental exposure to sex hormones in drugs, vitamins, or skin creams. A history of birth trauma or anoxia and encephalitis or meningitis should be sought. The growth pattern is reconstructed from previous measurements to display growth acceleration, and the status of sexual development and the sequence and rate of progression through stages of sexual development are recorded. The family pattern of sexual development should be noted.

*Physical examination* should include measurements of height, weight, and body proportion. A thorough and careful neurologic examination must be performed, including visual fields and fundus examination. The stage of sexual maturation should be judged using Tanner's criteria (see Chapter 5) and careful examination of the testes should be performed in boys, judging size by means of the Prader orchidometer (see Chapter 5). A rectal–abdominal examination should be performed in a girl to determine uterine and ovarian size (most ovarian tumors are palpable). On occasion anesthesia may be required to perform an adequate pelvic examination.

Skeletal maturation (bone age) should be estimated from appropriate x-ray (see Chapter 7) and compared to the growth pattern and degree of sexual maturation. Skull x-rays may show enlargement or erosion of the sella turcica, increased intracranial pressure, or intracranial calcification. In a CNS lesion is suspected, a CT scan or pneumo-encephalography may be needed.

In *girls*, isolated thelarche or pubarche raises the suspicion of premature incomplete puberty. The vaginal smear provides a physiologic marker of effects of estrogen in the female. The external genitalia should be examined carefully for signs of estrogen effect and a vaginal smear obtained for histologic study for estrogen effect. If there are no changes of the vaginal epithelium, it is unlikely that the premature thelarche represents pathologic precocious puberty. We have generally been able to obtain adequate samples for vaginal smears from even very small girls without undue discomfort with the use of a veterinary otoscope head introduced into the vagina (Figure 10-3). If vaginal bleeding is the initial and only complaint, speculum examination of the vagina under anesthesia should be performed to look for injury, foreign body, or tumor.

Cyclic menstruation occurs only in hypothalamic–pituitary forms of puberty; with ovarian tumors irregular vaginal bleeding occurs. Ovarian tumors are generally palpable on physical examination and the estrogen levels are high in serum or urine while gonadotropin levels are low. Enlargement of an ovary by tumor may be identified by pelvic ultrasound, CT scan or pneumoperitoneography. In trophoblastic gonadotropin-producing tumors, irregular menstrual bleeding also occurs and high levels of hCG are found in urine and blood.

True hypothalamic–pituitary precocity with normal pubertal levels of gonadotropins and estrogen demands consideration of lesions of the central nervous system and related disorders listed in Table 10-4. Girls with McCune–Albright syndrome and hormonal overlapping should be distinguishable on the basis of specific identifying characteristics. X-rays of long bones will be required to identify polyostotic fibrous dysplasia. Note should be taken of skin lesions, including acne and cafe-au-lait markings seen in neurofibromatosis (smooth edges) or polyostotic fibrous dysplasia (irregular edges). Thyroid function tests, $T_4$ and TSH, should be performed in a girl with suspected hypothyroidism whose bone-age is delayed and whose growth has not accelerated. One must look carefully for CNS signs, including headache, impaired vision, and seizures, and pay particular attention to neurologic, ophthalmalogic, and radiographic studies. If no pathologic findings emerge, the diagnosis of idiopathic precocious puberty is justified. Idiopathic precocious puberty is by far the commonest

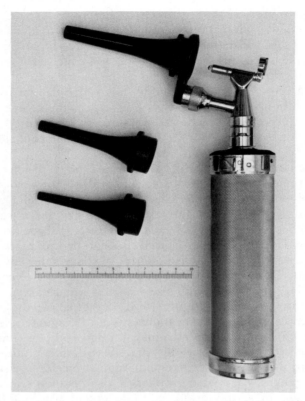

**Figure 10-3.** Device for obtaining vaginal smear in infants with premature thelarche suspected of precocious puberty. Depicted is an otoscope using veterinary speculae for vaginal examination of very young infants and collection of vaginal or cervical cells for examination for estrogen effect.

form of precocity in females. This is a diagnosis made by exclusion of all other known causes of hypothalamic–pituitary precocity and must be viewed as a potential reservoir of many yet-to-be-identified specific causes. The major differential considerations of precocious puberty in girls are outlined in Table 10-6.

For *boys*, the initial step in diagnosis should be to determine whether anabolic hormones or hCG have been administered. Isolated pubarche is rare and may simply represent the early onset of normal puberty. In contrast to females, incomplete forms of precocious puberty are common among males. The *adrenogenital syndrome* (AGS) accounts for approximately one-third of the cases of isosexual precocious puberty in boys. This can sometimes be identified from the disparity between advanced virilization and small testes. Characteristic hormonal patterns and response to cortisone allow definitive diagnosis. Urinary 17-ketosteroids and pregnanetriol

**Table 10-6. Sexual Precocity in Girls**

| | Hormone Determinations | | | Sexual Development, Breast, Menses | Pubic Hair |
|---|---|---|---|---|---|
| | Increased Gonadotropins | Increased 17-Oxysteroids | Increased Estrogens | | |
| **1. Hypothalamic Precocity** | | | | | |
| Idiopathic | + | + | + | + | + |
| Weil–Albright syndrome | + | + | ++ | ++ | ++ |
| Organic brain lesions | + | + | ++ | ++ | ++ |
| Hormonal overlapping | + | + | + | + | + |
| **2. Gonadotropin-Producing Tumors** | | | | | |
| Chorioepithelioma, teratoma | +++ | +/++ | +/++ | + | + |
| **3. Tumors and Hyperplasia Producing Sex Hormones** | | | | | |
| Adrenal cortex (AGS) | 0 | +++ | + | 0 | + |
| Ovaries | 0 | +/++ | ++ | + | + |
| **4. Exogenous Hormone Administration** | | | | | |
| Estrogens | 0 | 0/+ | ++ | + | 0/+ |
| Anabolic steroids | 0 | 0/+ | 0/+ | 0 | + |

Reproduced by permission from Prader, arranged in tabular form by Bierich JR: Sexual precocity. *Clin Endocrinol Metabol* **4**:107–142, March 1975.

and serum 17-OH-progesterone are elevated. If the hormonal pattern suggests an adrenal origin, suppression with corticosteroid should be performed (dexamethasone suppression test). Adrenal tumors may be identified by intravenous pyelography or abdominal CT scan. Uneven enlargement of the testes suggest either adrenal-rest tumor or Leydig-cell adenomas. With adrenal-rest tumors there will be elevated cortisol precursors, which are suppressible with corticoids.

Cerebral disorders are encountered more often in boys than in girls, occurring as often as idiopathic precocious puberty (35–50%) in some series (19, 56). The Weil–Albright syndrome does not occur in boys and hormonal overlapping occurs only rarely. Pinealomas seem to cause precocious puberty only in boys. This makes examination of the CNS and adrenals of great importance in boys. Idiopathic precocious puberty is, as with girls, a diagnosis by exclusion. The main differential considerations of precocious puberty in boys are outlined in Table 10-7.

## Management of Precocious Puberty

The management of precocious puberty depends on the cause of the accelerated sexual development. Isolated premature thelarche or adrenarche require no therapy except reassurance. Observation on a regular basis reinforces the reassurance and allows gradual interpretation of the phenomenon and psychological support. Cessation of exogenous hormonal administration or removal of an environmental source of hormones usually allows regression of some secondary sexual development, although it may be incomplete. In the hormonal overlap syndromes, treatment of hypothyroidism or adrenal insufficiency results in regression of precocious sexual development. Virilization from congenital adrenal hyperplasia can be controlled with hydrocortisone (25 mg/m²/day orally), but if skeletal maturation has progressed to the adolescent age range, normal pubertal changes may follow adequate glucocorticoid therapy.

Ovarian, testicular and adrenal neoplasms should be surgically removed. If discovered at an early age, regression of sexual precocity may be expected, but if advanced skeletal-age has already been attained, normal puberty may supervene after surgery. Although ovarian and testicular tumors are usually benign, adrenal tumors are often malignant and metastasize readily producing recurrence of the virilization. Gonadotropin-producing tumors are generally malignant and should be managed by surgical removal and subsequent irradiation. Early occurrence of metastases is generally unfavorable (56).

In patients with defined lesions of the central nervous system such as neoplasms, congenital cysts, or hydrocephalus, surgical management may be appropriate and helpful (18). However, the risk in surgical removal of a hamartoma of the hypothalamus or other cryptic lesions may outweigh potential benefits. If sexual precocity is the only symptom of a cerebral lesion, a clinical trial of medical management may be justified (56).

**Table 10-7. Sexual Precocity in Boys**

| | Hormone Determinations | | Size of Testes | Histology of Testes T:Tubuli and Spermatogenesis L:Leydig Cells |
|---|---|---|---|---|
| | Increased Gonadotropins | Increased 17-Oxysteroids | | |
| **1. Hypothalamic Precocity** | | | | |
| Idiopathic | + | + | Small to markedly increased | T immature to mature |
| Organic brain lesions | + | + | | |
| Hormonal overlapping | + | + | | L + |
| **2. Gonadotropin-Producing Tumors** | | | | |
| Chorioepithelioma | +++ | +/+++ | Small or moderately increased | T mostly immature |
| Hepatoma | +++ | +/+++ | | ·L + |
| **3. Tumors and Hyperplasia-Producing Sex Hormones** | | | | |
| Adrenal cortex (AGS) | 0 | +++ | Small or increased | T immature, L 0 |
| Testes | 0 | +++ | Unilateral enlargement | T immature, L 0 |
| **4. Exogenous Administration of Hormones** | | | | |
| Chorionic gonadotropin (HCG) | + | ++ | Moderately increased | T immature, L + |
| Androgenic and anabolic steroids | 0 | +/+++ | Small | T immature, L + |
| Estrogens | 0 | + | Small | T immature, L + |

Reproduced by permission from Prader, arranged in tabular form by Bierich JR: Sexual precocity. *Clin Endocrinol Metabol* **4**:107–142, March 1975.

The natural history of idiopathic precocious puberty is extremely variable. Such children may progress to full maturation slowly or very rapidly. They may remain at a particular level for a prolonged period or even regress spontaneously only to progress again at a later time (18). By contrast, girls with Weil–Albright syndrome or cerebral lesions tend to progress relentlessly toward full maturity (18). Because of the natural variability of progression in idiopathic precocious puberty, an initial observation period of 6–12 months may be warranted. Observations of changes in growth, sexual maturation, skeletal maturation, and hormonal levels can be made and psychological support provided to help the family and child understand the nature of the disorder.

If sexual maturation progresses rapidly, consideration should be given to medical intervention. The most widely used preparation in the United States is medroxyprogesterone acetate (MPA) which may be administered intramuscularly in doses of 100–300 mg every 2–4 weeks (18, 19) or orally, 10 mg every 8 hours (19). Medroxyprogesterone is a strong anti-gonadotropin progestin which has no androgenic or estrogenic side effects. With this preparation, one can arrest further breast development or cornification of the vaginal epithelium and prevent or stop menstruation. In the boy, further growth of the penis is prevented and spermatogenesis is suppressed (56, 84). Medroxyprogesterone acetate has mild glucocorticoid activity, usually inapparent clinically, but with excessive dosage, mild adrenal suppression occurs which disappears soon after cessation of therapy (85). Amenorrhea after cessation of medroxyprogesterone treatment may be prolonged (we have observed amenorrhea extending for longer than 5 years in one patient), however, in the long run menstruation returns spontaneously (84).

The original hope that progestins would not only arrest premature sexual development but would also slow down the accelerated growth and skeletal maturation has not been fulfilled. Although Schoen reported some slowing of skeletal maturation in one of three boys and suggested that early administration of progestin might prevent accelerated skeletal maturation and dwarfism (86), most investigators have reported no effect of progestins on either accelerated growth patterns or accelerated skeletal maturation (56, 84, 87). Skeletal maturation tends to progress more rapidly than the rate of linear growth so that ultimate height prognosis becomes progressively worse (56). Not only does growth prognosis deteriorate in the course of precocity, but accurate predictions of adult height may not be possible, especially in younger children (88).

In Europe, cyproterone acetate, an antiandrogenic steroid with inhibitory effects on gonadotropin secretion, has been used extensively in the treatment of precocious puberty. Theoretically, an antiandrogenic preparation has considerable appeal. Some of the acceleration of growth and skeletal maturation that occurs in precocious development is the consequence of premature androgen secretion from the adrenals, especially in girls. So far, there is no satisfactory preparation which selectively suppresses adrenal androgenic secretion, although in animal studies, cyproterone acetate slowed down both puberty and bone maturation (89). Cyproterone has a glucocorticoid effect (similar to that observed with MPA), causing ACTH suppression and significant adrenal hypofunction (90). In children with precocious puberty, cyproterone acetate appears to be as effective as medroxyprogesterone acetate in slowing pubertal events (56), but there is still controversy over whether it is more effective in slowing somatic growth. Several investigators have reported favorable responses (91, 92), although others have concluded that it is without effect on growth (93). The latter authors suggest that bone maturation may be more sensitive to the action of androgens and less suppressible than secondary sex characteristics (93).

Recent interest in analogues of GnRH provides another possible form of intervention therapy. GnRH analogues have been shown to be capable of binding to receptor sites for GnRH in the pituitary, diminishing noticeably gonadotropin secretion, an effect desired in the treatment of precocious puberty (94). Although still under investigation, GnRH analogues have been shown to be both effective and free of many undesirable side effects in preliminary testing (95). GnRH analogues have also been tested successfully in combination with the antiandrogen, cyproterone acetate (96). GnRH analogues may well become the preferred treatment of idiopathic precocious puberty in the near future.

In boys with idiopathic isosexual precocity repeated neurologic examination and periodic skull films (or CT scan) should be performed because of the high likelihood of cerebral lesions as a cause of precocious puberty and because of the slow or late manifestations of many small CNS lesions.

# REFERENCES

1. Barnes HV: The problem of delayed puberty. *Med Clin North Am* **59**:1337–1347, 1975.

2. Prader A: Delayed adolescence. *Clin Endocrinol Metab* **4**:143–155, 1975.

3. Horner JM, Thorsson AV, Hintz RL: Growth deceleration patterns in children with constitutional short stature: An aid to diagnosis. *Pediatrics* **62**:529, 1978.

4. Illig R, Bambach M, Pluznik S, et al: Die Wirkung von synthetischem LH-RH auf die Freisetzung von LH und FSH bei Kindern und Jugendlichen. *Schweiz Med Wochensch* **103**:840, 1973.

5. Job JC, Chaussain JL, Garnier PW, et al: Effect of synethetic luteinizing hormone-releasing hormone on the release of gonadotropins in hypophysogonadal disorders of children and adolescents. VII. Constitutional delay of puberty in males. *J Pediatr* **88**:494, 1976.

6. Roth JC, Grumbach MM, Kaplan SL: The effect of synthetic luteinizing hormone-releasing factor on serum testosterone and gonadotropins in pre-pubertal, pubertal, and adult males. *J Clin Endocrinol Metab* **37**:680–686, 1973.

7. Schneider J, Lee PA: Decreased LH response to the second of consecutive day luteinizing hormone releasing hormone (LHRH) infusions among patients with constitutional delay of puberty: A phenomenon of pubertal maturation? *Clin Endocrinol* **12**:467, 1980.

8. Lee PA, Hogan MJ: Constitutional delay of growth and adolescence. *Growth* **44:**147, 1980.

9. Root AW: Hormonal changes in puberty. *Pediatr Ann* **9**(October):365–375, 1980.

10. Foss G: The influence of androgen treatment on ultimate height in males. *Arch Dis Child* **40:**66, 1965.

11. Kaplan JG, Moshang T Jr, Bernstein R, et al: Constitutional delay of growth and development: Effects of treatment with androgens, *J Pediatr* **82:**38–44, 1973.

12. Martin LG, Grossman MS, Conner TB: Effect of androgens on growth hormone secretion and growth in boys with short stature. *Acta Endocrinol* **91:**201, 1979.

13. Van den Bosch JSG, Smals AGH, Valk IM, et al: Lack of difference in growth stimulating effect between weekly single and multiple human chorionic gonadotropin administration in boys with delayed puberty. *Clin Endocrinol* **16:**1, 1982.

14. Kulin AG, Reiter EO: Delayed sexual maturation with special emphasis on the occurrence of the syndrome in the male, in Grumbach MM, Grave GD, Mayer FE (eds): *The Control of the Onset of Puberty*. New York, Wiley, 1974, pp 238–270.

15. Tanner JM, Whitehouse RH, Takaishi M: Standards from birth to maturity for height, weight, height velocity and weight velocity: British children, 1965, Part 2. *Arch Dis Child* **41:**454, 613, 1966.

16. Marshall WA and Tanner JM: Variations in pattern of pubertal changes in girls. *Arch Dis Child* **44:**291–303, 1969.

17. Marshall WA and Tanner JM: Variations in the pattern of pubertal changes in boys. *Arch Dis Child* **45:**13–23, 1970.

18. Root AW: Endocrinology of puberty: II. Aberrations of sexual maturation. *J Pediatr* **83:**187–200, 1973.

19. Ducharme JR, Collu R: Pubertal development: Normal, precocious and delayed. *Clin Endocrinol Metab* **11:**57, 1982.

20. Reindollar RH, McDonough PG: Etiology and evaluation of delayed sexual development. *Pediatr Clin North Am* **28:**267, 1981.

21. Styne DM, Kaplan SL: Normal and abnormal puberty in the female. *Pediatr Clin North Am* **26:**123, 1979.

22. Kallmann F, Schonfeld WA, Barrera SE: Genetic aspects of primary eunuchoidism. *Am J Ment Defic* **48:**203, 1944.

23. Prader A, Labhart A, Willi H: Ein Syndrom von Adipositas, Kleinwuchs, Kryptorchismus and Oligophrenie nach hypotonieartigen Zustand im Neugeborenenalter. *Schweiz Med Wochenschr* **86:**1260, 1956.

24. Bauman ML, Hogan GR: Laurence–Moon–Biedl syndrome, *Am J Dis Child* **126:**119, 1973.

25. Costin G: Endocrine disorders associated with tumors of the pituitary and hypothalamus. *Pediatr Clin North Am* **26:**15–31, 1979.

26. Latorre H, Kenny FM, Lahey ME, et al: Short stature and growth hormone deficiency in histiocytosis-X. *J Pediatr* **85:**813, 1974.

27. Koenig WP, Zuppinger K, Liechti B: Hyperprolactinemia as a cause of delayed puberty: Successful treatment with bromocriptine. *J Clin Endocrinol Metab* **48:**825, 1977.

28. Rappaport R, Branner R, Czernichow P, et al: Effect of hypothalamic and pituitary irradiation on pubertal development in children with cranial tumors. *J Clin Endocrinol Metab* **54:**1164, 1982.

29. Ratcliffe SG, Bancroft J, Axworthy D, et al: Klinefelter's syndrome in adolescence. *Arch Dis Child* **57:**6, 1982.

30. Sizonenko PC: Pre-adolescent and adolescent endocrinology: Physiology and physiopathology. Section 2. Hormonal changes during abnormal pubertal development. *Am J Dis Child* **132:**797–805, 1978.

31. Smith DW: Klinefelter syndrome, XXY syndrome, in *Recognizable Patterns of Human Malformation*, ed. 3. Philadelphia, WB Saunders and Co, 1982, p 64.

32. Smith DW: Turner (XO) syndrome, in *Recognizable Patterns of Human Malformation*, ed 3. Philadelphia, WB Saunders and Co, 1982, pp 72–75.

33. Brook CGD, Gasser T, Werder EA, et al: Height correlation between parents and mature offspring in normal subjects and in subjects with Turner's and Klinefelter's and other syndromes. *Ann Hum Biol* **4**:17–22, 1977.

34. Conte FA, Grumbach MM, Kaplan SL: A diphasic pattern of gonadotropin secretion in patients with the syndrome of gonadal dysgenesis. *J Clin Endocrinol Metab* **40**:670, 1975.

35. Simpson JL: Gonadal dysgenesis and abnormalities of the human sex chromosomes: Current status of phenotypic–karyotypic correlations, in *Genetic Forms of Hypogonadism*. Birth Defects Conference, Bergsma O (ed): New York, Grune and Stratton, 1975, p 23.

36. Abeyaratne MR, Aherne WA, Scott JES: The vanishing testis. *Lancet* **22**:822, 1969.

37. Pinsky L: Sexual differentiation, in Coller R, Ducharme JR, Guyda H (eds), *Pediatric Endocrinology*, New York, Raven Press, 1981, pp 231–292.

38. Hay ID, Smail PH, Forsyth CC: Familial cytomegalic adrenocortical hypoplasia: An X-linked syndrome of pubertal failure. *Arch Dis Child* **56**:715, 1981.

39. Vigersky R, Anderson AR, Thompson RH, et al: Hypothalmic dysfunction in secondary amenorrhea associated with simple weight loss. *New Engl J Med* **297**:1141, 1977.

40. Burbige EJ, Huang SH, Bayless TM: Clinical manifestations of Crohn's disease in children and adolescents. *Pediatrics* **55**:866, 1975.

41. Sobel EH, Silverman FU, Lee CM Jr: Chronic regional enterities and growth retardation. *Am J Dis Child* **103**:569, 1962.

42. Ferraris J, Saenger P, Levine L, et al: Delayed puberty in males with chronic renal failure. *Kidney Int* **18**:344, 1980.

43. Warren MP, van de Wiel RL: Clinical and metabolic features of anorexia nervosa. *Am J Obstet Gynecol* **117**:435, 1973.

44. Conte FA, Grumbach MM, Kaplan SL, et al: Correlation of luteinizing hormone releasing factor-induced luteinizing hormone and follicle-stimulating hormone release from infancy to 19 years with the changing pattern of gonadotropin secretion in agonadal patients: Relation to restraint of puberty. *J Clin Endocrinol Metab* **50**:163, 1980.

45. Harman SM, Tsitouvas PD, Costa PT, et al: Evaluation of pituitary gonadotropic function in men: Value of luteinizing hormone-releasing hormone response versus basal luteinizing hormone level for discrimination of diagnosis. *J Clin Endocrinol Metab* **54**:196, 1982.

46. Bourguignon JP, Vanderscheuren-Lodewyckx M, Wolter R, et al: Hypopituitarism and idiopathic delayed puberty: A longitudinal study in an attempt to diagnose gonadotropin deficiency before puberty. *J Clin Endocrinol Metab* **54**:733, 1982.

47. Kelch RP, Hopwood NJ, Marshall JC: Diagnosis of gonadotropin defiancy in adolescents: Limited usefulness of a standard gonadotropin-releasing hormone in obese boys. *J Pediatr* **97**:820, 1980.

48. Cohen HN, Wallace AM, Beastall GH, et al: Clinical value of adrenal androgen measurement in the diagnosis of delayed puberty. *Lancet* **1**:689, 1981.

49. Zachmann M: The evaluation of testicular endocrine function before and in puberty. The effect of a single dose of human chorionic gonadotropin on urinary steroid excretion under normal and pathological conditions. *Acta Endocrinol* **2**(suppl):1–94, 1972.

50. Gendrel D, Roger M, Choussain JL, et al: Correlation of pituitary and testicular responses to stimulation tests in cryptorchid children. *Acta Endocrinol* **86**:641, 1977.

51. Perheentupa J, Lenko HL, Nevalainen I, et al: Hormonal treatment of Turner's syndrome. *Acta Paediatr Scand* suppl **256**:24, 1975.

52. Moore DC, Tattoni DS, Ruvalcaba RH, et al: Effect of prolonged administration of oxandrolone on growth in children and adolescents with gonadal dysgenesis. *J Pediatr* **90**:462, 1977.

53. Brook CGD: Adolescence: Delayed puberty. *Brit J Hosp Med* **26**(Dec):573, 1981.

54. Abrams CAL, Grumbach MM, Dyrenfurth I, et al: Ovarian stimulation with human menopausal and chorionic gonadotropins in a pre-pubertal hypophysectomized femal. *J Clin Endocrinol Metab* **27**:467, 1967.

55. Keller PJ: Induction of ovulation by synthetic luteinizing-hormone releasing factor in infertile women. *Lancet* **2**:570, 1972.

56. Bierich JR: Sexual precocity. *Clin Endocrinol Metab* **4**:107–142, 1975.

57. Prader A: Pubertas Praecox, in Labhart A (ed): *Klinik der Inneren Sekretion.* Berlin, Springer-Verlag, 1971.

58. Blunck W, Bierich JR, Bettendorf G: Ueber Frühreife, III. Mitteilung. Idiopathische Pubertas Praecox, temporäre Frühreife und prämature Thelarche. *Montasschr Kinderheilkd* **115**:555–563, 1967.

59. Odell WD: The physiology of puberty: Disorders of the pubertal process, in DeGrott LJ, et al (eds): *Endocrinology.* New York, Grune and Stratton, 1979, vol 3, pp 1363–1379.

60. Mills JK, Stolley PD, Davies J, et al: Premature thelarche: Natural history and etiologic investigation. *Am J Dis Child* **135**:743, 1981.

61. Collett-Solberg PR, Grumbach MM: A simplified procedure for evaluating estrogenic effects and the sex chromatin pattern in exfoliated cells in urine: Studies in premature thelarche and gynecomastia of adolescence. *J Pediatr* **66**:883, 1965.

62. Bidlingmaier F, Wagner-Barnack M, Butenandt T, et al: Plasma estrogens in childhood and puberty under physiologic and pathologic conditions. *Pediatr Res* **7**:901, 1973.

63. Kenny FM, Midgley AR, Jaffe RB, et al: Radioimmunoassayable serum LH and FSH in girls with sexual precocity, premature thelarche and adrenarche. *J Clin Endocrinol Metab* **29**:1272, 1969.

64. Perloff WH, Nodine JH: The association of congenital spastic quadriplegia and androgenic precocity in four patients. *J Clin Endocrinol Metab* **10**:721, 1950.

65. Visser HKA, Degenhart HJ: Excretion of six individual 17-ketosteroids and testosterone in four girls with precocious sexual hair (premature adrenarche). *Helv Paediatr Acta* **21**:409, 1966.

66. Rosenfeld RL, Rich BH, Lucky AW: Adrenarche as a cause of benign pseudopuberty in boys. *J Pediatr* **101**:1005, 1982.

67. Grumbach MM, Richards GE, Conte FA, et al: Clinical disorders of adrenal function and puberty: An assessment of the role of the adrenal cortex in normal and abnormal puberty in man and evidence for an ACTH-like pituitary adrenal androgen stimulating hormone, in Serio M (ed): *The Endocrine Function of the Human Adrenal Cortex*, Serono Symposium. New York, Academic Press, 1977.

68. Murram D, Dewhurst J, Grant DB: Premature menarche: A follow-up study. *Arch Dis Child* **58**:142, 1983.

69. Solyom AE, Anstad CC, Sherick I, et al: Precocious sexual development in girls: The emotional impact on the child and his parents. *J Pediatr Psychol* **5**:385, 1980.

70. Liu N, Grumbach MM, DeNapoli RA, et al: Prevalence of electroencephalographic abnormalities in idiopathic precocious puberty and premature pubarche. *J Clin Endocrinol Metab* **25**:1296, 1965.

71. Blunck W: Sexual precocity. *Pediatr Ann* **3**(July):30–46, 1974.

72. Weil D: Neun-jähriges Madchen mit Pubertas Praecox und Knochenbruchigkeit, *Klin Wochenschr*, 1922, cited by Bierich JR: Sexual precocity. *Clin Endocrinol Metab* **4**:107–142, 1975.

73. Grant DB, Martinez L: The McCune-Albright syndrome without typical skin pigmentation. *Acta Paediatr Scand* **72**:477, 1983.

74. Hall R, Warrick C: Hypersecretion of hypothalamic releasing hormones: A possible explanation of the endocrine manifestations of polyostotic fibrous dysplasia. *Lancet* **1**:1313, 1972.

75. Silver HK: Asymmetry, short stature, and variations in sexual development: A syndrome of congenital malformations. *Am J Dis Child* **107**:495, 1964.

76. Huseman CA, Kelch RP, Hopwood NJ, et al: Sexual precocity in association with septo-optic dysplasia and hypothalamic hypopituitarism. *J Pediatr* **92**:748, 1978.

77. Van Wyk JJ, Grumbach MM: Syndrome of precocious menstruation and galactorrhea in juvenile hypothyroidism: An example of hormonal overlap in pituitary feedback. *J Pediatr* **57**:416, 1960.

78. Marilus R, Dickerman Z, Kaufman H, et al: Addison's disease associated with precocious sexual development in a boy. *Acta Paediatr Scand* **70**:587, 1981.

79. Eberlein WR, Bongiovanni AM, Jones IT, et al: Ovarian tumors and cysts associated with sexual precocity. *J Pediatr* **57**:484, 1960.

80. Towne BH, Mahour GH, Woolley MM, et al: Ovarian cysts and tumors in infancy and childhood. *J Pediatr Surg* **10**:311, 1975.

81. Siegler RL, Rallison ML: Hypertension with virilizing adrenal tumor. *Pediatrics* **61**:925, 1978.

82. Moreira AC, Verissimo JMT, Foss MC, et al: Pubertal maturation of the LH stimulatory response to clomiphene citrate in congenital virilizing adrenal hyperplasia. *Clin Endocrinol* **17**:441, 1982.

83. Lamb DR: Anabolic steroids in athletes: How well do they work and how dangerous are they? *Am J Sports Med* **12**:31, 1984.

84. Kaplan SA, Ling SM, Irani NG: Idiopathic isosexual precocity therapy with medroxyprogesterone. *Am J Dis Child* **116**:591, 1968.

85. Sadeghi-Nejad A, Kaplan SL, Grumbach MM: The effect of medroxyprogesterone acetate on adrenocortical function in children with precocious puberty. *J Pediatr* **78**:616, 1971.

86. Schoen EJ: Treatment of idiopathic precocious puberty in boys. *J Clin Endocrinol Metab* **26**:363, 1966.

87. Menking M, Blunck W, Wiebel J, et al: Ueber Frühreife: IV. Mitteilung: Therapie der Pubertas Praecox. *Montasschr Kinderheilkd* **119**:19–22, 1971.

88. Kirkland JL, Gibbs AR, Kirkland RT, et al: Height predictions in girls with idiopathic precocious puberty by the Bayley–Pinneau method. *Pediatrics* **68**:251, 1981.

89. Steinbeck H, Neumann F: Effect of cyproterone acetate on puberty in rats. *J Reprod Fertil* **26**:59, 1971.

90. Savage DCL, Swift PGF: Effect of cyproterone acetate on adrenocortical function in children with precocious puberty. *Arch Dis Child* **56**:218, 1981.

91. Bossie E, Zurbrugg RP, Joss EE: Improvement of adult height prognosis in precocious puberty by cyproterone acetate. *Acta Paeditr Scand* **62**:405, 1973.

92. Rager K, Huegnes R, Gupta D, et al: The treatment of Precocious puberty with cyproterone acetate. *Acta Endocrinol* **74**:399, 1973.

93. Werder EA, Murset G, Zachmann M, et al: Treatment of precocious puberty with cyproterone acetate. *Pediatr Res* **8**:248–256, 1974.

94. Comite F, Cutler GB, Rivier J, et al: Short-term treatment of idiopathic precocious puberty with a long-acting analogue of luteinizing hormone-releasing hormone. *N Engl J Med* **305**:1546, 1981.

95. Crowley WF, Comite F, Vale W, et al: Therapeutic use of pituitary desensitization with a long-acting LHRH agonist: A potential treatment for idiopathic precocious puberty. *J Clin Endocrinol Metab* **52:**370, 1981.

96. Laron Z, Kauli R, Zeev ZB, et al: D = Trp$^6$-analogue of luteinizing hormone-releasing hormone in combination with cyproterone acetate to treat precocious puberty. *Lancet* **2:**955, 1981.

# 11
# Nutritional Problems in Children

We recognize the central role played by nutrition in the growth process and the effect on growth of nutritional disturbances, but optimal nutrition is difficult to define. The difficulty in tracing the effect of nutrition on growth stems not so much from our lack of appreciation of the interrelationships between substrate provision (nutrition) and metabolic regulation by the endocrine system as from our uncertainty about what constitutes an "adequate" diet. We acknowledge that there is variability in nutritional requirements and that each individual may have unique nutritional needs. "Minimal" or "recommended" daily allowances of calories and specific nutrients allow comparison of the individual with "group" needs and serve, in many instances, to alert us to probable nutritional excesses or deficiencies (1). We cannot, however, predict that a given nutritional intake will invariably lead to a specific growth abnormality, nor conversely, that a given growth excess or deficiency occurred because of nutritional excess or deficiency.

In this chapter we discuss failure to thrive as a nutritional aberration resulting from nutritional deficiency and obesity as nutritional excess emphasizing the effects on growth produced by these disorders of nutrition.

## FAILURE TO THRIVE

Failure to thrive is a descriptive term used to describe children who fail to gain weight at an adequate rate. Implicit in the definition of failure to thrive is the assumption that a child who fails to thrive fails to receive or utilize adequate nutrients to allow normal growth. Undernutrition may be indicated first by a reduction in weight velocity, although, a reduction of height velocity can be expected to accompany undernutrition as well (2). The Ten State Nutrition Survey documents a clear relationship between poverty (undernutrition) and lower growth achievements of children (3).

## How Failure to Thrive is Defined

Failure to thrive is defined as a failure to gain weight (or length) at the rate expected for an infant or child; that is, a weight (or length) gain falling below the 3rd percentile on weight (or length) velocity charts or tables, for at least 3 months. We are hampered in this definition by lack of access to growth tables and charts that will allow rapid and accurate assessment of rate of weight gain or length increments. Tanner and Whitehouse have constructed height and weight *velocity charts* for boys and girls, but the extreme percentiles (3rd and 97th) for weight become precise enough for our use only after the first year of life and for height only after the second year (4). We are obliged, therefore, to derive velocity of weight gain (or length increment) for infants from *longitudinal charts* or tables (Appendix Figures A-5, A-6, and Tables A-3, A-5). Most infants with failure to thrive, will eventually be found below the 3rd percentile line on achievement charts because of their low velocity of growth, but this does not improve much on the definition of failure to thrive attributed to an ancient Arabic physician . . . "a child . . . thin and delicate and weak, so that he has nothing but skin and bones . . ." (5).

## Causes of Failure to Thrive

Because weight loss or failure to thrive may be a presenting complaint for a large number of infancy and childhood disorders, we must formulate a plan to discover the cause without an unnecessarily long and costly investigation. In 832 children hospitalized for failure to thrive, from six published surveys (6–12), a diagnosis of constitutional small size was reported in 20% (range 4–32%), environmental or nonorganic causes were cited in 27% (range 15–55%), and organic causes were discovered in 53% (range 18–85%). Of the organic causes, gastrointestinal and neurologic causes accounted for about half (13% each); cardiac lesions were responsible in 10%, although there was a very wide range (1–31%), and genitourinary (4%) and endocrine (3%) causes were found least frequently. The remaining 11% were not categorized (12).

An approach to failure to thrive should allow the practitioner to detect normal low weight infants and those with nonorganic failure to thrive with minimal observation and testing, while allowing the recognition and correction of the organic disturbances leading to failure to thrive. Figure 11-1 displays the approach to children with failure to thrive developed by the Division of Pediatric Gastroenterology at the University of Utah. It is similar to the approach published by Green which has served as a diagnostic guide to failure to thrive for many years (13). Most of the information needed for discovering the area of concern can be obtained from history, examination, and observation of the infant.

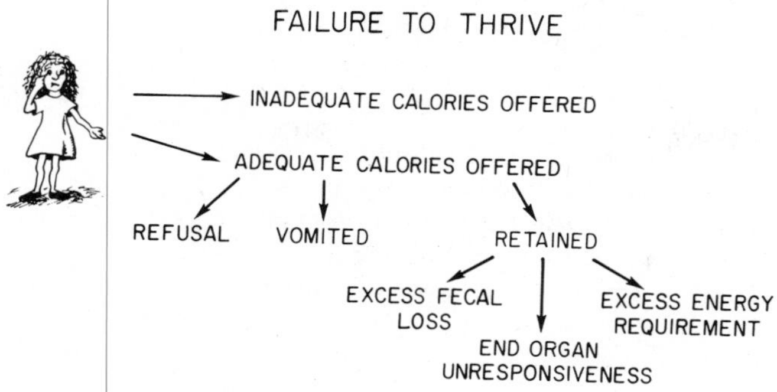

FAILURE TO THRIVE

**Figure 11-1.** Outline of causes for failure to thrive. (Courtesy of Dr. Linda S. Book, Division of Pediatric Gastroenterology, University of Utah.)

In the first step, we evaluate adequacy of calories offered. Inadequate calories may be offered because of poverty, poor feeding technique, or child neglect which focuses the attention on social or environmental issues. If adequate calories are offered, they may be refused, vomited or retained. Refusal may direct attention to neuromuscular disorders, malignancy, or anorexia nervosa. Vomiting will direct attention to intestinal obstruction, GE reflux, and so on. If calories are retained, they may be lost as diarrhea, consumed by excessive energy requirement, or be ineffective because of end organ unresponsiveness. Excess fecal loss should direct attention to malabsorptive disturbances. Excess energy requirement may be seen in chronic infections, cardiac disorders, or hyperthyroidism. End organ unresponsiveness may be due to systemic diseases or hormonal disorders. This scheme allows us to rapidly identify the area of concern most likely responsible for failure to thrive and directs our attention to a finite number of disorders which need be considered in discovering the cause of failure to thrive.

### Inadequate Calories Offered

Worldwide, the most common cause of failure to thrive is starvation or protein-calorie malnutrition, a consequence of unavailability of adequate food. In developed countries, poverty among small segments of the population may contribute to undernutrition, although malnutrition may also be a consequence of poor eating habits, food fads, or emotional aberrations which limit food intake (Table 11-1).

*Severe malnutrition* (marasmus) occurs in infants who are chronically deprived of adequate calories. Failure to gain weight is followed by progressive weight loss to the point of emaciation. Loss of subcutaneous fat leads to loss of skin turgor and wrinkling of the skin. Although sucking pads in the cheeks are retained for a considerable time, the face also eventually becomes sunken and wizened. The abdomen may be distended

### Table 11-1. Failure to Thrive Caused by Inadequate Calories Offered

Protein-calorie malnutrition
Improper feeding techniques
   Calorically inadequate formula
   Inadequate mothering
   Inadequate breast milk supply
Psychosocial deprivation
Child neglect

or sunken and the intestinal pattern may be visible because of subcutaneous fat and muscle atrophy. Generalized edema may be present. The child, although fretful early in the course, gradually becomes listless. Terminally, starvation diarrhea may occur (14).

Inadequate protein in food will produce *protein-calorie malnutrition* (*kwashiorkor*) in an infant or child. This state may also occur with abnormal protein loss or faulty protein absorption. Kwashiorkor is the most prevalent form of malnutrition in the world today. Infants in underdeveloped countries thrive as long as they receive their major nutrition from breast milk, but when they are weaned from the breast, their diet commonly contains inadequate protein and kwashiorkor (meaning the deposed child) develops. The child becomes lethargic, apathetic, and irritable. There is poor growth, atrophy of muscles, flabbiness of subcutaneous tissues, edema, and an increased susceptibility to infection. The hair is sparse, thin, and depigmented. Infestation with parasites is common. If unchecked, the disorder progresses to stupor, coma, and death. Treatment requires gradual increase in calories and gradual introduction of protein. If the protein is reintroduced too rapidly, liver enlargement and failure will ensue. If the malnutrition has been present from early infancy, some physical and mental retardation may be permanent (14, 15).

*Underfeeding* because of calorically inadequate formula may lead to a fretful infant with failure to thrive. Persistent underfeeding will cause irritability, restlessness, failure to sleep, excessive crying, constipation, loss of subcutaneous tissue, and weight loss. Increasing fluid and caloric intake and/or instructing the mother in infant feeding skills will produce gratifying results. Occasionally in breast-fed infants, the milk supply becomes inadequate. If the infant nurses avidly and after emptying both breasts is not satisfied, becomes restless, irritable, sleeps fitfully, and fails to gain weight, then the milk supply is probably inadequate. Supplementation will usually correct the inadequate supply of calories.

Abnormal maternal–child interaction may lead to a spectrum of disorders of nutrition which range from inadequate maternal–infant bonding

## Table 11-2. Failure to Thrive Caused by Inadequate Calories Accepted

Congenital anomalies of upper digestive system
  (cleft palate, glossoptosis, etc.)
Dyspnea due to congenital heart disease
Diabetes insipidus
Macroglossia of congenital hypothyroidism
Neuromuscular disorders (developmental retardation)
Malignancy (anorexia)
Recurrent or chronic illness
Anorexia nervosa

to psychosocial deprivation, to unequivocal child neglect. The failure to thrive in each of these disorders is, at least partly, a lack of adequate calories offered (16) (See nonorganic failure to thrive.)

### Inadequate Calories Accepted (Refusal of Adequate Calories)

Conditions, in which adequate calories are offered but are not accepted or are refused, range from purely mechanical inability to accept food to emotional rejection of nutrients (Table 11-2).

Anomalies of the upper digestive tract such as cleft palate, glossoptosis, or esophageal atresia, usually present no difficulties in recognition. Esophageal stenosis or atresia may present with dysphagia, regurgitation, and vomiting especially pronounced with solid foods. Oral malformations, major features of a number of syndromes, may interfere with the ability of the infant to suck or swallow food, resulting in inadequate intake of calories. Most malformations can be surgically corrected or can be ameliorated by careful feeding techniques so that adequate nutrition is possible (17). Intermittant upper airway obstruction has also led to poor growth and eventually to cardiovascular complications (cor pulmonale). Correction of the upper airway obstruction results in dramatic improvement in growth (18).

Caloric intake of children with developmental retardation, cerebral damage, or cerebral palsy is often less than that of normal children (13). Dyspnea, due to pulmonary or cardiac disease, may cause difficulty in the feeding of an infant. In diabetes insipidus, food intake is reduced to reduce the solute load presented to the kidney in order to preserve fluid otherwise lost by osmotic diuresis. Reduction of the solute load leads to a calorically inadequate intake and failure to grow (19). Infants with congenital hypothyroidism will frequently present in early infancy with failure to thrive because of feeding difficulties caused by the macroglossia. Malignancy or chronic illness may produce anorexia and refusal of adequate calories. Failure of weight gain or weight loss may be the initial manifestation of malignancy or chronic illness and always deserves careful investigation.

Voluntary starvation and severe weight loss in girls of adolescent age is characteristic of *anorexia nervosa*. Voluntary weight reduction is begun because the subject views herself as "too fat", although weight may be normal. Refusal of food and weight loss continue beyond acceptable limits and in even a near emaciated state the subject still may consider herself "overweight". The subject usually denies that she is trying to starve herself and generally claims to feel fine even when emaciated. Strength and muscle mass are retained to a remarkable degree despite loss of subcutaneous tissue. She may be athletically active and even excell while losing weight. Many subjects with anorexia nervosa are well-behaved, obedient, and good students, although they tend to be perfectionistic, obsessive–compulsive, and have limited affect. Sexual development is usually suspended; genitalia may become atrophic and amenorrhea is nearly universal. Refusal of food is persistent and malignant. Food may be hidden, or if ingested, vomited back up voluntarily. Enemas and laxatives may be used to further prevent nutrient absorption. The subject views her emaciated state as desirable and is repulsed by the idea of a normal adolescent figure with usual amounts of adolescent fat (15).

The diagnostic criteria for anorexia nervosa from DSM III include (a) intense fear of becoming obese, which does not diminish as weight loss progresses, (b) disturbance of body image, claiming to "feel fat" even when emaciated, (c) weight loss of at least 25% of original body weight, adjusted for projected growth for children, (d) refusal to maintain body weight over a minimal normal weight for age and height, and (e) no known physical illness that would account for the weight loss (20). Irwin questions whether the DSM III criteria are appropriate for younger children, particularly criteria (c) and (d), which deal with weight loss and failure to maintain minimal weight. He feels that anorexia may be present in many preteenagers who do not fit the DSM III criteria (21). The diagnosis of anorexia nervosa is not always simple. Excessive weight loss in the adolescent through restricted food intake to enhance athletic abilities is a common occurrence, and it is sometimes difficult to distinguish simple misguided enthusiasm from anorexia nervosa (22). A variation of this theme is reported by Pugliese et al., who report growth failure due to self-imposed restriction of caloric intake arising from a fear of becoming obese (23). Such behavior may actually fulfill the criteria for anorexia nervosa, being a self-inflicted weight loss with a morbid fear of becoming too fat (24).

Growth arrest may be the most striking observation in some girls with anorexia; suboptimal nutrition may be manifested only by little or no weight gain (25). Severe protein-calorie malnutrition lowers somatomedin levels despite high growth hormone levels (26). In anorexia nervosa, growth hormone levels tend to be elevated, while somatomedin levels are

**Table 11-3. Failure to Thrive Caused by Loss
of Calories by Chronic Vomiting**

Esophageal stenosis
Gastroesophegeal reflex
Intestinal obstruction (chronic and recurrent)
Toxic enteropathy (celiac syndrome)
Rumination (maternal–infant interaction)

low or normal (24). Loss of circadian fluctuations in the 24–hour secretion of LH and amenorrhea are seen in nearly every adolescent with anorexia nervosa and are somewhat independent of weight or nutritional status (27). This reversion to an immature pattern of LH secretion may represent a biologic "marker" of active anorexia nervosa (27).

Anorexia nervosa is a devastating illness for the patient and family (28). Treatment requires psychotherapy. Traditional psychoanalysis is rather ineffective, whereas an approach evoking active participation on the part of the patient leads to better results (29). Before proceeding with psychiatric therapy, it is important to exclude the possibility of hypopituitary cachexia, chronic infection, or malignancy, which can produce emaciation and the symptom complex of anorexia. If the emaciation is extreme and life-threatening, hospitalization will be required to reverse the weight loss. Treatment may include behavioral modification, forced nasogastric tube feedings, hyperalimentation, and psychopharmacotherapy with antidepressants, chlorpromazine, cyproheptadine, or diphenylhydantoin (28). Starvation to the point of death is possible, and death occasionally occurs unexpectedly even without extreme emaciation. Mortality from anorexia nervosa has been reported to be as low as 2% (30), but as high as 22% (28). Recovery from an acute episode of starvation is generally possible, but restoration to normal weight and psychological well-being with appropriate body image requires intensive long-term therapy (15, 28).

### Chronic Vomiting

Vomiting is a prominent symptom of disorders of the esophagus and stomach, of bowel obstruction at any level, and of systemic illnesses which can cause reflex vomiting. Dysphagia, regurgitation, and vomiting with chronic loss of calories leads to poor weight gain and failure to thrive (Table 11-3).

Congenital stenosis, atresia of the esophagus, or external compression of the esophagus from a vascular ring, cardiac malformation, mediastinal tumor, or nodes may present with chronic or recurrent regurgitation. Disorders of the gastroesophageal junction such as hiatus hernia and achalasia (lack of relaxation of the lower esophageal sphincter) may lead to chronic vomiting and weight loss as can strictures at the cardioesophageal junction from reflux esophagitis or ingestion of a corrosive substance (17). In the infant, pyloric stenosis, congenital stricture, or web within the duodenum may be responsible for persistent vomiting and weight loss, but the symptoms are usually sufficiently urgent that chronic obstruction is not allowed to occur (17).

*Gastroesophageal (GE) reflux* (chalasia) represents the most common gastrointestinal disorder, leading to vomiting and failure to thrive in the infant. Incompetence of the cardioesophageal sphincter, frequently in association with hiatal hernia, leads to GE reflux. Vomiting usually begins within the first week of life and is present in 95% by 6 weeks of age (31). Vomiting may be forceful because of pylorospasm and esophageal irritation. Growth and weight gain are adversely affected in over two-thirds. Diagnosis may be suspected from the clinical history of vomiting with recurrent pneumonitis and confirmed by esophogram, fluoroscopy, or scintiscan. Probes to detect pressure and acidity in the lower esophagus have been found to be helpful, especially in cases with episodic reflux (31).

Without treatment, symptoms in the majority of children ameliorate by age 2 as they assume an upright position for eating. Propping the child upright during and after feedings and burping carefully may be sufficient treatment for mild cases. Most of the remaining children improve spontaneously by 4 years. Use of a reflux board to maintain an angle of 30–50% may be required in more persistent cases. Thickened foods are also often helpful. Use of antacids for esophagitis may be necessary. Esophageal strictures occur in about 5% and death occurs from peptic esophagitis, aspiration, and inanition in an additional 5%. If intensive medical therapy is ineffective, surgical bouginage of strictures and/or gastropexy or fundoplication are necessary for relief (31).

Chronic or recurrent intestinal obstruction, below the level of the stomach, may also present with vomiting, although there will usually be additional signs to suggest a lower level of obstruction. Celiac syndrome and other disorders, characterized primarily by diarrhea, may present with vomiting. Any chronic illness which may cause anorexia may also cause reflex vomiting and lead to weight loss apart from the systemic illness.

### Excess Fecal Loss

Although adequate calories may be offered and accepted, they may be lost in excessive amounts from diarrhea. In Table 11-4, are listed representative disorders associated with chronic diarrhea (fecal loss of nutrients) and failure to thrive.

*Inadequate digestion* of food because of unavailability of digestive enzymes results in excess fecal loss of partially digested food. *Malabsorption*, failure of absorption and transport of nutrients from the bowel into the blood stream, is characterized by increased fecal loss of nutrients, abdominal

**Table 11-4. Excess Fecal Losses
in Failure to Thrive**

Inadequate digestion (maldigestion)
    Cystic fibrosis of pancreas
    Pancreatic insufficiency and neutropenia
    Digestive enzyme deficiencies
Inadequate absorption (malabsorption)
    Celiac syndrome (gluten-induced enteropathy)
    Giardiasis (parasitic infestation)
    Gastrointestinal allergy
Inflammatory bowel disease
    Ulcerative colitis
    Crohn's disease (ileitis)
Biliary tract disease
Protein-losing enteropathy
Hirschprung's disease
Idiopathic prolonged (secretory) diarrhea

distention, and failure to thrive. The stool may be watery, bulky and fatty, or even normal, depending on the cause of the malabsorption (32) (Table 11-5).

In *cystic fibrosis of the pancreas*, the single most common cause of chronic malabsorption in children, lack of pancreatic digestive enzymes leads to maldigestion of all classes of food, most notably protein and fat. Malnutrition may be severe despite a good appetite and apparently adequate nutritional intake. The abdomen is distended. The stools are frequent, bulky, greasy, and foul smelling. Failure to thrive may be primarily due to the nutritional disorder, but pulmonary infection and insufficiency may contribute to growth failure as well. Pancreatic insufficiency, malabsorption, and growth failure are also seen with chronic severe neutropenia in

**Table 11-5.  Types of Stools in Malabsorption Syndromes**

| Watery | Fatty | Normal |
|---|---|---|
| Milk allergy | Cystic fibrosis | Malabsorption of |
| Parasites (giardia, etc.) | Pancreatic insufficiency |    aminoacids |
| Sugar enzyme | Celiac syndrome (sprue) | Vitamin B$_{12}$ deficiency |
|    deficiencies | Biliary tract disorders | Folic acid deficiency |
| Intestinal kinase | A-betaliproproteinemia | |
|    deficiencies | Lymphangiectasia | |

Reproduced by permission from Ament ME: Intestinal malabsorption, in Vaughan VC, McKay RJ, Behrman RE (eds), *Nelson's Textbook of Pediatrics*, ed 11. Philadelphia, WB Saunders Co, 1979, p 1076.

the Bodian–Schwachman syndrome, a rare familial disorder, characterized by atrophy and fatty replacement of the pancreas, malabsorption, and diarrhea (33). Specific digestive enzyme deficiencies, such as, disaccharidase, enterokinase, lactase, or sucrose-isomaltase, can cause malabsorption of a specific class of food and lead to diarrhea and failure to thrive. Lack of the specific enzyme leads to accumulation of sugar within the bowel; water accumulates because of the osmotic gradient and a watery diarrhea ensues.

*Celiac syndrome* (nontropical sprue or gluten-induced enteropathy) is said to be a rare cause of chronic malabsorption, although its frequency may have been underestimated (34). Celiac syndrome is caused by a hereditary intolerance for gluten—a protein fraction of wheat, barley, rye, and oats. The gliadin fraction of gluten causes progressive damage to the surface epithelium and gradual disappearance of villi. The mechanism of injury appears to involve an immunologic reaction (35). Absorptive surface is greatly diminished, leading to malabsorption and diarrhea.

Chronic diarrhea, irritability, vomiting, and failure to grow may occur any time after introduction of gluten-containing foods, most commonly within the first 2 years of life. Stools are bulky, poorly formed, and foul-smelling; food intake is often reduced by anorexia. Abdominal distention, wasted musculature, decreased subcutaneous fat, and dependent edema produce a child with an emaciated, malnourished appearance (Figure 11-2). Growth failure is common at all ages and anemia may be present in the older child as well. Failure to grow and delayed puberty may be the only manifestations of the syndrome in a few patients (32, 36).

The diagnosis of celiac syndrome requires demonstration of impaired intestinal absorption, characteristic histologic changes in duodenojejunal mucosa, and a beneficial response to a gluten-free diet. Impaired absorption of fat may be shown by measurement of fecal fat in a 72-hour stool collection, or absorption of an orally administered Lipiodol meal. A mucosal biopsy specimen shows loss of villi, increased mononuclear cells in the lamina propia, and damaged surface epithelial cells. Restoration of the gut mucosa to normal occurs with institution of a gluten-free diet (32). A diet free of gluten is necessary for life, since the gluten intolerance is a permanent condition (37). Catch-up growth can be expected to occur when the malabsorption is corrected (Figure 11-2). Return to gluten-containing foods will result in suboptimal growth, chronic fatigue, and anemia (32).

Many foods are capable of provoking an *allergic response in the gastrointestinal tract*, but milk is the most common offender among children who fail to thrive. Most infants fed cow's milk develop circulating cow's milk antibodies, but only a few exhibit systemic or intestinal symptoms. Diarrhea occurs often with vomiting and abdominal pain, beginning within the first few weeks or months of life. The stools are watery and contain excessive mucus, and frequently blood. Chronic diarrhea with loss of intestinal villi

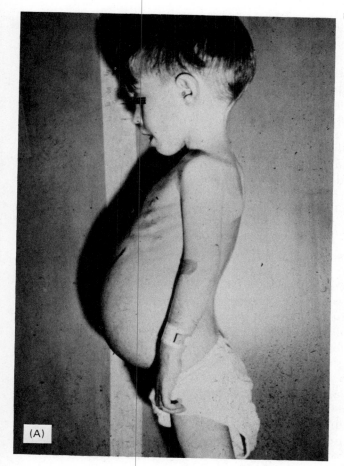

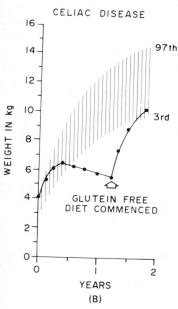

(A)

**Figure 11-2.** Child with celiac syndrome (A) demonstrating characteristic emaciation and protuberant abdomen. (B) Weight loss with catch-up growth upon treatment with gluten-free diet is shown on the growth chart. (Courtesy of Dr. Linda S. Book.)

may mimic celiac syndrome (38). The diagnosis of food (milk) allergy is based on clinical criteria. Symptoms should subside within 48 hours after removal of milk from the diet and recur within 48 hours after a trial feeding. If identified by clinical trial, the offending allergen should be removed from the diet. Calcium supplements may be required for an infant who must use milk substitutes indefinitely (39).

Although formerly a disease of the tropics, *giardiasis* has been introduced into the watersheds of an increasing number of localities so that in some areas infestation with *Giardia lamblia* must be considered in children with malabsorption and failure to thrive. Among campers and hikers the most common complaint has been severe and persistent diarrhea; conditions resembling celiac syndrome have been described. The parasite may be eradicated with quinacrine hydrochloride or metronidazole.

Regional or granulomatous enteritis (*Crohn's disease*) is a slowly progressive, relentless, and persistent inflammatory disorder of the gastrointestinal tract characterized by monocytic inflammation of the mucosa and submucosa of the bowel wall. Granulomas, composed of epithelial and giant cells, are found in mucosa and in lymph nodes (40). The appearance of the disease is usually insidious. Early symptoms include anorexia, bloating, lethargy, fatigue, intermittent cramping, abdominal pain, and diarrhea. On occasion the onset may be abrupt and severe, suggesting appendicitis or bowel perforation, but pain is more commonly a constant aching or soreness. Watery diarrhea, occasionally with gross blood, is present in 90% of patients at the time of diagnosis and fever in about one-third. Weight loss, short stature, abdominal tenderness, anemia, clubbing of the fingers, and gall or kidney stones may be found on examination (41). Puberty is usually delayed in the adolescent (42) and small size and delayed puberty may be the presenting complaint (43).

Many simultaneous processes lead to failure to thrive in granulomatous inflammatory bowel disease. The inflammatory process may produce anorexia and malaise while increasing metabolic needs. The thick, inflamed portion of the bowel interferes with mobility and produces a "functional" bowel obstruction, causing postprandial pain, a feeling of satiety, or anorexia. Protein may be lost in large amounts from the inflamed mucosa (protein-losing enteropathy) (44). Involvement of the ileum may lead to bile salt loss and impaired fat absorption. Together these factors produce undernutrition and failure to thrive (17).

No treatment is entirely effective in Crohn's disease. Acute, inflammatory attacks may respond to corticosteroids or salicylazosulfapyridine, but prolonged use of steroids will further interfere with growth. Use of low dose or alternate day steroids may be effective without causing growth failure. In patients who fail to respond to medication, total parenteral nutrition may be necessary. Surgery must be performed for massive uncontrolled bleeding or toxic megacolon, but elective surgery for removal of affected bowel offers limited relief (45).

In its active state, *ulcerative colitis* may interfere temporarily with growth and be a cause of failure to thrive, but it only occasionally produces permanent growth failure (46). Children with severe disease have a bloody diarrhea, abdominal cramps, fever, anemia, weight loss, and peripheral edema (47). Shortness of stature occurs if the disease continues untreated for a sufficient length of time (41). Arthritis may be a prominent symptom and erythema nodosum, pyoderma gangrenosum, or iritis may occur occasionally. Proctosigmidoscopy in subjects suspected of ulcerative colitis will allow recognition of the typical crypt abcesses, diffuse colonic inflammation, friability, and ulceration (17).

A nutritious diet, avoiding foods which cause exacerbations, and counseling to reduce life's pressures and anxieties are basic to all other care. Adrenocorticosteroids may be used rectally as an enema or systemically, during the acute phase of the disease. For control of the colitis, systemic steroids are generally required in high dosage for several weeks, after which they may be tapered and replaced with salicylazosulfapyradine (45). Growth retardation may be expected from this level of steroid administration, but catch-up growth should occur once the colitis is controlled and the steroids discontinued. If steroid therapy is ineffective, parenteral alimentation may be needed. Colectomy may be advised for profuse hemorrhage, perforation, obstruction, toxic megacolon, malignancy, or for chronic failure to grow and thrive. Total colectomy generally restores the growth to normal and may allow catch-up growth if performed before pubertal events limit achievable growth (42).

Failure to thrive in *biliary atresia* or *chronic liver ailments* may stem from diminished food intake due to lack of appetite, nausea and vomiting, or from malabsorption and diarrhea due to faulty fat absorption. In addition to the impairment of fat absorption, there may also be deficiences of fat soluble vitamins (A, D, E, K,). If there is severe hepato-cellular damage, the liver may fail to carry out efficiently its many metabolic activities, resulting in inappropriate or wasteful utilization of substrate from food (17).

*Congenital megacolon* (Hirschsprung's disease) is the most common cause of chronic intestinal obstruction in children. The disease results from lack of ganglion cells in a portion of the bowel wall, which results in abnormal peristalsis and functional obstruction. Episodes of constipation and diarrhea alternate with periods of apparently normal bowel function. The diarrhea may become a fulminant enterocolitis, causing profound dehydration and shock (toxic megacolon). Large amounts of fluid and electrolytes are lost into the bowel sufficient to produce vascular collapse and death if not energetically treated. Chronic constipation, abdominal distention, and growth failure are common complaints in the older child. Subcutaneous tissue may be diminished so that the child resembles the chronically malnourished child with malabsorption (Figure 11-2). Diagnosis is made by rectal biopsy and roentgenographic studies of the bowel. Anorectal manometry may show the characteristic increased sphincter pressure. Following preliminary colostomy, the aganglionic segment of bowel is excised and anastamosis of functional bowel segments performed. Most children regain normal bowel function and catch-up in their growth (48).

Diarrhea beginning shortly after birth may become prolonged and intractable (*intractable secretory diarrhea*). Small bowel mucosa is flattened and malabsorption occurs. Some children improve slowly after many months of total parenteral nutrition (hyperalimentation), but many still die in spite of all therapeutic efforts (49, 50).

### Table 11-6. Failure to Thrive
### Secondary to Excess Energy
### Requirements

Excessive crying or restlessness
Prolonged fever
Repeated acute or chronic infection
Inflammatory bowel disease
Arthritis and other inflammatory disorders
Malignancy
Cardiac disorders
Hyperthyroidism
Diabetes mellitus

## Excess Energy Expenditure

It is logical to assume that an infant or child will fail to gain or even lose weight if energy expenditure exceeds that of intake, but it is difficult to demonstrate excess energy expenditure as the probable cause of failure to thrive. In many circumstances in which excess energy expenditure is suspected, anorexia and decreased food intake may contribute to the failure to thrive. In Table 11-6, are listed some disorders in which excess energy requirements seem to be major factors in the failure to thrive. Perhaps only in hyperthyroidism is this clearly the major factor, but it appears to be important in most of the others as well.

*Excessive crying or restlessness* in an infant may expend sufficient calories that weight gain is suboptimal, but a fussy baby may also refuse adequate calories. One feels a little uncomfortable attributing failure to thrive to nonspecific excessive and persistent fussiness, but clinically experienced physicians attest to the reality of such an entity (13).

*Recurrent or prolonged fever* may require excess energy, however, the disease state which produces the fever may also cause malaise and anorexia, leading to decreased food intake or may interfere with food utilization by vomiting or diarrhea. Any disease state characterized by prolonged fever is capable of interfering with growth and only correction of the fever-producing disease will assure resumption of normal growth. Excess caloric utilization may be combined with anorexia or failure to utilize nutrients in *repeated acute or chronic infections* (Table 11-6). Urinary tract infections may present simply as a chronically ill child with failure to thrive. Likewise, the symptoms of sepsis are often nonspecific in the neonate and the temperature may be subnormal instead of elevated. Any infant with failure to thrive, loss of vigor, poor feeding and irritability should be suspected of sepsis (13).

*Inflammatory bowel disease* can contribute to failure to thrive in several ways; there may be excess fecal loss, but there may also be anorexia and excess energy expenditure because of the indolent inflammatory process.

A similar wasting of energy and failure of weight gain can be seen in the *inflammatory arthritides* such as juvenile rheumatoid arthritis. *Malignancies* commonly present with weight loss and unexplained listlessness. There may be subtle evidences of widespread nutritional deficiency, such as anemia, osteopenia, and loss of subcutaneous tissue. Increased metabolism by the tumor may be merely additive to interference with food utilization by vital organs or anorexia in producing the failure to thrive.

Failure to thrive in *congenital cardiac disease* is multifactorial. It occurs in infants with congestive failure or cyanotic heart defects for which cellular hypoxia seems to be the common denominator. In addition, there is a reduction in food intake and a relative or absolute hypermetabolism. There is an increased metabolic requirement of the myocardium and respiratory muscles and increased formation of red blood cells for carrying oxygen. Hypoxia and acidosis, common in cyanotic heart disease, may also contribute to the failure to thrive (51).

*Hyperthyroidism* represents the prototype for failure to thrive due to hypermetabolism. In the neonatal period the hypermetabolic state is characterized by restlessness, irritability, tachypnea, tachycardia, and sometimes fever. The hypermetabolic state is fueled by a super-sensitivity to sympathetic stimulation, and even increased food intake fails to prevent emaciation. Untreated congenital hyperthyroidism may result in cardiac failure and death. In the older child, weight loss and restlessness or emotional lability may be the presenting complaints, and unless proptosis draws attention to the possibility of Graves' disease, the failure to thrive may become quite severe before the hyperthyroidism is suspected. Children with hyperthyroidism may have advanced skeletal maturation in addition to their weight loss. Control of the hypermetabolism produces a restoration of normal growth, although the advanced skeletal maturation is not reversible and ultimate height may be compromised. Insulin deficiency, in *diabetes mellitus,* leads to a catabolic state, producing rapid weight loss and inanition in addition to dehydration from the polyuria.

### End Organ Unresponsiveness

Failure to thrive, which may have its origin in end organ unresponsiveness, is the most varied and most nebulous of the causes of failure to thrive. It is sometimes difficult to demonstrate the defect of nutrient utilization so there may only be tacit assumption that there is interference with the usual metabolic processes of growth. As can be seen from Table 11-7, end organ unresponsiveness embraces causes as disparate as hypercalcemia, galactosemia, metabolic acidosis, and maternal cigarette smoking.

Failure to thrive in *chronic lung disease* is attributed to tissue anoxia, though infection, anorexia, increased metabolic needs of muscles of respiration, and acid–base disturbances may also contribute to end organ unresponsiveness and failure to thrive.

**Table 11-7. Failure to Thrive**
**End Organ Unresponsiveness**

Chronic lung disease (hypoxia)
Renal disease
   Chronic renal insufficiency (metabolic acidosis)
   Renal tubular acidosis
   Urinary tract anomalies
     Hydronephrosis
     Polycystic disease of the kidneys
Idiopathic hypercalcemia
Hepatic insufficiency
Bartter's syndrome (hypokalemic alkalosis)
Chronic anemia
Endocrine disorders
   Congenital hypothyroidism
   Congenital adrenal hyperplasia
   Diabetes insipidus
Storage diseases
   Lysosomal storage disease
   Mucopolysaccharidoses
   Mucolipidoses
Inborn errors of metabolism
   Galactosemia
   de Toni–Fanconi syndrome (cystinosis)
   Hypophosphatasia
   Fructose intolerance
   Homocystinuria
   Kinky hair disease
   Other inborn errors
Chondrodystophies—congenital
Chromosomal anomalies
Fetal environmental toxin syndromes
   Alcohol, smoking and drugs
Diencephalic syndrome

Children with *chronic renal failure* often fail to ingest adequate amounts of food (anorexia) or protein leading to a protein-calorie malnutrition (52). However, even with correction of dietary deficiencies, normal growth may not be achieved. Acidosis has a retarding effect on growth and appears to be the major cause of failure to thrive in renal tubular acidosis, although secondary imbalances in calcium and phosphorus metabolism lead to rickets as well. Somatomedin levels are low in renal failure, although plasma growth hormone levels are often high. The similarity of hormonal and metabolic changes to malnutrition has led to the suggestion that this represents a "deficit in cellular energy supply" (52). Glucocorticoids, often employed in management of renal disease, may contribute directly to failure to grow with their retarding effect on cartilage proliferation (53).

Abnormalities in metabolism of substrate or disturbances of electrolyte and acid–base balance seem to contribute to growth failure in hepatic insufficiency, storage diseases, hypercalcemia, Bartter's syndrome and inborn errors of metabolism. Tissue anoxia may contribute to growth failure in chronic anemia. In utero, insults from viral infections or from maternal ingestion of alcohol, drugs, or maternal cigarette smoking seem to affect fundamental growth regulating processes and render tissues thereafter incapable of normal growth. (The ultimate in end organ unresponsiveness?)

*Endocrine disorders* are a relatively infrequent cause of failure to thrive, although there are a few disturbances which result in characteristic patterns of growth failure. Congenital hypothyroidism is characterized by slow development and delayed growth, poor feeding, and at times slow weight gain. Congenital hypopituitarism is characterized by growth failure, microphallus, and hypoglycemia in infancy. Diabetes insipidus should be considered in an infant with dehydration, fever, and failure to thrive, although polydipsia or polyuria may not be readily evident in infancy. Salt-losing adrenogenital syndrome may present abruptly in the newborn period with an adrenal crisis, but may be preceded by several weeks of weight loss, vomiting, diarrhea, and failure to thrive. Immediate recognition and treatment are essential to prevent death from shock or electrolyte disturbances. Chronic adrenal insufficiency (Addison's disease), although rare in childhood, is characterized by anorexia, vomiting, diarrhea, intermittent fever, dehydration, and weight loss. A pheochromocytoma can also be the cause of profound weight loss (54).

The *diencephalic syndrome* is characterized by poor weight gain and loss of subcutaneous fat but normal or accelerated linear growth (55). Most cases of the diencephalic syndrome are due to tumors in the floor of the third ventricle (56). Failure to thrive is usually evident within the first year of life, leading to extreme emaciation. Despite the emaciated appearance, most infants have a pleasant or euphoric temperament. The poor weight gain cannot be explained simply on the basis of inadequate caloric intake. Tumors are generally inoperable, but radiotherapy may palliate symptoms and some children survive for several years (57).

## Nonorganic Failure to Thrive

Adequate nutrition, especially for the infant, requires a healthy interaction between mother and child. The development of abnormal maternal–child interaction may lead to "nonorganic" failure to thrive. This form of failure to thrive may be seen in a variety of psychosocial situations ranging from improper feeding techniques to physical and psychological abuse (See Table 11-8). Environmental or nonorganic failure to thrive may be

### Table 11-8. Nonorganic Failure
### to Thrive

Abnormal maternal–child interaction
   Inadequate mother–child bonding
   Improper feeding techniques
   Inadequate mothering
Psychosocial deprivation
   Maternal deprivation
   Emotional deprivation
   Environmental deprivation
Child abuse
   Physical
   Psychological

recognized by the following criteria: (a) the child has a low weight which improves noticeably with appropriate nurturing; (b) there is no evidence of systemic disease or an organic cause for the failure to thrive; (c) developmental retardation improves with appropriate stimulation and feeding; (d) signs of social or intellectual deprivation improve with better nurturing in a new environment; (e) the family environment shows signs of psychosocial disruption (58).

"Bonding" between mother and child appears to be a basic need for normal growth and development of the child. Observations among primate infants (monkeys) have shown the necessity for a "mother" to provide contact-comfort and to promote early growth and development (59) and normal behavior in adolescence (60). If the baby is placed with the mother even for a short time immediately after birth, "bonding" and subsequent growth and development are noticeably improved. Failure to develop maternal–infant bonding leads to a variety of deficiencies in growth and personality development.

The adverse effect of abnormal maternal–child interaction on growth and nutrition represents the most common cause of failure to thrive with the exception of worldwide protein-calorie malnutrition (12). In the first decade of this century, Chapin described growth failure in hospitalized children, which he called the "cachexia of hospitalism"; he attributed it to poor physical conditions within the hospital and lack of nurturing (61). The role of lack of nurturing in producing failure to thrive in institutionalized infants and children, was emphasized by Renee Spitz, who followed the progress of infants raised in a foundling home compared to infants raised by their mothers in prison and to infants raised in their own homes. Children raised in the foundling home had a higher mortality rate, deficient neurologic and social achievement, and failed to develop warm, loving personalities (62). Failure to thrive from lack of "nurturing" (i.e., maternal deprivation) is still with us, although the scene has changed from the institution or hospital to the home. The social and emotional environment of the child in the home must now be thoroughly investigated to identify this common source of failure to thrive.

Improper feeding technique or inadequate mothering represents the simplest *abnormal maternal–child interaction.* Fussy eaters may spit up, vomit, turn away from the feeding, or fall asleep during feedings. Many have loose, foul-smelling stools, abdominal distention, and appear sick and pale or simply "will not grow" (6). The mother may not understand simple fundamentals in infant feeding and may be offering too much or too little, through a nipple with holes too large or too small, of a formula which is too rich or too poor. The more fussy and fretful the baby, the less likely the distraught, undertaught mother will be able to improve the maternal–child interaction.

Ineffective maternal behavior may be subtle. Failure to thrive with severe congenital disorders or acquired diseases may be due, in part, to a breakdown of mothering caused by the mother's attitudes toward the defective child. Barbero describes a child with a small congenital heart defect who failed to thrive until mother became convinced that the child was not defective and going to die (58). Similar problems have been seen with infants with tracheoesophageal fistula and gastrostomy, (63) mental retardation, and other disorders (60).

*Psychosocial deprivation* represents a more serious disruption of the maternal–child bond and has been variously termed *maternal deprivation, emotional deprivation, or environmental deprivation.* All of the terms imply a gross disturbance of the normal maternal–child interaction, resulting in disordered growth and development. The deprivation may include "withholding of calories, protein, or other essential nutritional elements, . . . harsh physical environment, trauma, social isolation and disruption of physical and emotional bonds between infant and mother" (60). Environmental situations contributing to psychosocial deprivation include poor child-rearing practices, separation experiences, social isolation, institutional life style, neglect or cruelty, and socioeconomic deprivation (64).

Original observations of "maternal deprivation" were made in infants in foundling homes exposed to the emotionally sterile atmosphere of the "caretaker". The institutionalized infant is described as listless, apathetic, and depressed with failure to thrive despite access to adequate food, and subject to frequent stools, persistent respiratory infections, and unexplained fevers, all of which disappear upon the return of the infant to home and mother (65). This need for love and attention, in addition to adequate food, has led some observers to nod in affirmation to the proverbial advice: "Better is a dinner of herbs where love is than a stalled ox and hatred therewith" (Proverbs Ch. XV: 17). Spitz and Wolff describe the foundling home infant as dejected, withdrawn, not responding to the environment, slow in movement, and stuperous; exhibiting anorexia, weight loss, insomnia, and frequent respiratory infections. Without intervention, the children assumed a posture of "frozen rigidity" and "cachexia" and death were frequent (66). The "institutional syndrome" is characterized by head-rolling, stereotyped behavior, and refusal to show recognition of surrounding objects or persons, considered to be a form of sensory deprivation (67). Lack of warm, affectionate relationships in infancy or childhood may result in aggressive, negativistic behavior with eneuresis and speech defects (68) or a "psychopathic personality" with superficial emotional reponses, asocial behavior, and limited capacity for affective relations (69, 70). Intelligence also appears to be profoundly affected by psychosocial deprivation, especially if it occurs in early infancy. Perhaps the most eloquent description of environmental failure to thrive is attributed to a Dr. Barnardo: "a glazed stupor, a vacant stare, a sullen apathetic fear and misery that goes to the heart. A little lamp with the light gone out" (71).

In children suffering from psychosocial deprivation there may be failure to provide adequate calories, protein or other essential nurients, deliberate or otherwise. Reduced appetite or refusal to feed may also contribute to inadequate nutrition. Assimilation of nutrients may be affected by changes in intestinal motility or rate of absorption of nutrients. Several observers have noted pituitary deficiencies in psychosocial deprivation and suggested that transient or reversible pituitary deficiency may be a major cause of growth failure in children with psychosocial deprivation (72–74). Release of hGH, FSH, LH, TSH, and ACTH are all controlled by hypothalamic factors which appear to be deficient in many subjects with psychosocial deprivation (and anorexia nervosa). Frasier and Rallison describe a 6-year-old girl with growth hormone deficiency who failed to respond to growth hormone therapy. When her home environment was discovered to be emotionally injurious and her mother admitted to rejecting behavior, she was sent to live with an aunt. Soon after the change in environment, she began to grow at an accelerated rate and growth hormone levels were restored to normal (75). Perhaps the lack of response to administered growth hormone represents a lack of somatomedin production or activity brought on in some as yet undefined way by the psychosocial deprivation, similar to that seen with malnutrition (76).

The most severe form of nonorganic failure to thrive is displayed in forms of *child abuse* in which the child is viewed by the parents as "bad" and physically or emotionally segregated within the family. In this extreme form of psychosocial deprivation the child is frequently subjected to physical abuse and separated from any intercourse with others. The children may be deliberately starved (77) leading to bizarre eating habits including scavenging or binge eating and vomiting. Failure to grow can be extreme, as can intellectual retardation and language communication, but the behavior pattern may reflect the need to survive. The child becomes wary and withdrawn but resourceful in obtaining food rather than apathetic. Restoration of such abused children to a warm accepting atmosphere and adequate nutrition may result in some catch-up growth, but ultimate height attainment is likely to be impaired. Similarly, intellectual status may improve, but ultimate intellectual attainment is limited and bizarre behavior patterns may persist (78).

## Assessment of Failure to Thrive

The first step in the assessment of a child with suspected failure to thrive should be the accurate reconstruction of recent and remote growth patterns so that it can be determined whether the growth is normal or sufficiently aberrant to warrant a consideration of failure to thrive.

### Clues from History and Physical Exam

A careful history and physical examination should identify the most likely cause of the failure to thrive, following the scheme outlined in the beginning of this section. One should determine if adequate calories are offered or refused, if there is loss attributed to vomiting or excess fecal loss, evidence of excess energy requirements or end organ unresponsiveness, or if there is evidence of nonorganic failure to thrive.

Since in most recent series, nonorganic failure to thrive is the most common cause of failure to thrive, it is prudent to seek historical or physical evidence of abnormal maternal–child interaction as an affirmative diagnosis, rather than relegating it to a diagnosis of exclusion (12). Children with nonorganic failure to thrive tend to be the youngest in the family, born within 18 months of the next oldest sibling and manifest growth failure before their first birthday. They often come from single parent, low income homes, and present with vomiting and diarrhea (12). Nonorganic failure to thrive has usually been characterized by a rapid reversal of weight loss during a visit to the hospital or removal of the child from the malignant environment (58), but Berwick points out that "severely deprived infants may take several weeks to establish healthy feeding patterns even in a quiet and consistent hospital environment and . . . (many) infants with nonorganic failure to thrive have either lost weight or remained unchanged in hospitalizations as long as two weeks" (12).

During the taking of a history in a child with failure to thrive, particular attention should be paid to parental strengths and weaknesses. Nonorganic failure to thrive represents a continuum of interactional disorders and may concern a severely disturbed or ill child who taxes even a competent parent or a mentally ill parent unable to respond to the needs of even an undemanding baby (79). Mothers of infants who fail to thrive tend to be depressed, angry, and lack self-esteem (80). Mothers of infants with maternal deprivation may have had a disturbed early childhood, exhibit poor performance in usual daily activities, have limited capacity for abstract thinking, and display evidence of psychopathology or depression (81).

Berkowitz and Sklaren emphasize the need to carefully evaluate the family profile of the infant with failure to thrive. A child's needs may be neglected if mother is severely depressed or if the home environment is totally inadequate. The most threatening home environment is the one in which the nurturing of the child is inadequate because of parental anger or hostility. Children in this latter situation are often subject to emotional and physical abuse; their failure to thrive will only be corrected by aggressive intervention (82).

## Help from the Laboratory

The search for a physical basis of failure to thrive should be based on the clues provided by the history and physical examination. A careful neurological examination with transillumination of the skull in infants should be part of the physical evaluation. An assessment of development should be performed by means of a test such as the Denver Developmental Screening Test (DDST) (83). A few laboratory tests which reflect general health may be useful; these may include CBC, urinalysis, electrolytes, BUN or creatinine, stool examination for reducing substances and fat, urine culture, chest x-ray, and bone-age estimate. In addition, if indicated by the history or physical examination, electrocardiogram, gastrointestinal x-ray series, sweat test, IVP or VCUG, and thyroid function tests ($T_4$, $T_3$ resin uptake, TSH) may be useful (83). In the absence of strongly suggestive evidence from history and physical examination, there is little likelihood that extensive laboratory examination will prove fruitful (84).

After the initial laboratory tests, it is informative in most cases to cease invasive tests and allow a period of adjustment to the hospital. During this time a feeding trial and calorie count may be carried out to discover changes in feeding patterns in a new environment. During this time the psychodynamics of the home environment can be more thoroughly explored based on clues obtained from the history. It is important both during the diagnostic period and later, during the treatment of the failure to thrive, that the parents be involved in all steps and that all appropriate medical–social personnel be involved from the beginning (social worker, developmental specialist, nutritionist, etc.). Much valuable treatment can actually be started during the diagnostic evaluation, especially during the "nontesting" observation period (12).

## Treatment of Failure to Thrive

The treatment of failure to thrive must fit the diagnosis, and the list of potential causes is very long. Failure to thrive may involve any organ system—the correction of which may require medication, surgery, or adaptation to the defect. The treatment of nonorganic failure to thrive may require the most skill and understanding. Child and parent should be treated as a unit to help mother develop nurturing skills or resolve her interaction problems (11). Treatment often requires services of physician, nurse, psychiatrist, social worker, and nutritionist. The climate of care should be conducive to natural parent–child interaction, and the therapeutic team should avoid expressing hostility toward the parents who may already suffer from low self-esteem (17).

Goldbloom emphasizes the role of insufficient caloric intake in the pathogenesis of failure to thrive and the need to provide extra calories to allow catch-up growth (84). After initial measurement of caloric intake, Goldbloom recommends diagnostic provision of a daily intake of 50% greater than the usual requirement for growth of a child of same height, together with a program of environmental stimulation and affection (84). The progress of the child is checked daily through charted weight, 24-hour caloric intake, calculated kcal per kg of ideal weight, and weight chart for displaying short-term gain (84).

Regular follow-up by concerned observers appears helpful, although in some instances the total environment of the child must be changed, at least temporarily. Every effort should be made through a "team" of providers to enable the mother and child to improve their interaction and reestablish the nurturing capacities of the mother. For most children with failure to thrive in infancy and early childhood, the outlook for physical recovery is good, provided aggressive feeding and stimulation are carried out; the outlook for intellectual or behavior recovery is less certain (84).

## OBESITY

Fat is a normal body constituent. When excessive amounts of fat are deposited within the adipose organ we say the individual is *obese*. The definition of "excessive" fat is arbitrary, however, because we are dealing with an accumulation of a "normal" tissue. A child is said to be obese if body weight exceeds "ideal" weight (adjusted for age, sex, height and body build) by 20% (85–87), or if skin fold thickness exceeds the 90th percentile adjusted for age and sex (85, 87) (Appendix Tables A-4, A-6). For practical purposes, Dietz suggests that visual assessment is clinically satisfactory (87). Most studies suggest that there is a high likelihood that a child who becomes obese will remain obese throughout childhood and adolescence (85, 88, 89). Approximately 80% of obese adolescents become obese adults; obesity of later onset or increasing severity stands a higher risk of persistence (87).

Although a number of health problems have been cited to occur more readily in obese individuals to shorten the lifespan and increase morbidity from illness (hypertension, diabetes, etc.), only a few have actually stood the test of time and skeptical review. Life insurance mortality statistics show that life expectancy is increased in individuals lighter than average, but significant morbidity and mortality from obesity are difficult to demonstrate until the individual is more than 20% overweight (90).

For children, obesity represents primarily a psychologic or social handicap. "The obese child often has a poor body image, a sense of failure, and a passive approach to life situations" (85). The lot of fat children, as described by Bruch, is a sad one. "They are bashful and ashamed of their shapeless figures yet unable to conceal them. Wherever they go they attract attention because they look ungainly, awkward and slow. . . . Obesity is a serious handicap in the social life of a child, even more so of a teenager. It interferes with the child's ability to mix freely with others and enjoy their activities and interests. . . . They become the laughing stock of their peers. . . . Quite often they are passive and fearful, incapable of defending themselves against their tormentors" (91).

## Factors Predisposing Toward Obesity

From a thermodynamic viewpoint, fat accumulation (obesity) takes place if caloric input is increased, caloric utilization is reduced, or if calories ingested are somehow more efficiently utilized. Studies of concordance in monozygotic versus dizygotic twins, of twins reared in different environments, and of adopted and natural children raised in the same family, tend to support genetic factors as providing the basis for obesity in children (92, 93), but observations are equally persuasive in support of environment influences (94, 95) (Figure 11-3).

Commonly, fat accumulation is attributed to malfunction of the endocrine "glands"; however, attempts to link obesity to glandular dysfunction have never produced unequivocal affirmation of the role of endocrine malfunction in the genesis of obesity. There are a number of metabolic aberrations which tend to perpetuate the obesity. Excess insulin, decreased human growth hormone, and increased adrenal hormones can contribute to obesity; but except for Cushing's syndrome, hormonal aberrations appear to be secondary to obesity rather than causative (96, 97). In considering the role of metabolic efficiency of obese subjects, the basal metabolic rate and oxygen consumption of obese subjects are comparable to those in normal subjects and obese subjects mobilize fat normally (87, 98). Diet induced thermogenesis (DIT) in brown adipose tissue represents a mechanism of "wasting" energy not needed for activity or storage in mice (99). Differences in diet-induced thermogenesis (or brown adipose tissue) could account for differences in weight gain among individuals with essentially identical intake of calories. However, neither reduced metabolic rate nor a decrease in thermogenic response to carbohydrate or overfeeding has been convincingly demonstrated in obese humans (87).

The hypothalamus may act as a "ponderostat"—a neurologic mechanism capable of detecting whether the organism is at its "set-point" for weight (100). Implicit in this suggestion is the assumption that there may be different set-points for different individuals; for an obese individual a high "ponderostat" setting (obese state) may be the natural state (101). The existence of a ponderostat has not been proved, however, the role which the central nervous system plays in the regulation of food intake behavior must be considered seriously (100).

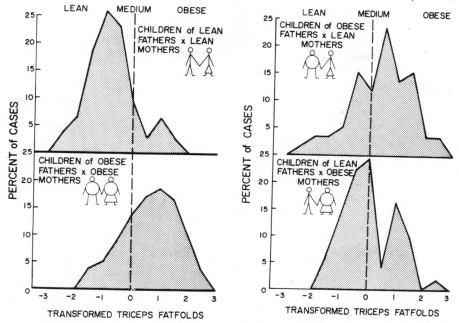

**Figure 11-3.**   Fat fold histograms of the children of lean parents (upper left panel) and obese parents (lower left panel), showing segregation in the offspring along the lines of parental fatness. In the right panels comparison of children of obese fathers and lean mothers (above) and obese mothers and lean fathers (below) showing that an obese father seems to have more influence on the level of fatness of his progeny than the fat mother. (Reproduced by permission from Garn SM, Clark DC: Trends in fatness and the origins of obesity. Report from ad hoc committee to review the 10-state nutrition survey. *Pediatrics* **57:**443, 1976, copyright American Academy of Pediatrics 1976.)

Behavioral and social factors may contribute to obesity in several ways (87). Poor children receive fewer calories and are generally thinner. In women, an inverse relationship between obesity and socioeconomic status is seen (102). Eating may be a means to show affection or to get attention. There may even be anxiety in some mothers to prevent brain damage in infants by assuring adequate nutrition (85). The obese individual tends to eat more food and more rapidly at mealtime. His eating pattern is similar to that of the individual who is constantly hungry. In a series of elegant behavioral experiments, Schachter showed that the eating behavior of nonobese subjects was ruled by physiologic cues and of obese subjects by external cues such as food availability, fear, taste, sight of others eating, and so on, in determining the amount of food eaten (103).

Obesity can occur only when calories consumed are greater than calories expended, but the relative importance of increased food intake and

### Table 11-9. Causes of Obesity in Childhood

| | |
|---|---|
| Idiopathic (exogenous) obesity | Common |
| Hormonal disturbances | Rare |
|   Hypothyroidism | |
|   Cushing's syndrome | |
|   Hyperinsulinism | |
|   Hypopituitarism (hypothalamic) | |
|   Hypogonadism | |
|   Estrogen therapy | |
| Malformation syndromes | Rare |
|   Prader–Labhart–Willi syndrome | |
|   Lawrence–Moon–Biedl | |
|   Fröhlich's adiposogenital syndrome | |
|   Albright hereditary osteodystrophy | |
|   Alstrom's syndrome | |

Reproduced by permission after Barnes HV, Berger R: An approach to the obese adolescent. *Med Clin North Am* **59**:1507, 1975.

decreased physical activity in the development of obesity is still hotly debated (85). Most studies of activity levels in obese children or adults do affirm a reduced activity level (104, 105), but whether this represents the cause of the obesity or its perpetuation is uncertain. Nonobese individuals tend to outwalk obese subjects (104), and obese girls are less active than their nonobese counterparts when engaged in sports (105). It is, however, common experience to find that obese individuals actually eat less than nonobese counterparts and the reduced activity may actually serve only to perpetuate the obese state.

### Differential Considerations of Obesity

Over 95% of obesity in childhood or adolescence represents *idiopathic or exogenous obesity* (Table 11-9). Children with moderate to severe idiopathic (exogenous) obesity generally have a family history of obesity and have been overweight from childhood, often from the pre school years (106). General health is good, although obese adolescents are prone to slipped capital femoral epiphyses. As a rule the exogenously obese child tends to be taller and matures faster than average (107). Pubertal development may be accelerated, but final height achieved is within the height predicted by the mid-parent height (106). This pattern of growth is in sharp contrast to that seen in Cushing's syndrome, hypothyroidism, and malformation syndromes in which the children tend to be short and weak with delayed skeletal maturation and delayed puberty.

Hormonal disturbances are frequently invoked as a cause of obesity, but, in fact, they represent a rare cause of obesity. Accumulation of myxedematous fluid in *hypothyroidism* can give the impression of obesity.

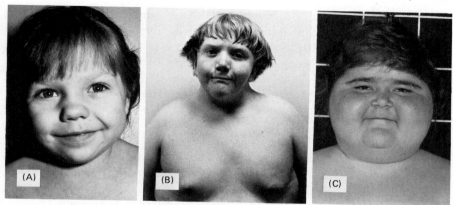

**Figure 11-4.**   Facial appearance of children with (A) hypothyroidism, (B) exogenous obesity, and (C) Cushing's syndrome. In hypothyroidism (A) there is puffiness of the face (and eyes) and a younger than stated age appearance (child in figure is 10 years of age). In Cushing's syndrome (C), the face and neck are full and rounded (moon shaped) with a deep flush on the cheeks and often associated with acne and hirsutism.

However, myxedematous facial features, delayed growth, short stature, sluggish activity, and dry skin should serve to distinguish the hypothyroid child or adolescent from the child with idiopathic (exogenous) obesity (Figure 11-4). Presentation of hypothyroidism may at times be subtle and search for hypothyroidism may be justified in any *short* obese individual. Children with *Cushing's syndrome*, display a striking facial and truncal obesity which tends to spare the extremities (Figure 11-4). Linear growth is suppressed by excess glucocorticoid, and therefore, such children suffer from growth retardation and delay in skeletal maturation; musculature becomes wasted and they become weak, especially in proximal girdle muscles. This contrasts to the child with exogenous obesity who retains normal strength and displays an accelerated growth pattern. Moderate generalized obesity may be found in children with *hyperinsulinism* secondary to an insulin-producing tumor. Many *hypopituitary* (growth hormone deficient) subjects become modestly obese, particularly in the truncal or pectoral region. A similar type of obesity has been described for *hypogonadal* adolescents (86).

The *malformation syndromes* associated with obesity are rare and may be recognized by characteristics of the dysmorphism. Short stature and mental retardation are usually present, providing a distinction from idiopathic or exogenous obesity. Children with *Prader–Labhart–Willi syndrome* become obese in infancy or early childhood. They are often unable to control appetite and vigorously and persistently pursue food to produce progressive obesity. Following a central nervous system infection, tumor or degeneration, a child may rarely become obese, which together with short stature and hypogonadotropic hypogonadism (hypogenitalism) may lead to consideration of *Fröhlich's* syndrome which is now generally considered to be an extreme presentation of the obesity of hypopituitarism (108). Moderate obesity may be a feature of *Albright's hereditary osteodystrophy*, characterized by short stature, rounded facies, mental deficiency, extraskeletal calcification, and hypocalcemia (86).

## Management of Obesity

The management of obesity as a growth aberration can be derived from recent reviews (85–87, 109, 110). We will sketch only the essentials of management here. Although in an occasional subject, correction of the hypothyroid state or treatment of Cushing's syndrome may require specific medical or surgical intervention, the mainstay of nearly all treatment of obesity is a shift in energy balance which requires a decrease in caloric intake, an increase in energy expenditure, or both. Caloric restriction to produce weight *loss* should not be used for children; statural growth and CNS development could be impaired by a prolonged catabolic state (88).

A program of weight containment for the individual with obesity should include nutritional education of the family and individual, restriction of calories consumed, modification of eating behavior, and increase in physical activity (111). This generally means a change in lifestyle for both the individual and family, and must be approached thoughtfully and decisively. A family-based approach to therapy offers the greatest likelihood of achieving compliance (87). Much encouragement will be required for acceptance of the altered lifestyle, but no permanent effect can be achieved without such commitment. In its simplest form, behavior modification during treatment of the obese child consists of setting realistic goals, practical nutritional education, and persistent encouragement with positive reinforcement of progress, however slight (112). In many instances, optimistic and realistic encouragement is sufficient to help the family to healthier attitudes and improved eating habits (113).

We avoid drug therapy of obesity in children (114, 115), although we are aware of its occasional value as an adjunct therapy. We are unconvinced of the efficacy or practicality of thyroid, growth hormone, or hCG in the treatment of most obesity in children (115, 116). Most of the weight lost with thyroxine is lean body mass (117) and the long term success in maintaining weight loss is essentially nil. Unless thyroid deficiency is demonstrable in the obese child, thyroid hormone has no place in the therapy of obesity. Collip claims that caloric restriction may "unmask" subclinical hypothyroidism in obese children, reflected in a brisk rise of TSH to >20 $\mu$U/mL after TRH in youngsters who fail to lose weight on adequate caloric restriction. He reports an enhanced weight loss when such children are given 25 $\mu$g of $T_3$ (Cytomel) daily, proposing that the "acquired" hypothyroidism is a result of reduced peripheral conversion of $T_4$ to $T_3$ (118).

The use of severe caloric restriction (total fast or ketogenic diet) or of surgical procedures such as bowel bypass or stomach plication have very little place in the treatment of obesity in children and should be considered only if the obesity is *progressive* and *intractable* or if the obesity is interfering substantially with physical health (87, 88). Given the problems of indiscriminate catabolism with total fasting, there seems to be little justification for this form of therapy in a growing subject (119).

For most children, realistic goals of weight control can be satisfied by teaching the child appropriate nutrition habits and improving habits of physical activity. The child's weight gain should be limited to expected increase in lean body mass (88). In this way the effects on total body growth are minimal and not destructive and normal growth of the child will be encouraged.

## REFERENCES

1. Weaver DS, Owen GM: Nutrition and short stature. *Postgrad Med* **62**(Dec):93, 1977.
2. Tanner JM: Growth as a monitor of nutritional status. *Proc Nutr Soc* **35**:315, 1976.
3. Garn SM, Clark DC (Ad Hoc Committee to review Ten State Nutrition Survey): Nutrition, growth, development, and maturation: Findings from the Ten State Nutrition Survey of 1968–1970. *Pediatrics* **56**:306–319, 1975.
4. Tanner, JM: *Fetus into Man: Physical Growth from Conception to Maturity.* Cambridge, Harvard University Press, 1978, pp 167–205.
5. Levine MI: Failure to thrive: Introduction. *Pediatr Ann* **7**(November):8/737, 1978.
6. English PC: Failure to thrive without organic reason. *Pediatr Ann* **7**(November):83/774, November, 1978.
7. Sills RH: Failure to thrive: The role of clinical and laboratory evaluation. *Am J Dis Child* **132**:967, 1978.
8. Hannaway PJ: Failure to thrive: A study of 100 infants and children. *Clin Pediatr* **9**:96, 1970.
9. Riley RL, Landwirth J, Kaplan SA, et al: Failure to thrive: An analysis of 83 cases. *California Med* **108**:32, 1968.
10. Shaheen E, Alexander D, Truskowsky M, et al: Failure to thrive: A retrospective profile. *Clin Pediatr* **7**:255, 1968.
11. Ambuel JP, Harris B: Failure to thrive. *Ohio State Med J* **59**:997, 1963.
12. Berwick DM: Nonorganic failure to thrive. *Pediatrics in Review* **1**(March):265, 1980.
13. Green M: Why some infants fail to thrive: A problem with serious implications. *J Indiana State Medical Assoc* **71**(December):1129–1132, 1978.
14. Barness L: Protein malnutrition, in Vaughan VC, McKay RJ, Behman RE (eds). *Nelson's Textbook of Pediatrics*, ed 11, Philadelphia, WB Saunders Co, 1979, pp 212–215.
15. Gardner LI: Endocrine aspects of under-nutrition: Protein-calorie malnutrition, psychosocial deprivation, and anorexia nervosa, in Gardner LI (ed). *Endocrine and Genetic Diseases of Childhood and Adolescence*, ed 2. Philadelphia, WB Saunders Co, 1975, pp 1174–1180.
16. Whitten CF, Pettit MG, Fischoff J: Evidence that growth failure from maternal deprivation is secondary to under-eating. *JAMA* **209**:1675, 1969.

17. Lavy U, Bauer CH: Pathophysiology of failure to thrive in gastrointestinal disorders. *Pediatr Ann* **7**(November):20/743, 1978.

18. Osborn LM, Metcalf T: Failure to thrive secondary to upper respiratory tract obstruction and corpulmonale. *J Fam Prac* **15**:71, 1982.

19. Vest M, Talbot NB, Crawford JD: Hypocaloric dwarfism and hydronephrosis in diabetes insipidus. *Am J Dis Child* **105**:175, 1963.

20. *Diagnostic and Statistical Manual for Mental Disorders*, ed 3 (DSM III). Washington, D.C., American Psychiatric Association, 1980, p 69.

21. Irwin M: Diagnosis of anorexia nervosa in children and the validity of DSM-III. *Am J Psychiatry* **138**:1382, 1981.

22. Chipman JJ, Hogan RD, Edlin JC, et al: Excessive weight loss in the athletic adolescent: A diagnostic dilemma. *J Adol Health Care* **3**:247, 1983.

23. Pugliese MT, Lifshitz F, Grad G, et al: Fear of obesity. A cause of short stature and delayed puberty. *N Engl J Med* **309**:513, 1983.

24. Lucas AR: Undernutrition and growth. *N Engl J Med* **309**:550, 1983.

25. Root AW, Powers PS: Anorexia nervosa presenting as growth retardation in adolescents. *J Adol Health Care* **4**:25, 1983.

26. Daughaday WH, ed, *Endocrine Control of Growth*. New York, Elsevier Press, 1981, pp 1–24.

27. Gold MS, Pottash AC, Martin D, et al: The 24–hour LH test in the diagnosis and assessment of response to treatment of patients with anorexia nervosa. *Intl J Psych Med* **11**:245, 1981–82.

28. Maloney ML, Klykylo WM: An overview of anorexia nervosa, bulimia and obesity in children and adolescents. *J Am Acad Child Psych* **22**(2):99, 1983.

29. Bruch H: Anorexia nervosa: Therapy and theory. *Am J Psych* **139**:1531, 1983.

30. Crisp AH: Therapeutic outcome in anorexia nervosa. *Can J Psych* **26**:232, 1981.

31. Herbst JJ: Gastroesophageal reflux (chalasia), in Vaughan VC, McKay RJ, Behrman RE (eds), *Nelson's Textbook of Pediatrics*, ed 11. Philadelphia, WB Saunders Co, 1979, pp 1044–1048.

32. Ament ME: Malabsorption syndrome, in Vaughan VC, McKay RJ, Behrman RE (eds), *Nelson's Textbook of Pediatrics*, ed 11. Philadelphia, WB Saunders Co, 1979, pp 1080–1090.

33. Schwachman H, Diamond LK, Oski FA, et al: The syndrome of pancreatic insufficiency and bone marrow dysfunction. *J Pediatr* **65**:645, 1964.

34. Lebenthal E, Branski D: Childhood celiac disease—A reappraisal. *J Pediatr* **98**:681, 1981.

35. Anderson CM, Gracey M, Burke V: Celiac disease—Some still controversial aspects. *Arch Dis Child* **47**:292, 1972.

36. Young WF, Pringle EM: 110 children with celiac disease—1950–1969. *Arch Dis Child* **46**:421, 1971.

37. Hamilton JR, McNeill LK: Celiac disease—Duration of therapy. *J Pediatr* **81**:885, 1972.

38. Hamilton JR: Gastrointestinal allergy caused by food, in Vaughan VC, McKay RJ, Behrman RE (eds), *Nelson's Textbook of Pediatrics*, ed 11. Philadelphia, WB Saunders Co, 1979, pp 1091–1092.

39. Lebenthal E: Cow's milk protein allergy. *Ped Clin North Am* **22**:827, 1975.

40. Ament ME: Crohn disease (regional enteritis), in Vaughan VC, McKay RJ, Behrman RE (eds), *Nelson's Textbook of Pediatrics*, ed 11. Philadelphia, WB Saunders Co, 1979, pp 1095–1098.

41. McCaffery JD, Naskr K, Lawrence AM, et al: Severe growth retardation in children with inflammatory bowel disease. *Pediatrics* **45**:386, 1970.

42. Doyle PH, McKay AJ, Browne MK: Failure to thrive in adolescence due to inflammatory bowel disease. *Practioner* **222**:253–259, 1979.

43. Sobel EH, Silverman FN, Lee AN: Growth failure as the presenting feature in regional enteritis. *Am J Dis Child* **103**:569, 1962.

44. Beeken WL, Busch HJ, Sylvester DL: Intestinal protein loss in Crohn disease. *Gastroenterology* **62**:207, 1972.

45. Grand RJ, Homer DH: Approaches to inflammatory bowel disease in childhood and adolescence. *Pediatr Clin North Am* **22**:835, 1975.

46. Berger M, Gribetz D, Korelitz B: Growth retardation in children with ulcerative colitis: The effect of medical and surgical therapy. *Pediatrics* **55**:459, 1975.

47. Ament ME: Inflammatory disease of the colon. *J Pediatr* **86**:322, 1975.

48. Shandling B: Congenital megacolon (Hirschsprung disease), in Vaughan VC, McKay RJ, Behrman RE (eds), *Nelson's Textbook of Pediatrics*, ed 11. Philadelphia, WB Saunders Co, 1979, pp 1057–1060.

49. Avery GB, Villaviciencio O, Lilley JR, et al: Intractable diarrhea in early infancy. *Pediatrics* **41**:712 1968.

50. Greene HL, McCabe DR, Merenstein GB: Protracted diarrhea and malnutrition in infancy: Changes in intestinal morphology and disaccharidase activities during treatment with total intravenous nutrition or oral elemental diet. *J Pediatr* **87**:695, 1975.

51. Ehlers KH: Growth failure in association with congenital heart disease. *Pediatr Ann* **7**(November):35/750, 1978.

52. Holliday MA, Chantler C: Metabolic and nutritional factors in children with renal insufficiency. *Kidney Int* **14**:306, 1978.

53. Friedman J, Lewy JE: Failure to thrive associated with renal disease. *Pediatr Ann* **7**(November):73/767, 1978.

54. Abrams CAL: Endocrinologic aspects of failure to thrive. *Pediatr Ann* **7**(November):58/760, 1978.

55. Fishman MA, Peake GT: Paradoxical growth in a patient with diencephalic syndrome. *Pediatrics* **45**:973, 1970.

56. Addy DP, Hudson FP: Diencephalic syndrome of infantile emaciation. *Arch Dis Child* **47**:338, 1972.

57. Smith DW: Diencephalic syndrome of infantile emaciation, in *Growth and Its Disorders*. Philadelphia, WB Saunders Co, 1977, p 111.

58. Barbero GJ, Shaheen E: Environmental failure to thrive: A clinical view. *J Pediatr* **71**:639, 1967.

59. Harlow HF, Zimmerman R: Affectional responses in the infant monkey. *Science* **130**:421, 1959.

60. Patton RT, Gardner LI: Deprivation dwarfism (psychosocial deprivation): Disordered family environment as cause of so-called idiopathic hypopituitarism, in Gardner LI (ed), *Endocrine and Genetic Diseases of Childhood and Adolescence*, ed 2. Philadelphia, WB Saunders Co, 1975, pp 85–98.

61. Chapin HD: A plan of dealing with atrophic infants and children. *Arch Pediatr* **25**:491, 1908.

62. Spitz R: Hospitalism: A follow-up report. *Psychoanal Study Child* **2**:113–117, 1946.

63. Engel GL, Reichsman F: Spontaneous and experimentally-induced depressions in an infant with a gastric fistula—A contribution to the problem of depression. *J Am Psychoanal Assoc* **4**:428, 1956.

64. Clarke ADB, Clarke AM: Some recent advances in the study of early deprivation. *J Child Psychol Psychiatry* **1**:26, 1960.

65. Bakwin H: Emotional deprivation in infants. *J Pediatr* **35:**512, 1949.

66. Spitz RA, Wolff K: Anaclitic depression. *Psychoanal Study Child* **2:**313, 1946.

67. Gesell A, Amatruda T: *Developmental Diagnosis.* New York, Paul B Hoeber Inc, 1941.

68. Lowrey LG: Personality distortion and early institutional care. *Am J Orthopsychiatry* **10:**576, 1940.

69. Bowlby J: The nature of a child's ties to his mother. *Int J Psychoanal* **39:**350, 1958.

70. Bowlby J: *Attachment.* New York, Basic Books, 1969.

71. Williams AE: *Barnardo of Stepney,* London, Allen and Unwin, 1943, quoted by J Goodall, *Proceed Nutr Soc* **38:**17, 1979.

72. Powell GF, Brasel JA, Blizzard RM: Emotional deprivation and growth retardation simulating idiopathic hypopituitarism, Part 1. *N Engl J Med* **276:**1271, 1967.

73. Powell GF, Brasel JA, Raiti S, et al: Emotional deprivation and growth retardation simulating idiopathic hypopituitarism, Part 2. *N Engl J Med* **276:**1279, 1967.

74. Thompson RG, Parra A, Schultz RB, et al: Endocrine evaluation in psychosocial dwarfism. *Clin Res* **17:**592, 1969.

75. Frasier SD, Rallison ML: Growth retardation and emotional deprivation: Relative resistance to treatment with human growth hormone. *J Pediatr* **80:**603, 1972.

76. Underwood LE, D'Ercole AJ, Van Wyk JJ: Somatomedin-C and the assessment of growth. *Ped Clin North Am* **27:**771, 1980.

77. Krieger I: Food restriction as a form of child abuse in ten cases of psychosocial deprivation dwarfism. *Clin Pediatr* **13:**127, 1974.

78. Money, J: The syndrome of abuse dwarfism (psychosocial dwarfism or reversible hyposomatotropism. *Am J Dis Child* **131:**508, 1977.

79. Pollitt E, Eichler A: Behavioral disturbances among failure to thrive children. *Am J Dis Child* **130:**24, 1976.

80. Barbero GJ, Morris MG, Redford M: The neglected, battered child syndrome: Role reversal in parents malidentification of mother–baby–father relationships expressed in infant failure to thrive. New York, Child Welfare League of America, 1963.

81. Fischoff J, Whitten C, Pettit M: A psychiatric study of mothers of infants with growth failure secondary to maternal deprivation. *J Pediatr* **79:**209, 1971.

82. Berkowitz CD, Sklaren BC: Environmental failure to thrive: The need for intervention. *Am Fam Prac* **29:**191, 1984.

83. Barbero GJ, McKay RJ: Failure to Thrive, in Vaughan VC, McKay RJ, Behrman RE (eds), *Nelson's Textbook of Pediatrics,* ed 11. Philadelphia, WB Saunders Co, 1979, pp 311–312.

84. Goldbloom RB: Failure to thrive. *Ped Clin North Am* **29**(Feb):151, 1982.

85. Weil WB Jr: Current controversies in childhood obesity. *J Pediatr* **91:**175, 1977.

86. Barnes HV, Berger R: An approach to the obese adolescent. *Med Clin North Am* **59:**1507, 1975.

87. Dietz WA: Childhood obesity: Susceptibility, cause, and management. *J Pediatr* **103:**676, 1983.

88. Committee on Nutrition, Am. Acad. Pediatr.: Nutritional aspects of obesity in infancy and childhood. *Pediatrics* **68:**880, 1981.

89. Charney E, Goodman HC, McBride M, et al: Childhood antecedents of adult obesity: Do chubby infants become obese adults? *N Engl J Med* **295:**6, 1976.

90. Seltzer CC: Some re-evaluation of the build and blood pressure study, 1959, as related to ponderal index, somatotype and mortality. *N Engl J Med* **274:**254, 1966.

91. Bruch H: Emotional aspects of obesity in children. *Pediatr Ann* **4**(May):91/290, 1975.

92. Borjeson M: The etiology of obesity in children: A study of 101 twin pairs. *Acta Paediatr Scand* **65:**279, 1976.

93. von Verschuer O: Die vererbungsbiologische Zwillingsforschung: Ihre biologische Grundlagen: Studien an 102 eineiigen and 45 gleichgeschlechtlichen zweieiigen Zwillinge und an 2 Drillingspaaren. *Ergeb Inn Med Kinderheilkd* **31:**35, 1927.

94. Shenker IR, Fisichelli V, Lang J: Weight differences between foster infants of overweight and non-overweight foster mothers. *J Pediatr* **84:**715, 1974.

95. Garn SM, Clark DC: Trends in fatness and the origins of obesity, Report from Ad Hoc Committee to review the Ten State Nutrition Survey. *Pediatrics* **57:**443, 1976.

96. Cahill GF Jr: Obesity and insulin levels. *N Engl J Med* **284:**1268, 1971.

97. Kalkhoff R, Ferrou C: Metabolic differences between obese overweight and muscular overweight men. *N Engl J Med* **284:**1236, 1971.

98. Nelson RA, Anderson LF, Gastineau CF, et al: Physiology and natural history of obesity. *JAMA* **223:**627, 1973.

99. Rothwell NJ, Stock MJ: A role for brown adipose tissue in diet-induced thermogenesis. *Nature* **281:**31, 1979.

100. Hirsch J: Hypothalamic control of appetite. *Hosp Pract* **19**(Feb):131, 1984.

101. Nisbett RE: Hunger, obesity and the ventromedial hypothalamus. *Psychol Rev* **79:**433, 1972.

102. Goldblatt PB, Moore ME, Stunkard AJ: Social factors in obesity. *JAMA* **192:**1039, 1965.

103. Schachter S: Some extraordinary facts about obese humans and rats. *Am Psychol* **26:**129, 1971.

104. Chirico A, Stunkard AJ: Physical activity and human obesity. *N Engl J Med* **263:**935, 1960.

105. Bullen BA, Reed RB, Mayer J: Physical activity of obese and non-obese adolescent girls appraised by motion picture sampling. *Am J Clin Nutr* **14:**211, 1964.

106. Smith DW: Adipose tissue and obesity, in *Growth and Its Disorders*. Philadelphia, WB Saunders Co, 1977, pp 140–144.

107. Hammar SL, Campbell MM, Campbell VA, et al: An interdisciplinary study of adolescent obesity. *J Pediatr* **80:**373, 1972.

108. Bray GA: Syndromes of hypothalamic obesity in man. *Pediatr Ann* **13**(July):525, 1984.

109. Golden MP: An approach to the management of obesity in childhood. *Pediatr Clin North Am* **26:**187, 1979.

110. Merritt RJ: Obesity. *Curr Prat Pediatr* **12**(Sep):1–58, 1982.

111. Kahle EB, Walker RB, Eisenmann PA, et al: Moderate diet control in children: The effects on metabolic indicators that predict obesity-related degenerative diseases. *Am J Clin Nutr* **35:**950, 1982.

112. Brownell KD, Wadden TA: Confronting obesity in children: Behavioral and psychological factors. *Pediatr Ann* **13**(Jun):473, 1984.

113. Stuart RB, Davis B: *Slim Chance in a Fat World: Behavioral Control of Obesity*. Champaign, IL, Research Press, 1982.

114. Grollman A: Drug therapy of obesity in chidren. *Pediatr Ann* **4**(May):39/265, 1975.

115. Rivlin RS: Therapy of obesity with hormones. *N Engl J Med* **292:**26, 1975.

116. Birmingham CL, Smith KC: Human chorionic gonadotropin is of no value in the management of obesity. *Can Med Assoc J* **128:**1156, 1983.

117. Bray GA, Raben MS, Londono J, et al: Effects of triiodothyronine, growth hormone, and anabolic steroids on nitrogen excretion and oxygen consumption of obese patients. *J Clin Endocrinol Metab* **33:**293, 1971.

118. Collip PJ: New developments in medical therapy of obesity: Thyroid and zinc. *Pediatr Ann* **13**(Jun):465, 1984.

119. Alpers DH: Surgical therapy for obesity. *N Engl J Med* **308:**1026, 1983.

# 12
# Psychological Problems in Children with Growth Disorders

Most children prefer to be like their peers. Any deviation from peer group standards, whether in size, appearance, or fashion, is viewed as undesirable. Approval or acceptance by peers is very important and noticeable deviations from "normal" growth patterns is viewed as endangering peer acceptance. The physician should be aware of the wide variation of normal growth patterns, and appreciate how much height, sexual maturity, and appearance mean to a child or adolescent (1).

## PSYCHOLOGICAL IMPACT OF GROWTH DISTURBANCES

Children who are noticeably shorter or taller than their peers become self-conscious of their deviation from mean height. The same is true of the child who is obese or very thin. The child who remains sexually infantile while most peers are experiencing sexual development is acutely aware of his or her deficiency and the child who matures early feels equally conspicuous and embarrassed. Such variations, while normal and hence only temporary, are very disturbing to the child or adolescent. If medical authority suggests the condition may be more or less permanent, the effect on the morale of the child or adolescent may be devastating (1).

When the child's self-image is distorted by a growth disorder, he or she may become introverted, withdrawn, depressed, or may try to compensate for the distorted self-image by exaggerated or deviant behavior in order to gain approval or at least attention. Either is characterized by confusion of feelings which can have profound long-term effects on the psychological growth of the individual and require careful counseling to avoid permanent emotional scars (1).

## COUNSELING A CHILD OR ADOLESCENT WITH GROWTH PROBLEMS

Growth problems which are temporary and which do not produce gross deviations from "normal" may be handled by simple explanation and reassurance, but continued observation and reassurance are important to emphasize to the child or adolescent that the physician and parents recognize the concern of the child or adolescent and are doing all they can to assure a "normal" outcome (1). Many growth deviations cannot be readily or completely corrected and for many children living with a growth pattern which is noticeably deviant may be a fact of life. In such cases simple reassurance is not enough and more elaborate counseling is necessary to help the child or adolescent adapt to the growth deviation. The following suggestions are derived from discussions of the psychological impact of growth disturbances on children by Gallagher, Smith, and Money (1–3).

1.   The parents and the child should be encouraged to talk about the child's growth and how the growth pattern affects lifestyle of the child or adolescent so the physician can assess the child's self-image and feelings about the growth deviation. The physician should display genuine interest in the child's feelings and a sympathetic understanding of how the child feels about him or herself.

2.   The physiologic basis for the child's growth deviation should be explained in simple terms, avoiding terms which tend to stigmatize growth deviations, such as "midget", "dwarf", or "giant". It is appropriate to share with the child or adolescent usual ranges of variability in growth or puberty and to demonstrate (e.g., by hand x-ray) the developmental level achieved by the child and expectations of growth. It is important to point out probable limitations in the child's growth pattern and express sympathetic understanding of how the child may feel about limitations. Adequate time must be given for the child or adolescent to express his or her feelings about the diagnosis and to ask questions, not just hear explanations.

3.   It is important to treat the child in age-appropriate rather than size-appropriate manner. Although strangers may be expected to treat a child according to height or general appearance, the physician, parents, and close friends or associates should treat the child or adolescent in an age-appropriate manner at all times.

4.   The types of treatment which would *not* be effective should be reviewed. Most youngsters come to the doctor hoping for a magic cure for their growth problems, but fearing that the doctor will dash their hopes. It requires time for the youngster (and parents) to adjust to the reality of adaptation rather than remedy. The child must be helped to understand that although the growth problem cannot be completely corrected, the worth of the child or adolescent is not diminished.

5. The expected physical and endocrine responses to the treatment should be reviewed. The limitations as well as the risks of the treatment should be carefully stated. It is important that the physician be realistic in describing the probable response to the treatment. If the child has unrealistic expectations which fail to materialize, the subsequent depression and frustration may produce severe emotional scars.

6. The child's expectations should be discussed and if they are unrealistic, substitute activities should be encouraged which would fit the child's physical limitations and yield satisfaction and acceptance by peers. There are many activities and vocations in which size is no consideration or in which size is a distinct advantage.

7. A child or adolescent should not be abandoned after he or she has been confronted with the probable limitations in remedy of the growth deviation. Continued interest in the progress of the child and sympathy and understanding for his or her limitations are most important. This may be the only treatment possible or necessary for adjustment to the growth problem.

8. In providing support for the child, one must not overlook the needs of other members of the family. During the initial evaluation, family strengths or weaknesses should be explored. If serious weaknesses in the family's ability to cope with the child's reactions to his or her growth problems are perceived, it may be appropriate to seek counseling for the family.

## PSYCHOLOGICAL STRESSES IN SPECIFIC GROWTH PROBLEMS

Understanding the nature and natural history of specific growth problems can suggest specific help in handling the psychological pressures likely to occur.

### Constitutional Delay of Growth and Adolescence

Constitutional delay in growth and adolescence represents a normal growth variant, however, if the delay is extreme, there may be psychological problems because of small size and sexual infantilism. The reason for seeking medical advice is usually concern whether the growth pattern is normal and when or whether sexual maturation will take place. Teasing from peers, because of the small size and the sexual immaturity, may heighten the anxiety.

It is important to appreciate how much height, sexual maturity, and appearance mean to a child or adolescent and to approach the anxiety created by the constitutional delay with understanding and thoroughness (1). Once the diagnosis of constitutional delay is reasonably established, the child should be reassured of the normal status of his or her growth pattern. This should include a careful explanation of the physiology of growth and the effect of timing on growth and sexual maturation. We find the velocity growth curves prepared by Tanner to be particularly helpful in displaying the expected rate of growth and the expected growth spurt and events of puberty. A late maturing curve drawn over the "usual" curve will help the child to understand why his growth is so slow, especially when compared to peers who are following curves with normal or even accelerated timing.

The maturational status of the child should be explained to the child (and parents). This may include a demonstration of skeletal maturation from x-rays and of sexual maturation using Tanner's standards. Predicted adult height using the child's skeletal maturation level may be particularly comforting, especially if it is in the normal range. Explanation of genetic potential and expected height achievement helps the child to see his growth in relation to his family, as well as compared to that of his peers. Time must be allowed for questions from the child and parents and for consideration of the implications for current and future growth. Most children and parents will be reassured by a full explanation and reassurance of the normal status of the delayed growth process (4).

In those youngsters who request hormonal intervention, there should be a careful and complete discussion of benefits and risks. The decision to apply hormonal stimulation of growth (testosterone for the male or estrogen for the female) should be made only after sufficient time has been allowed for careful consideration of the normal physiology of growth and of the psychological pressures perceived by the child and parents. It should be made perfectly clear that hormonal therapy will not increase ultimate height achievement and, may in fact, compromise final height at the expense of a hormonally induced growth spurt and initiation of secondary sexual changes. Whether hormonal therapy is pursued or simple assurance is accepted, it is important for the physician to display continued interest in the child's maturation and to provide opportunities for follow-up examinations and counsel until full maturity is achieved (1).

## Excessive Height, Familial

Concern about excessive height is usually confined to girls of tall parents or to girls with accelerated growth patterns, though occasionally rapidly growing boys may need some assurance that they will not become outlandishly tall. For the girl of tall parents, the issue is generally anxiety over social acceptance of excessive height and depends upon the previous experience of the parents (especially the mother) and of the current social climate regarding height.

It is important to establish the usual growth patterns of the family, including early or late sexual maturation patterns. From the child's height, skeletal-age, and status of puberty a predicted mature height can be derived. The normal nature of the child's growth pattern should be emphasized and a full discussion of growth potential encouraged. If the height prediction falls within a range acceptable to the child and parents, nothing further need be done, although it is desirable to offer yearly follow-up examinations and counsel to assure the child and family of the physician's continued interest and to discuss changes in height prediction which frequently occur. It has been our philosophy to encourage acceptance of natural height whenever possible, and to encourage the girl to consider her height as an advantage. Most naturally tall girls are slim and considered physically attractive. If as much time and effort is spent in reassurance and support of the tall girl as might be expended through hormonal intervention therapy, it is our view that most girls would be able to adjust comfortably to their natural height.

If the predicted height is viewed as unacceptable by the child or parents, the reasons for the unacceptability should be thoroughly discussed. If hormonal therapy is desired to limit excessive height, the physician must realistically describe probable results achievable and the risks of such therapy. The risks of thromboembolism, relative infertility, and increased breast and uterine cancer risks must be frankly discussed and carefully weighed against the expected benefits from limitation of excessive height. Only if the parents view the predicted height as clearly threatening to their child's social and psychological well-being, is hormonal intervention acceptable. The physician should play the role of interested counselor in helping the family arrive at an acceptable decision. We generally discourage hormonal treatment in all but the most persuasive circumstances.

In those girls who choose hormonal intervention, we provide frequent follow-up during treatment and long-term follow-up into adulthood. Most girls who have chosen therapy have achieved an acceptable result and are satisfied with their adult height. Fortunately, we have not yet encountered any serious side effects (5). Among those who have chosen not to undergo hormonal therapy, we have seen only occasional unhappiness and chagrin at not attempting hormonal therapy.

## Short Stature

Though some short stature is correctible either by patience (constitutional delayed growth pattern) or hormonal replacement (hypothyroidism) most youngsters must learn to adapt to permanent short stature of varying degree. The nature of the growth problem, the anticipated natural growth, and probable ultimate height achievement should be carefully explained to the child and parents, with care taken to be neither unduly pessimistic nor unrealistically optimistic. From observation and questioning, one should determine how the child and the family view the problem of short stature.

Treatment, which might be effective in correcting some of the shortness, should be reviewed, with care taken to be realistic in outlining probable response to treatment. It is equally important to review those treatments which would *not* be effective and to explain why they would not be effective. "It is important to emphasize to the parents that a small child who is growing at a slow rate . . . needs less caloric intake than usual . . . smaller food intake is usually secondary to the slow growth and not the cause of it" (2). The addition of vitamins or energy-rich foods will not improve the stature of a small child, but may lead to excessive weight gain.

Most people who do not know the child with short stature can be expected to treat the child according to apparent age as judged by height. Small children are commonly carried about and babied because of their small size and this may lead to less than optimal social and intellectual maturation. Parents, family members, and friends should avoid overprotective behavior. The small child should be treated with age-appropriate language, clothing, and responsibilities (2). Unless the child is extremely gifted intellectually, it may be desirable to wait a year before introducing him or her into the school system. The teacher should be encouraged to treat the child in an age-appropriate manner. Teachers can be helpful in protecting the child from teasing. Most peer groups will accept a simple explanation of the problem associated with short stature and will befriend the small child. If there are physical stigmata which can be corrected by surgery (ptosis, webbed neck, epicanthal folds, etc.), these should be corrected as early as practicable. Judicious use of clothing may mask some disfiguring stigmata, but clothes should be appropriate for age. Use of hormones at the usual time of puberty provide natural changes helpful in reducing the stigma of sexual infantilism.

Since the small child cannot hope to escape notice in a group, he or she may become a willing or unwilling "celebrity". Some children adapt well to this celebrity role and are able to turn it to their advantage in school elections and in making friends (2, 3). Some find themselves befriended by larger children who become their protectors from those who would tease them. Such a mascot-like role can be healthy and desirable (2, 3). An unprotected small child may need to develop a "joking relationship" to protect him- or herself against unremitting teasing (3). Most bullies will stop short of inflicting actual physical harm on small children, but the teasing can become intense. In such situations, Money has suggested that the small child be encouraged to learn the game of one-upmanship to cut his or her opponent down to size (3). The child may be helped to discover a weakness in the culprit, such as personal behavior, appearance, or even an imaginative behavior, as long as it might be true, for example, bed-wetter, rat teeth, monkey ears, nose-picker, and so on. These weapons can then be used in a "joking relationship" to elevate the status of the small child to the detriment of his or her detractor. According to Money, for those small children whose disposition allows them to use joking, this can be remarkably effective (3).

In counseling small children, one should emphasize the ways in which small size can be of advantage. If athletic aspirations of the child are unrealistic, the child should be directed into activities which would be more fulfilling. Swimming, wrestling, tennis, gymnastics, skiing, golf, and baseball usually can be enjoyed regardless of size. Many school activities, such as acting, debating, playing musical instruments, singing, leading cheers, and so on, place no limits on size and, in some instances, small size can be an advantage. Choosing a career may be difficult for some small people, but introduction to groups of small people such as "Little People of America" may be of help. There are examples of small people who have achieved success in nearly all trades and professions (2).

### Hypopituitarism

The effects of pituitary hormone deficiencies on growth, sexual development, and fertility should be discussed with the patient with hypopituitarism and his or her parents. The expected results from hormonal replacement should be shared with the family without arousing unrealistic expectations. Even with human growth hormone readily available, it is unlikely that most children with hypopituitarism will reach heights in excess of 65 inches. There will, therefore, need to be some counseling to help the child adapt to being small, as suggested in the section dealing with short stature.

Even though secondary sex characteristics can be stimulated with androgen and/or estrogen, the likelihood of infertility is still very great. Judicious use of gonadotropins during child-bearing years has occasionally resulted in fertility, but it is a rare occurrence. Small size and sexual immaturity may also interfere with romantic physical love, but the desire and need for intimate companionship should be recognized and fostered. The hypopituitary subject tends to exhibit aggressive behavior, become depressed or withdrawn, or suffer self-image problems. If simple reassurance does not correct the aberrant personality traits, more intensive counseling may be needed. It is sometimes helpful for such individuals to help each other with questions of adaptation, vocational opportunities, and so on, by meeting with a group such as Little People of America (2).

### Hypothyroidism

Most youngsters with hypothyroidism in whom delay in growth is the chief complaint will be suffering from acquired hypothyroidism in childhood or adolescence, due to chronic lymphocytic thyroiditis. Although growth is delayed during the thyroid deficiency, with adequate therapy catch-up growth can be expected, unless therapy is not begun until late in puberty. Most physiologic effects of subdued metabolism are rapidly restored to normal. Though mental dullness is characteristic while thyroxine levels are low, intellectual function is maintained remarkably well and complete recovery is usually assured.

We have found that school performance does not always respond to treatment in a salutary fashion. While hypothyroid the school-age child may become phlegmatic and dull; this may be translated into persistent application to school chores and win approval of teachers. When the child is rendered suddenly euthyroid with thyroxine therapy, the attention span shortens noticeably and school chores suffer because of the child's distractability. It takes some time, a great deal of patience, and often a lower, gradually increasing thyroxine medication level to allow the child to regain his previous level of performance.

Intellectual impairment may occur in children with congenital hypothyroidism. The degree of impairment appears to be related to the time of the onset of the deficiency, the duration and degree of thyroid deficiency, time of onset of therapy, and the adequacy of the therapy. With so many variables, it is patently impossible to predict with accuracy what degree of deficiency an individual child is apt to experience, but one can speak of high or low risk for encountering intellectual deficit. Even if some deficit of intellectual function seems certain, it may be reassuring to the parents to learn that, contrary to pessimistic views previously held, there is some tendency for the intelligence quotient to improve moderately (20–40 points) with treatment (3). The psychological problems surrounding the intellectually deficient hypothyroid child are not related to growth as much as they are to the mental slowness and may require the services of school counselors or psychologists as well as special class placement.

### Primordial Dwarfism

In children with primordial dwarfism, with or without other congenital defects, there are neither nutritional nor endocrine deficiencies and the cells seem to resist any efforts to make them change their predetermined size and number. With this group of youngsters, it is important to share with the parents what we currently understand of their expected growth patterns and emphasize why treatment with hormones or vitamins would not be effective. Recently this thesis has been challenged by a study showing more than expected gains in growth in children with intrauterine growth retardation treated with human growth hormone over a 3-year period (6). It may be that as hormones, such as pituitary growth hormone or somatomedin, become available for wider clinical usage that various forms of primordial dwarfism will in fact, be found to be more or less responsive. Presently, children with primordial dwarfism, must be counseled to adapt to their small size. There may also be psychological stresses related to intellectual deficit and infertility, depending on the nature of the growth problem and the associated defects.

### Turner's Syndrome

For girls with Turner's syndrome, short stature appears to be the feature most often of concern. Many of the suggestions for handling problems relating to short stature described in the section on short stature are appropriate for the girl with Turner's syndrome. When the diagnosis has been established, the nature of the growth and gonadal problems should be discussed with the parents and with the girl, if she is of an age when a discussion of short stature and gonadal dysgenesis would be understandable. Many parents are willing to have the girl learn of the growth limitations at any age, but wish to defer discussion of infertility until adolescence because of family taboos concerning discussion of sexual function. Tact and the passage of time may be required before the parents feel at ease in discussing the implications of gonadal dysgenesis.

Height achievement is generally under 60 inches in the adult female with Turner's syndrome and, according to Smith, is related more to parental height than to medication used to bring about secondary sexual characteristics (2). Human growth hormone is of limited value in treating the short stature of Turner's syndrome and the short supply of human growth hormone has precluded any large scale test of its efficacy (7). Although some increase in predicted mature height has been claimed from combined androgen–estrogen therapy (8), the achievements in height are still severely limited. Major psychological support should be geared to helping the girl with Turner's syndrome to adapt to the inevitability of short stature. Physical stigmata of Turner's syndrome can to some extent be ameliorated by plastic surgery, which should be performed as early as is practicable to avoid the feeling of being "different" in the child.

When the child arrives at the usual age of puberty, either chronologically or, more commonly, developmentally, replacement endocrine therapy is offered. The probability of gonadal dysfunction should be introduced at the time the diagnosis is made and reviewed at the time of puberty to justify and explain the need for hormonal therapy. In some girls with Turner's syndrome (especially those with mosaicism) some spontaneous secondary sexual development does occur, but it is seldom complete, and supplemental therapy is usually required. Money suggests that the probable status of the ovaries can be tactfully and positively introduced by suggesting that the probability of adoptive motherhood is close to 100% while that of natural pregnancy is near 0 (3). With hormonal therapy the girl can be assured that she will achieve natural sexual development and adoptive motherhood implies a normal, happy marriage. Girls with Turner's syndrome have normal intelligence, although they may have specific learning disabilities. They tend not to be aggressive, are relatively unperturbed by the stigmata of their condition, and are not usually "celebrities" (3). Most have a pleasant, friendly disposition and make good "mothers."

## Klinefelter's Syndrome (47 XXY)

Excessive height in the male adolescent with Klinefelter syndrome is not usually a source of concern, but behavior problems may occur because of intellectual impairment and lack of impulse control. Sexual infertility may provoke psychological problems in the young adult.

## Sexual Precocity

Children with accelerated or precocious maturity are generally large for their chronologic age and often of above average intelligence, but are emotionally near their chronologic age. They may choose friends who are a little older, but nearer their size, but they are often unable to compete with them socially or emotionally and may be teased because of apparent social immaturity (3). Despite rather large size, the accelerated or precocious child may be shy, retiring, and awkward, feeling unacceptable to both his age group and his physique group. Vulnerability to teasing only exacerbates their natural shyness.

To help the child and his or her family adapt to the stresses of precocious development, it is important that they understand the natural sequence of maturation and the reason for early sexual development. It should be stressed that the sequence of maturation is normal, only the timing is unusual, and that fertility is usually undiminished by precocious development. Correction of the cause by surgery or medication will interrupt the progress of the maturation but not eliminate maturation already achieved. In children with idiopathic sexual precocity, use of medication may slow the rate of sexual maturation but accelerated growth tends to continue. There is, therefore, nearly always a disparity between physique or developmental age and chronologic age, even with treatment. Parents and close friends should be encouraged to treat the child in an age-appropriate manner; others may be expected to be excessively demanding until they discover the nature of the problem. Some students may tease the precocious child, but school teachers should be careful to treat the child in age-appropriate manner.

Full sexual maturity and fertility will be achieved at a young age in the child with precocious puberty, usually long before social or emotional maturity has been achieved. The child may, therefore, be sexually vulnerable and may need protection from those who would take advantage of them. Use of loose fitting clothes to obscure breast and hip development and use of a training bra in the young girl may be cosmetically helpful in diverting attention from the developing secondary sex characteristics. Early sex education, geared to the intellectual and emotional level of the child, will be necessary with continual updating of information, as the child's level of sophistication increases. Some have suggested contraceptive protection for girls who prove to be vulnerable despite educational and counseling efforts.

## Sexual Infantilism (Delayed Puberty)

Adolescents with delayed puberty or sexual infantilism are often short and the psychological stresses may originate from either short stature or lack of sexual development. It is important, therefore, to explore carefully the feelings which the young person has about his or her condition (especially their "body image") and to allow them time to vent their feelings and fears. The natural sequence of sexual development should be reviewed with the subjects and parents and the reason for their late sexual development clearly explained. It is important to do this in a way which expresses understanding of the feelings of the young person and sympathy for his or her fears and expectations.

Ehrhardt et al. suggest the following criteria for recommending hormonal treatment of delayed puberty: symptoms of emotional tension, irritability and depression; psychosomatic complaints (e.g., abdominal pain); inferiority feelings; symptoms of overcompensation (e.g., fighting, extreme competitiveness in sports, etc.); regression in or withdrawal from peer contacts and lack of social participation in peer group activities (parties, teams, and clubs); rejection by and/or withdrawal from the other sex; poor school performance due to emotional rather than intellectual problems; dropping out of sports and teams because of emotional problems; much school absenteeism; age-inadequate lack of vocational-educational goals and plans; and dependence on parents, possibly combined with parental overprotection (9).

The limits of effectiveness of hormonal therapy should be carefully outlined. Expectations should be reasonable and reassurance given when appropriate. Continued interest should be shown by carefully following the progress of the endocrine therapy. The probability of full sexual development and of fertility should be discussed with the young person and/or parents giving realistic probabilities, being careful not to raise expectations unreasonably and run the risk of later adjustment reactions. When infertility is likely, it may be well to emphasize attainment of normal sexual characteristics and discuss the feasibility of adoptive parenthood.

## Obesity

The obese child is often described as unhappy, depressed and withdrawn, with a poor body image, and the continual target of teasing. Psychological or emotional problems may be involved in the genesis or the perpetuation of the obese state and in either context must be discovered and corrected before obesity can be effectively controlled. It is important to explore the family's attitudes toward obesity and toward the child, including a review of how the child gets along at school and at play and of interpersonal relations with friends, parents, and siblings.

Any plan for treatment of obesity must take into consideration the emotional impact of the obesity on the child and the motivation of child and family to remedy the condition. This will require frequent reassurance from dietician and physician, but may also require intervention by behavioral counselor, medical social worker, psychologist, or psychiatrist. Permanent control of obesity requires changing lifestyle and modifying behavior which may require specific counseling. Sometimes this can be accomplished through groups by common encouragement, but for others, individual encouragement or counsel is necessary. Clearly, any program of successful management of obesity must offer services of medical, nutritional, and behavioral counseling and all three must understand the unique contribution of each other to the welfare of the obese child.

### Anorexia Nervosa

Anorexia Nervosa represents a severe degree of disrupted body image in which the child (usually a preteen or teenage female) views any subcutaneous fat as undesirable. The pathologic aversion to food appears to represent a serious and sometimes malignant psychologic aberration. Milder forms of the disorder may be treated by attempting behavior modification of eating habits, setting goals, and defining either rewards or consequences (i.e., intravenous or naso-gastric supplements to compensate for failure to ingest adequate food). The aim of counseling is the restitution of the body image of the anorectic child toward normal. Often this can be accomplished only by intensive psychotherapy.

### Psychosocial Dwarfism

The behavior patterns which accompany the growth retardation in psychosocial (deprivation) dwarfism mark it as an unusual growth problem. The manner in which the psychological stresses affect growth independently of the nutritional deficiency have not been thoroughly explained, although interference with release of growth hormone or of somatomedin have been suggested. Recovery requires change of living place and a loving, accepting environment, as well as access to adequate food. In a new environment there is gradual disappearance of bizarre behavior, improved learning and speech, and elevation of the intelligence quotient (3). To achieve normal growth and emotional/social improvement requires continuing long-term care in an accepting, concerned environment.

### REFERENCES

1. Gallager JR: Short and tall stature in otherwise normal adolescents: Management of their medical and psychologic problems, Gardner LI (ed), *Endocrine and Genetic Diseases of Childhood and Adolescence*, ed 2. Philadelphia, WB Saunders Co, 1975, pp 99–105.
2. Smith DW: Psychologic aspects of short stature, *Growth and Its Disorders*. Philadelphia, WB Saunders Co, 1977, pp 118–119.
3. Money J: Psychologic aspects of endocrine and genetic disease in children, Gardner LI (ed), *Endocrine and Genetic Diseases of Childhood and Adolescence*, ed 2. Philadelphia, WB Saunders Co, 1975, pp 1207–1240.
4. Shenker IR, Nussbaum M, Kaplan E: Delayed puberty and short stature in adolescents. *Pediatric Annals* 7(September):56–66, 1978.
5. Rallison ML, Lester PD, Wood C: Management of excessive height in girls with familial tall stature. Unpublished observations.

6. Lanes R, Plotnick LP, Lee PA: Sustained effect of human growth hormone therapy on children with intrauterine growth retardation. *Pediatrics* **63:**731, 1979.

7. Tanner JM, Whitehouse RH, Hughes PCR, et al: Effect of human growth hormone treatment for 1 to 7 years on growth of 100 children with growth hormone deficiency, low birthweight, inherited smallness, Turner's syndrome and other complaints. *Arch Dis Child* **46:**745, 1971.

8. Moore DC, Tattoni DS, Ruvalcaba RH, et al: Effect of prolonged administration of oxandrolone on growth in children and adolescents with gonadal dysgenesis. *J Pediatr* **90:**462, 1977.

9. Ehrhardt AA, Meyer-Bahlburg HFL: Psychological correlates of abnormal pubertal development. *Clin Endocrinol Metab* **4**(March):207–222, 1975.

# Appendix

## Table A-1. Newborn Male Length, Weight, and Head Circumference by Gestational Age

| | Gestational Age—Weeks | | | | | |
|---|---|---|---|---|---|---|
| Percentiles | 37 | 38 | 39 | 40 | 41 | 42–43 |
| **Distribution of Crown–Heel Lengths (cm) of White Newborn Male Infants (controls) by Percentiles According to Their Gestational Ages** | | | | | | |
| 95 | 52.0 | 53.0 | 54.0 | 54.5 | 55.0 | 55.3 |
| 90 | 51.5 | 52.5 | 53.5 | 54.0 | 54.5 | 54.8 |
| 75 | 50.5 | 51.5 | 52.5 | 53.0 | 53.5 | 54.0 |
| 50 | 50.0 | 50.7 | 51.5 | 52.0 | 52.5 | 53.0 |
| 25 | 49.0 | 49.7 | 50.5 | 51.0 | 51.5 | 52.0 |
| 10 | 48.0 | 48.7 | 49.5 | 50.0 | 50.5 | 51.0 |
| 5 | 47.5 | 48.2 | 49.0 | 49.5 | 50.0 | 50.5 |
| **Percentile Distribution of Birth Weights (kg) of White First-Born Male Infants (controls) According to Their Gestational Ages** | | | | | | |
| 95 | 3.63 | 3.82 | 3.97 | 4.10 | 4.23 | 4.34 |
| 90 | 3.50 | 3.70 | 3.86 | 4.00 | 4.13 | 4.24 |
| 75 | 3.30 | 3.48 | 3.65 | 3.78 | 3.92 | 4.03 |
| 50 | 3.10 | 3.27 | 3.43 | 3.57 | 3.70 | 3.82 |
| 25 | 2.85 | 3.00 | 3.13 | 3.26 | 3.38 | 3.49 |
| 10 | 2.70 | 2.84 | 2.96 | 3.08 | 3.18 | 3.28 |
| 5 | 2.62 | 2.76 | 2.88 | 3.00 | 3.10 | 3.20 |
| **Percentile Distribution of Birth Weights (kg) of White Male Infants (controls) Born to Multiparas According to Infants' Gestational Ages** | | | | | | |
| 95 | 3.66 | 4.00 | 4.20 | 4.39 | 4.50 | 4.60 |
| 90 | 3.47 | 3.70 | 3.90 | 4.08 | 4.24 | 4.37 |
| 75 | 3.30 | 3.50 | 3.70 | 3.87 | 4.03 | 4.15 |
| 50 | 3.10 | 3.27 | 3.44 | 3.61 | 3.75 | 3.85 |
| 25 | 2.85 | 3.02 | 3.18 | 3.34 | 3.50 | 3.62 |
| 10 | 2.71 | 2.86 | 3.02 | 3.19 | 3.34 | 3.45 |
| 5 | 2.63 | 2.78 | 2.94 | 3.08 | 3.21 | 3.32 |
| **Distribution of Occipitofrontal Circumferences (cm) of White Newborn Male Infants (controls) by Percentiles According to Their Gestational Ages** | | | | | | |
| 95 | 35.5 | 36.0 | 36.4 | 36.8 | 37.2 | 37.4 |
| 90 | 35.2 | 35.6 | 35.9 | 36.3 | 36.7 | 37.2 |
| 75 | 34.6 | 34.9 | 35.3 | 35.7 | 36.0 | 36.2 |
| 50 | 34.0 | 34.3 | 34.6 | 34.9 | 35.2 | 35.5 |
| 25 | 33.4 | 33.7 | 34.0 | 34.3 | 34.7 | 35.0 |
| 10 | 32.8 | 33.2 | 33.5 | 33.8 | 34.2 | 34.5 |
| 5 | 32.4 | 32.7 | 33.1 | 33.4 | 33.8 | 34.2 |

(Reproduced by permission from Miller HC and Merritt TA: *Fetal Growth in Humans*. Chicago, Year Book Medical Publishers, Inc, copyright © 1979 by Year Book Medical Publishers, Chicago.)

## Table A-2. Newborn Female Length, Weight, and Head Circumference by Gestational Age

| | Gestational Age—Weeks | | | | | |
|---|---|---|---|---|---|---|
| Percentiles | 37 | 38 | 39 | 40 | 41 | 42–43 |
| **Distribution of Crown–Heel Lengths (cm) of White Newborn Female Infants (controls) by Percentiles According to Their Gestational Ages** | | | | | | |
| 95 | 51.5 | 52.5 | 53.5 | 54.0 | 54.5 | 54.5 |
| 90 | 51.0 | 52.0 | 53.0 | 53.5 | 54.0 | 54.0 |
| 75 | 50.0 | 51.0 | 52.0 | 52.5 | 52.8 | 53.1 |
| 50 | 49.0 | 50.0 | 50.7 | 51.3 | 51.7 | 52.0 |
| 25 | 48.0 | 48.9 | 49.5 | 50.0 | 50.5 | 51.0 |
| 10 | 47.5 | 48.5 | 49.0 | 49.5 | 50.0 | 50.5 |
| 5 | 47.0 | 47.9 | 48.6 | 49.1 | 49.5 | 50.0 |
| **Percentile Distribution of Birth Weights (kg) of White First-Born Female Infants (controls) According to Their Gestational Ages** | | | | | | |
| 95 | 3.44 | 3.72 | 3.90 | 4.03 | 4.12 | 4.20 |
| 90 | 3.30 | 3.60 | 3.80 | 3.92 | 4.02 | 4.10 |
| 75 | 3.17 | 3.38 | 3.57 | 3.70 | 3.82 | 3.94 |
| 50 | 3.00 | 3.15 | 3.30 | 3.43 | 3.56 | 3.66 |
| 25 | 2.79 | 2.93 | 3.07 | 3.18 | 3.29 | 3.37 |
| 10 | 2.55 | 2.72 | 2.85 | 2.97 | 3.09 | 3.17 |
| 5 | 2.46 | 2.61 | 2.76 | 2.89 | 3.01 | 3.10 |
| **Percentile Distribution of Birth Weights (kg) of White Female Infants (controls) Born to Multiparas According to Infants' Gestational Ages** | | | | | | |
| 95 | 3.60 | 3.86 | 4.02 | 4.14 | 4.23 | 4.31 |
| 90 | 3.50 | 3.67 | 3.84 | 3.95 | 4.07 | 4.15 |
| 75 | 3.26 | 3.48 | 3.64 | 3.75 | 3.85 | 3.95 |
| 50 | 3.00 | 3.20 | 3.34 | 3.50 | 3.62 | 3.72 |
| 25 | 2.80 | 2.95 | 3.08 | 3.23 | 3.35 | 3.45 |
| 10 | 2.67 | 2.80 | 2.93 | 3.05 | 3.16 | 3.26 |
| 5 | 2.52 | 2.67 | 2.80 | 2.92 | 3.04 | 3.15 |
| **Distribution of Occipitofrontal Circumferences (cm) of White Newborn Female Infants (controls) by Percentiles According to Their Gestational Ages** | | | | | | |
| 95 | 35.0 | 35.5 | 35.9 | 36.2 | 36.5 | 36.8 |
| 90 | 34.5 | 35.0 | 35.4 | 35.7 | 36.1 | 36.3 |
| 75 | 33.9 | 34.3 | 34.7 | 35.1 | 35.5 | 35.8 |
| 50 | 33.2 | 33.6 | 34.1 | 34.5 | 34.8 | 35.2 |
| 25 | 32.5 | 32.9 | 33.4 | 33.8 | 34.2 | 34.5 |
| 10 | 32.0 | 32.4 | 32.8 | 33.2 | 33.6 | 33.9 |
| 5 | 31.8 | 32.2 | 32.6 | 32.9 | 33.3 | 33.6 |

(Reproduced by permission from Miller HC and Merritt TA: *Fetal Growth in Humans.* Chicago, Year Book Medical Publishers, Inc, copyright © 1979 by Year Book Medical Publishers, Chicago.)

## Table A-3. Mean and Standard Deviations for Height, Weight, Height Velocity, and Weight Velocity for Males

| Age | Length[a] and Height (cm) | | Weight (kg) | | Length and Height Velocity (cm/yr) | | Weight Velocity (kg/yr) | |
|---|---|---|---|---|---|---|---|---|
| | Mean | SD | Mean | SD | Mean | SD | Mean | SD |
| Birth | 50.0 | 1.94 | 3.50 | 0.53 | 47.00 | 3.00 | 8.93 | 1.80 |
| 1 mo | | | | | | | | |
| 3 mo | 60.7 | 2.16 | 5.93 | 0.66 | 36.00 | 2.63 | 9.85 | 2.38 |
| 6 mo | 68.2 | 2.34 | 7.90 | 0.80 | 24.00 | 2.34 | 6.80 | 1.61 |
| 9 mo | 72.7 | 2.52 | 9.20 | 1.15 | 16.25 | 2.15 | 4.30 | 1.22 |
| 12 mo | 76.3 | 2.69 | 10.20 | 1.01 | 13.40 | 1.98 | 3.33 | 0.93 |
| 1½ yr | 82.1 | 3.01 | 11.60 | 1.17 | 10.50 | 1.75 | 2.44 | 0.71 |
| 2 yr | 86.9/85.9 | 3.30/3.30 | 12.70 | 1.33 | 8.90/9.00 | 1.48/1.64 | 2.10 | 0.63 |
| 3 yr | 94.2 | 3.83 | 14.70 | 1.61 | 7.88 | 1.34 | 1.96 | 0.69 |
| 4 yr | 101.6 | 4.30 | 16.60 | 1.90 | 7.00 | 1.12 | 1.90 | 0.77 |
| 5 yr | 108.3 | 4.74 | 18.50 | 2.17 | 6.48 | 1.03 | 1.92 | 0.85 |
| 6 yr | 114.6 | 5.14 | 20.50 | 2.44 | 6.09 | 0.91 | 2.07 | 0.94 |
| 7 yr | 120.5 | 5.46 | 22.60 | 2.75 | 5.79 | 0.87 | 2.31 | 1.02 |
| 8 yr | 126.2 | 5.75 | 25.00 | 3.12 | 5.55 | 0.77 | 2.47 | 1.14 |
| 9 yr | 131.6 | 6.00 | 27.50 | 5.98 | 5.35 | 0.76 | 2.67 | 0.88 |
| 10 yr | 136.9 | 6.20 | 30.30 | 7.04 | 5.16 | 0.70 | 2.87 | 1.60 |
| 11 yr | 142.0 | 6.37 | 33.30 | 7.78 | 5.01 | 0.68 | 3.08 | 1.70 |
| 12 yr | 146.9 | 6.48 | 36.50 | 8.48 | 4.98 | 0.79 | 3.50 | 1.75 |
| 13 yr | 152.2 | 6.55 | 40.70 | 8.47 | 6.55 | 1.03 | 5.13 | 1.78 |
| 14 yr | 160.6 | 6.59 | 48.40 | 9.42 | 9.45 | 1.20 | 9.06 | 1.95 |
| 15 yr | 168.7 | 6.61 | 56.30 | 9.52 | 5.86 | 1.13 | 5.68 | 1.89 |
| 16 yr | 172.7 | 6.63 | 60.20 | 9.63 | 2.65 | 0.91 | 2.60 | 1.00 |
| 17 yr | 174.3 | 6.65 | 62.10 | 9.60 | 1.00 | 0.50 | | |
| 18 yr | 174.7 | 6.65 | 63.00 | 9.69 | 0.05 | 0.40 | | |
| 19 yr | | | | | | | | |

Reproduced by permission from Tanner JM, Physical growth and development, in Forfar JO, Arneil GC (eds) Textbook of Pediatrics. London, Churchill Livingstone, 1973.

[a] First 2 years.

**Table A-4. Mean and Standard Deviations for Head Circumference, Sitting Height, and Skin Fold Thickness for Males**

| Age | Head Circumference (cm) | | Crown–Rump[a] and Sitting Height (cm) | | Triceps Skinfold (mm log transf.) | | Subscapular Skinfold (mm log transf.) | |
|---|---|---|---|---|---|---|---|---|
| | Mean | SD | Mean | SD | Mean | SD | Mean | SD |
| Birth | 36.00 | 1.97 | | | | | | |
| 1 mo | 40.20 | 1.70 | 35.0 | 1.55 | 175.0 | 12.56 | 172.0 | 14.8 |
| 3 mo | 43.65 | 1.60 | 39.0 | 1.42 | 193.0 | 12.10 | 182.0 | 14.8 |
| 6 mo | 45.60 | 1.60 | 43.1 | 1.67 | 201.0 | 12.00 | 184.8 | 15.0 |
| 9 mo | 46.65 | 1.60 | 45.5 | 1.67 | 202.0 | 12.50 | 184.0 | 15.2 |
| 12 mo | 48.10 | 1.49 | 47.4 | 1.71 | 201.0 | 12.70 | 182.0 | 15.8 |
| 1½ yr | 49.03 | 1.49 | 50.2 | 1.83 | 198.3 | 12.90 | 173.0 | 15.6 |
| 2 yr | 50.37 | 1.41 | 52.7 | 1.95 | 195.8 | 13.10 | 168.0 | 15.2 |
| 3 yr | 51.12 | 1.36 | 56.0 | 2.25 | 191.0 | 10.40 | 162.0 | 15.5 |
| 4 yr | 51.60 | 1.33 | 59.2 | 2.33 | 187.0 | 13.50 | 158.3 | 16.2 |
| 5 yr | 51.88 | 1.33 | 62.0 | 2.38 | 183.5 | 13.90 | 155.2 | 16.6 |
| 6 yr | 52.12 | 1.33 | 64.7 | 2.40 | 181.4 | 14.70 | 153.4 | 16.8 |
| 7 yr | 52.29 | 1.33 | 67.2 | 2.45 | 180.3 | 15.60 | 153.0 | 17.5 |
| 8 yr | 52.43 | 1.36 | 69.5 | 2.55 | 180.0 | 17.00 | 153.8 | 18.3 |
| 9 yr | 52.70 | 1.49 | 71.7 | 2.70 | 180.8 | 18.70 | 155.5 | 19.9 |
| 10 yr | 53.10 | 1.46 | 73.8 | 2.90 | 182.4 | 20.70 | 158.0 | 23.4 |
| 11 yr | 53.60 | 1.54 | 75.7 | 3.13 | 184.4 | 22.40 | 162.0 | 26.0 |
| 12 yr | 54.10 | 1.54 | 77.6 | 3.39 | 186.0 | 23.00 | 165.8 | 26.5 |
| 13 yr | 54.59 | 1.54 | 80.1 | 3.72 | 184.4 | 23.70 | 187.0 | 25.2 |
| 14 yr | 54.85 | 1.49 | 83.2 | 4.18 | 181.0 | 23.50 | 186.0 | 23.1 |
| 15 yr | 55.00 | 1.46 | 86.5 | 4.52 | 178.4 | 23.20 | 188.0 | 20.7 |
| 16 yr | | | 89.6 | 4.12 | 178.8 | 23.40 | 179.6 | 18.7 |
| 17 yr | | | | | 182.0 | 21.70 | 185.7 | 17.8 |
| 18 yr | | | | | 185.7 | 21.50 | 190.4 | 17.5 |
| 19 yr | | | | | 188.8 | 21.20 | 192.3 | 17.5 |

Reproduced by permission from Tanner JM, Physical growth and development, in Forfar JO, Arneil GC (eds) *Textbook of Pediatrics.* London, Churchill Livingstone, 1973.

[a] First 2 years.

**Table A-5. Mean and Standard Deviations for Height, Weight, Height Velocity, and Weight Velocity for Females**

| Age | Length[a] and Height (cm) Mean | SD | Weight (kg) Mean | SD | Length and Height Velocity (cm/yr) Mean | SD | Weight Velocity (kg/yr) Mean | SD |
|---|---|---|---|---|---|---|---|---|
| Birth | 49.5 | 1.94 | 3.40 | 0.57 | 41.00 | 3.00 | 7.42 | 1.91 |
| 1 mo | 59.0 | 2.16 | 5.56 | 0.64 | 32.00 | 2.63 | 9.25 | 2.69 |
| 3 mo | 65.5 | 2.34 | 7.39 | 0.80 | 22.50 | 2.34 | 6.60 | 1.55 |
| 6 mo | 70.2 | 2.52 | 8.72 | 0.90 | 16.45 | 2.15 | 4.29 | 1.32 |
| 9 mo | 74.2 | 2.69 | 9.70 | 1.01 | 14.70 | 1.98 | 3.37 | 0.99 |
| 12 mo | 80.5 | 3.01 | 11.10 | 1.12 | 11.20 | 1.75 | 2.44 | 0.72 |
| 1½ yr | 85.6/84.6 | 3.3/3.3 | 12.20 | 1.33 | 9.15/9.30 | 1.43/1.64 | 2.08 | 0.57 |
| 2 yr | 93.0 | 3.83 | 14.30 | 1.54 | 7.90 | 1.34 | 2.00 | 0.73 |
| 3 yr | 100.4 | 4.30 | 16.30 | 1.69 | 7.03 | 1.15 | 2.00 | 0.78 |
| 4 yr | 108.3 | 4.74 | 18.30 | 2.65 | 6.48 | 1.09 | 2.05 | 1.10 |
| 5 yr | 114.6 | 5.17 | 20.40 | 3.39 | 6.09 | 0.95 | 2.17 | 1.22 |
| 6 yr | 120.5 | 5.46 | 22.60 | 4.23 | 5.82 | 0.87 | 2.30 | 1.34 |
| 7 yr | 125.0 | 5.73 | 25.10 | 5.24 | 5.55 | 0.80 | 2.54 | 1.38 |
| 8 yr | 130.5 | 5.86 | 27.70 | 6.34 | 5.47 | 0.78 | 2.81 | 0.96 |
| 9 yr | 136.0 | 5.94 | 30.70 | 7.72 | 5.47 | 0.83 | 3.16 | 1.56 |
| 10 yr | 141.7 | 5.96 | 34.20 | 8.68 | 6.50 | 1.01 | 4.05 | 1.65 |
| 11 yr | 149.5 | 5.98 | 39.60 | 9.52 | 8.33 | 1.10 | 7.43 | 1.42 |
| 12 yr | 156.8 | 6.00 | 47.80 | 9.79 | 5.50 | 1.05 | 7.25 | 1.40 |
| 13 yr | 160.6 | 6.00 | 53.00 | 9.79 | 2.36 | 0.84 | 3.55 | 1.30 |
| 14 yr | 161.9 | 6.00 | 55.20 | 9.79 | 0.60 | 0.52 | 1.48 | 1.41 |
| 15 yr | 162.2 | 6.00 | 56.00 | 9.79 | 0.20 | 0.52 | 0.22 | 1.11 |
| 16 yr | 162.2 | 6.00 | 56.40 | 9.79 | 0.00 | 0.50 | | |
| 17 yr | 162.2 | 6.00 | 56.60 | 9.79 | 0.00 | 0.40 | | |
| 18 yr | 162.2 | 6.00 | | 9.79 | | | | |
| 19 yr | | 6.00 | | | | | | |

Reproduced by permission from Tanner JM, Physical growth and development, in Forfar JO, Arneil GC (eds) *Textbook of Pediatrics*. London, Churchill Livingstone, 1973.

[a] First 2 years.

# Table A-6. Mean and Standard Deviations for Head Circumference, Sitting Height, and Skin Fold Thickness for Females

| Age | Head Circumference (cm) | | Crown–Rump[a] and Sitting Height (cm) | | Triceps Skinfold (mm log transf.) | | Subscapular Skinfold (mm log transf.) | |
|---|---|---|---|---|---|---|---|---|
| | Mean | SD | Mean | SD | Mean | SD | Mean | SD |
| Birth | 34.00 | 1.60 | | | | | | |
| 1 mo | 39.60 | 1.52 | 34.2 | 1.55 | 175.7 | 10.9 | 173.2 | 12.3 |
| 3 mo | 42.60 | 1.44 | 38.0 | 1.42 | 189.7 | 10.5 | 183.0 | 12.9 |
| 6 mo | 44.62 | 1.44 | 42.2 | 1.57 | 196.3 | 11.9 | 186.0 | 14.1 |
| 9 mo | 45.45 | 1.41 | 44.7 | 1.67 | 198.8 | 12.9 | 184.8 | 14.4 |
| 12 mo | 46.90 | 1.38 | 46.5 | 1.71 | 199.5 | 13.6 | 182.0 | 14.0 |
| 1½ yr | 47.90 | 1.37 | 49.4 | 1.83 | 199.4 | 13.8 | 177.3 | 14.4 |
| 2 yr | 49.33 | 1.25 | 51.8 | 1.95 | 198.7 | 13.7 | 173.8 | 14.8 |
| 3 yr | 50.20 | 1.28 | 55.2 | 2.25 | 196.8 | 13.6 | 169.0 | 16.3 |
| 4 yr | 50.80 | 1.28 | 58.5 | 2.34 | 194.7 | 13.4 | 166.0 | 17.5 |
| 5 yr | 51.20 | 1.28 | 61.4 | 2.50 | 192.5 | 13.9 | 163.4 | 18.5 |
| 6 yr | 51.50 | 1.28 | 64.4 | 2.70 | 190.7 | 14.7 | 162.0 | 19.1 |
| 7 yr | 51.70 | 1.28 | 66.9 | 2.90 | 190.0 | 16.1 | 162.1 | 20.7 |
| 8 yr | 51.90 | 1.28 | 69.1 | 3.08 | 191.7 | 17.6 | 164.2 | 23.2 |
| 9 yr | 52.15 | 1.30 | 71.3 | 3.22 | 194.6 | 18.7 | 167.8 | 25.5 |
| 10 yr | 52.65 | 1.33 | 73.4 | 3.36 | 197.0 | 19.4 | 172.2 | 27.7 |
| 11 yr | 53.20 | 1.33 | 76.3 | 3.50 | 198.7 | 19.8 | 178.0 | 28.0 |
| 12 yr | 53.62 | 1.28 | 79.6 | 3.70 | 199.8 | 20.1 | 184.0 | 26.5 |
| 13 yr | 53.97 | 1.20 | 82.3 | 3.88 | 201.5 | 19.9 | 188.3 | 24.7 |
| 14 yr | 54.18 | 1.14 | 84.6 | 3.40 | 205.3 | 19.2 | 193.0 | 22.6 |
| 15 yr | 54.27 | 1.14 | 86.2 | 3.18 | 209.8 | 18.2 | 198.7 | 19.9 |
| 16 yr | | | 87.0 | 3.10 | 213.4 | 17.4 | 201.5 | 19.0 |
| 17 yr | | | | | 215.0 | 16.6 | 202.8 | 18.3 |
| 18 yr | | | | | 215.5 | 16.4 | 203.0 | 18.7 |
| 19 yr | | | | | 215.5 | 16.4 | 203.0 | 18.7 |

Reproduced by permission from Tanner JM, Physical growth and development, in Forfar JO, Arneil GC (eds) *Textbook of Pediatrics*. London, Churchill Livingstone, 1973.

[a] First 2 years.

**Table A-7. Upper Segment and Lower Segment Ratios from Birth to 17 Years for Boys**

| Age | Height (cm) | Weight (kg) | Upper Segment (cm) | Lower Segment (cm) | U/L Ratio |
|---|---|---|---|---|---|
| Birth | 50.8 | 3.4 | 32.0 | 18.8 | 1.70 |
| $\frac{1}{12}$ | 53.6 | 4.3 | 33.5 | 20.3 | 1.67 |
| $\frac{2}{12}$ | 56.4 | 5.1 | 35.3 | 21.1 | 1.67 |
| $\frac{3}{12}$ | 59.2 | 6.0 | 36.8 | 22.4 | 1.64 |
| $\frac{4}{12}$ | 61.7 | 6.8 | 38.4 | 23.4 | 1.64 |
| $\frac{5}{12}$ | 64.5 | 7.6 | 39.9 | 24.6 | 1.62 |
| $\frac{6}{12}$ | 67.3 | 8.5 | 41.7 | 25.7 | 1.62 |
| $\frac{7}{12}$ | 68.8 | 8.9 | 42.4 | 26.4 | 1.61 |
| $\frac{8}{12}$ | 70.4 | 9.3 | 43.2 | 27.2 | 1.59 |
| $\frac{9}{12}$ | 71.9 | 9.6 | 43.9 | 27.9 | 1.57 |
| $\frac{10}{12}$ | 73.2 | 10.0 | 44.7 | 28.4 | 1.57 |
| $\frac{11}{12}$ | 74.7 | 10.4 | 45.5 | 29.2 | 1.56 |
| $\frac{12}{12}$ | 76.2 | 10.8 | 46.2 | 30.0 | 1.54 |
| $1\frac{1}{12}$ | 77.2 | 11.0 | 46.7 | 30.5 | 1.53 |
| $1\frac{2}{12}$ | 78.0 | 11.3 | 47.0 | 31.0 | 1.52 |
| $1\frac{3}{12}$ | 79.0 | 11.5 | 47.5 | 31.5 | 1.51 |
| $1\frac{4}{12}$ | 79.8 | 11.8 | 48.0 | 31.8 | 1.51 |
| $1\frac{5}{12}$ | 80.8 | 12.0 | 48.5 | 32.3 | 1.50 |
| $1\frac{6}{12}$ | 81.8 | 12.2 | 49.0 | 32.8 | 1.50 |
| $1\frac{7}{12}$ | 82.8 | 12.4 | 49.5 | 33.3 | 1.50 |
| $1\frac{8}{12}$ | 83.8 | 12.6 | 50.0 | 33.8 | 1.49 |
| $1\frac{9}{12}$ | 84.6 | 12.8 | 50.0 | 34.5 | 1.48 |
| $1\frac{10}{12}$ | 85.6 | 12.9 | 51.0 | 35.0 | 1.45 |
| $1\frac{11}{12}$ | 86.6 | 13.1 | 51.3 | 35.6 | 1.44 |
| $1\frac{12}{12}$ | 87.4 | 13.3 | 51.3 | 36.1 | 1.42 |
| $2\frac{6}{12}$ | 92.2 | 14.3 | 53.3 | 38.9 | 1.37 |
| 3 | 96.5 | 15.2 | 55.1 | 41.4 | 1.33 |
| $3\frac{6}{12}$ | 100.8 | 16.3 | 56.6 | 43.4 | 1.30 |
| 4 | 103.9 | 17.3 | 57.7 | 46.2 | 1.25 |
| $4\frac{6}{12}$ | 107.2 | 18.4 | 58.9 | 48.3 | 1.22 |
| 5 | 110.7 | 19.5 | 59.0 | 50.8 | 1.19 |
| $5\frac{6}{12}$ | 114.3 | 20.7 | 61.2 | 53.1 | 1.15 |
| 6 | 117.6 | 21.9 | 62.2 | 55.4 | 1.12 |
| $6\frac{6}{12}$ | 120.7 | 23.3 | 63.0 | 57.7 | 1.09 |
| 7 | 123.7 | 24.6 | 64.0 | 59.7 | 1.07 |
| $7\frac{6}{12}$ | 126.7 | 26.2 | 65.0 | 61.7 | 1.05 |
| 8 | 129.8 | 27.7 | 65.8 | 64.0 | 1.03 |
| $8\frac{6}{12}$ | 123.6 | 29.4 | 67.1 | 65.5 | 1.02 |
| 9 | 135.4 | 31.1 | 68.3 | 67.1 | 1.02 |
| $9\frac{6}{12}$ | 138.2 | 33.0 | 69.1 | 69.1 | 1.00 |
| 10 | 141.0 | 34.9 | 70.1 | 70.9 | 0.99 |
| $10\frac{6}{12}$ | 143.3 | 36.9 | 70.9 | 72.4 | 0.98 |

| Age | Height (cm) | Weight (kg) | Upper Segment (cm) | Lower Segment (cm) | U/L Ratio |
|---|---|---|---|---|---|
| 11 | 145.8 | 38.9 | 72.1 | 73.7 | 0.98 |
| $11\frac{6}{12}$ | 148.6 | 41.1 | 73.4 | 75.2 | 0.98 |
| 12 | 151.4 | 43.3 | 74.9 | 76.5 | 0.98 |
| $12\frac{6}{12}$ | 154.4 | 45.7 | 76.5 | 78.0 | 0.98 |
| 13 | 157.5 | 48.0 | 77.7 | 79.8 | 0.97 |
| $13\frac{6}{12}$ | 161.3 | 51.1 | 79.5 | 81.8 | 0.97 |
| 14 | 164.8 | 54.1 | 81.3 | 83.6 | 0.97 |
| $14\frac{6}{12}$ | 167.9 | 57.1 | 82.8 | 85.1 | 0.97 |
| 15 | 171.2 | 60.1 | 84.8 | 86.4 | 0.98 |
| $15\frac{6}{12}$ | 173.2 | 62.3 | 86.1 | 87.1 | 0.99 |
| 16 | 175.3 | 64.5 | 87.4 | 87.9 | 0.99 |
| $16\frac{6}{12}$ | 176.0 | 65.8 | 87.6 | 88.4 | 0.99 |
| 17 | 176.5 | 67.1 | 87.9 | 88.6 | 0.99 |

Reproduced by permission from Johns Hopkins Hospital: *The Harriet Lane Handbook*, ed 9, edited by Jeffrey A. Biller and Andrew M. Yeager, copyright © 1981 by Year Book Medical Publishers, Inc, Chicago.

**Table A-8. Upper Segment and Lower Segment Ratios from Birth to 17 Years for Girls**

| Age | Height (cm) | Weight (kg) | Upper Segment (cm) | Lower Segment (cm) | U/L Ratio |
|---|---|---|---|---|---|
| Birth | 50.8 | 3.2 | 32.0 | 18.8 | 1.70 |
| $\frac{1}{12}$ | 54.6 | 4.1 | 34.3 | 20.3 | 1.69 |
| $\frac{2}{12}$ | 57.2 | 5.0 | 36.1 | 21.3 | 1.68 |
| $\frac{3}{12}$ | 59.7 | 5.9 | 37.3 | 22.4 | 1.67 |
| $\frac{4}{12}$ | 62.0 | 6.6 | 38.6 | 23.4 | 1.65 |
| $\frac{5}{12}$ | 64.0 | 7.3 | 39.6 | 24.4 | 1.62 |
| $\frac{6}{12}$ | 65.5 | 7.7 | 40.4 | 25.1 | 1.61 |
| $\frac{7}{12}$ | 67.1 | 8.2 | 41.1 | 25.9 | 1.59 |
| $\frac{8}{12}$ | 68.6 | 8.6 | 41.9 | 26.7 | 1.57 |
| $\frac{9}{12}$ | 70.1 | 9.0 | 42.7 | 27.4 | 1.56 |
| $\frac{10}{12}$ | 71.4 | 9.3 | 43.2 | 28.2 | 1.53 |
| $\frac{11}{12}$ | 72.9 | 9.6 | 43.9 | 29.0 | 1.52 |
| $\frac{12}{12}$ | 74.2 | 10.0 | 44.7 | 29.5 | 1.52 |
| $1\frac{1}{12}$ | 75.2 | 10.2 | 45.2 | 30.0 | 1.51 |
| $1\frac{2}{12}$ | 76.2 | 10.5 | 45.7 | 30.5 | 1.50 |
| $1\frac{3}{12}$ | 77.2 | 10.7 | 46.2 | 31.0 | 1.49 |
| $1\frac{4}{12}$ | 78.2 | 10.9 | 46.7 | 31.5 | 1.48 |
| $1\frac{5}{12}$ | 79.2 | 11.1 | 47.2 | 32.0 | 1.48 |

| Age | Height (cm) | Weight (kg) | Upper Segment (cm) | Lower Segment (cm) | U/L Ratio |
|---|---|---|---|---|---|
| $1\frac{6}{12}$ | 80.0 | 11.4 | 47.5 | 32.5 | 1.46 |
| $1\frac{7}{12}$ | 81.0 | 11.6 | 47.8 | 33.3 | 1.44 |
| $1\frac{8}{12}$ | 82.0 | 11.8 | 48.3 | 33.8 | 1.42 |
| $1\frac{9}{12}$ | 83.1 | 12.0 | 48.8 | 34.3 | 1.42 |
| $1\frac{10}{12}$ | 84.1 | 12.2 | 49.3 | 34.8 | 1.42 |
| $1\frac{11}{12}$ | 85.1 | 12.4 | 49.8 | 35.3 | 1.41 |
| $1\frac{12}{12}$ | 86.1 | 12.5 | 50.3 | 35.8 | 1.40 |
| $2\frac{6}{12}$ | 91.2 | 13.7 | 52.3 | 38.9 | 1.35 |
| 3 | 95.5 | 14.8 | 54.1 | 41.4 | 1.31 |
| $3\frac{6}{12}$ | 99.6 | 15.9 | 55.6 | 43.9 | 1.27 |
| 4 | 103.4 | 16.9 | 56.9 | 46.5 | 1.22 |
| $4\frac{6}{12}$ | 107.2 | 18.2 | 58.4 | 48.8 | 1.20 |
| 5 | 110.5 | 19.2 | 59.2 | 51.3 | 1.15 |
| $5\frac{6}{12}$ | 114.1 | 20.6 | 60.5 | 53.6 | 1.13 |
| 6 | 117.6 | 22.0 | 61.7 | 55.9 | 1.10 |
| $6\frac{6}{12}$ | 120.7 | 23.4 | 62.7 | 57.9 | 1.08 |
| 7 | 123.7 | 24.8 | 63.8 | 59.9 | 1.06 |
| $7\frac{6}{12}$ | 126.8 | 26.5 | 64.8 | 62.0 | 1.05 |
| 8 | 129.8 | 28.1 | 66.0 | 63.8 | 1.04 |
| $8\frac{6}{12}$ | 132.6 | 29.9 | 67.3 | 65.3 | 1.03 |
| 9 | 135.4 | 31.6 | 68.3 | 67.1 | 1.02 |
| $9\frac{6}{12}$ | 138.2 | 33.5 | 69.6 | 68.6 | 1.01 |
| 10 | 141.0 | 35.5 | 70.6 | 70.4 | 1.00 |
| $10\frac{6}{12}$ | 144.3 | 37.8 | 72.1 | 72.1 | 1.00 |
| 11 | 147.6 | 40.2 | 73.4 | 74.2 | 0.99 |
| $11\frac{6}{12}$ | 150.9 | 42.9 | 75.2 | 75.7 | 0.99 |
| 12 | 154.2 | 45.6 | 76.7 | 77.5 | 0.99 |
| $12\frac{6}{12}$ | 157.0 | 47.9 | 78.2 | 78.7 | 0.99 |
| 13 | 159.5 | 50.2 | 79.8 | 79.8 | 1.00 |
| $13\frac{6}{12}$ | 161.0 | 52.4 | 80.5 | 80.5 | 1.00 |
| 14 | 162.8 | 54.6 | 81.8 | 81.0 | 1.01 |
| $14\frac{6}{12}$ | 163.8 | 56.0 | 82.3 | 81.5 | 1.01 |
| 15 | 164.8 | 57.5 | 82.8 | 82.0 | 1.01 |
| $15\frac{6}{12}$ | 165.1 | 58.4 | 83.1 | 82.0 | 1.01 |
| 16 | 165.6 | 59.3 | 83.3 | 82.3 | 1.01 |
| $16\frac{6}{12}$ | 165.6 | 60.0 | 83.3 | 82.3 | 1.01 |
| 17 | 165.6 | 60.7 | 83.3 | 82.3 | 1.01 |

## Table A-9. Fels Parent-Specific Standards for Height: Boys' Stature by Age and Mid-parent Stature

| Age | Parental Midpoint (cm) | | | | | | | | |
|---|---|---|---|---|---|---|---|---|---|
| | 163 | 165 | 167 | 169 | 171 | 173 | 175 | 177 | 178 |
| Birth | 47.1 | 49.7 | 50.3 | 50.0 | 48.3 | 50.7 | 50.0 | 51.5 | 51.4 |
| 0–1 | 52.7 | 54.6 | 54.7 | 57.6 | 53.2 | 53.6 | 52.2 | 55.6 | 55.9 |
| 0–3 | 58.9 | 60.8 | 60.0 | 62.2 | 57.4 | 60.8 | 61.2 | 61.4 | 62.6 |
| 0–6 | 65.1 | 66.2 | 66.8 | 67.4 | 65.8 | 70.2 | 69.0 | 70.2 | 70.3 |
| 0–9 | 70.7 | 72.9 | 73.8 | 73.2 | 71.0 | 74.8 | 75.2 | 77.1 | 75.7 |
| 1–0 | 73.1 | 75.6 | 75.7 | 75.1 | 73.4 | 76.6 | 77.1 | 79.6 | 77.8 |
| 1–6 | 79.9 | 82.4 | 81.7 | 82.0 | 81.2 | 82.6 | 83.4 | 86.8 | 85.2 |
| 2–0 | 85.4 | 87.2 | 87.0 | 87.4 | 87.8 | 88.0 | 88.9 | 92.0 | 91.3 |
| 2–6 | 88.8 | 91.3 | 92.0 | 92.1 | 93.2 | 93.5 | 94.0 | 96.7 | 96.0 |
| 3–0 | 93.2 | 94.9 | 96.1 | 96.0 | 97.2 | 98.1 | 98.3 | 100.7 | 99.9 |
| 3–6 | 96.3 | 98.4 | 100.0 | 99.5 | 101.0 | 102.3 | 102.6 | 104.5 | 103.5 |
| 4–0 | 99.5 | 102.2 | 103.5 | 103.1 | 104.6 | 106.0 | 106.3 | 108.0 | 107.0 |
| 4–6 | 102.7 | 105.4 | 107.1 | 106.6 | 108.0 | 109.6 | 109.6 | 111.4 | 110.4 |
| 5–0 | 105.6 | 108.5 | 110.6 | 110.0 | 111.5 | 113.2 | 112.7 | 114.6 | 113.8 |
| 5–6 | 108.3 | 111.3 | 113.4 | 112.7 | 114.5 | 116.3 | 115.8 | 117.4 | 116.8 |
| 6–0 | 110.9 | 114.1 | 116.4 | 115.4 | 117.4 | 119.4 | 118.7 | 120.4 | 119.8 |
| 6–6 | 113.6 | 116.9 | 119.3 | 118.4 | 120.3 | 122.4 | 121.7 | 123.4 | 122.8 |
| 7–0 | 116.2 | 119.7 | 122.3 | 121.3 | 123.2 | 125.6 | 124.6 | 126.4 | 125.6 |
| 7–6 | 118.9 | 122.5 | 125.1 | 124.3 | 126.1 | 128.8 | 127.6 | 129.5 | 128.4 |
| 8–0 | 121.6 | 125.0 | 127.8 | 126.8 | 128.8 | 131.6 | 130.4 | 132.8 | 131.6 |
| 8–6 | 124.2 | 127.6 | 130.7 | 129.3 | 131.5 | 134.9 | 133.2 | 135.9 | 134.6 |
| 9–0 | 126.9 | 130.4 | 133.3 | 131.9 | 134.1 | 138.0 | 136.0 | 138.8 | 137.5 |
| 9–6 | 129.9 | 132.9 | 136.1 | 134.6 | 136.9 | 141.0 | 138.8 | 142.0 | 140.5 |
| 10–0 | 132.5 | 135.8 | 138.8 | 137.4 | 139.8 | 143.8 | 141.5 | 145.3 | 143.2 |
| 10–6 | 135.6 | 138.8 | 141.5 | 140.3 | 142.6 | 146.8 | 144.3 | 148.6 | 146.0 |
| 11–0 | 138.5 | 141.8 | 144.1 | 143.0 | 145.4 | 149.9 | 146.8 | 151.9 | 148.9 |
| 11–6 | 141.6 | 144.9 | 146.9 | 145.6 | 148.3 | 152.8 | 149.6 | 155.4 | 151.6 |
| 12–0 | 144.7 | 148.0 | 149.7 | 148.4 | 151.4 | 155.7 | 152.4 | 158.8 | 154.5 |
| 12–6 | 147.7 | 151.1 | 152.6 | 151.6 | 154.6 | 158.3 | 155.8 | 162.6 | 157.5 |
| 13–0 | 151.0 | 154.2 | 155.7 | 154.9 | 158.0 | 161.7 | 159.6 | 166.3 | 160.5 |
| 13–6 | 154.5 | 157.7 | 158.9 | 158.1 | 161.6 | 164.6 | 163.6 | 170.1 | 163.8 |
| 14–0 | 158.8 | 161.7 | 162.3 | 161.6 | 165.7 | 167.6 | 167.8 | 173.4 | 166.9 |
| 14–6 | 162.6 | 164.9 | 165.9 | 164.8 | 169.6 | 170.3 | 172.0 | 175.2 | 171.3 |
| 15–0 | 165.8 | 168.1 | 169.1 | 167.9 | 172.9 | 173.0 | 174.7 | 176.4 | 175.2 |
| 15–6 | 168.0 | 171.3 | 172.0 | 170.6 | 174.5 | 175.6 | 175.8 | 177.0 | 178.6 |
| 16–0 | 169.4 | 173.3 | 174.3 | 172.8 | 177.3 | 177.5 | 176.6 | 177.4 | 181.2 |
| 16–6 | 170.3 | 174.2 | 175.8 | 174.4 | 178.4 | 178.7 | 177.3 | 177.4 | 182.8 |
| 17–0 | 170.9 | 174.7 | 176.8 | 175.4 | 179.2 | 179.4 | 177.8 | 177.5 | 184.3 |
| 17–6 | 171.2 | 174.9 | 174.4 | 176.0 | 180.0 | 179.9 | 178.2 | 177.6 | 185.4 |
| 18–0 | 171.5 | 175.0 | 177.9 | 176.2 | 180.5 | 180.2 | 178.6 | 177.6 | 186.3 |

Reproduced by permission from Garn SM, Rohmann CG: Interaction of nutrition and genetics in the timing of growth and development. *Pediatr Clin North Am* **13**:357, 1966.

## Table A-10. Fels Parent-Specific Standards for Height: Girls' Stature by Age and Mid-parent Stature

| Age | Parental Midpoint (cm) | | | | | | | | | |
|-----|-----|-----|-----|-----|-----|-----|-----|-----|-----|-----|
| | 161 | 163 | 165 | 167 | 169 | 171 | 173 | 175 | 177 | 178 |
| Birth | 47.3 | 48.9 | 49.0 | 49.2 | 49.2 | 48.8 | 49.7 | 49.1 | 49.0 | 47.5 |
| 0–1 | 53.0 | 53.4 | 54.2 | 52.0 | 53.3 | 53.1 | 53.5 | 53.2 | 55.8 | 52.8 |
| 0–3 | 57.4 | 58.4 | 59.6 | 57.4 | 59.4 | 59.6 | 59.4 | 58.0 | 61.5 | 57.6 |
| 0–6 | 64.4 | 64.7 | 65.6 | 65.7 | 64.6 | 66.5 | 66.6 | 67.4 | 67.3 | 65.8 |
| 0–9 | 68.2 | 69.0 | 70.2 | 70.1 | 69.8 | 71.5 | 71.5 | 71.0 | 72.2 | 69.8 |
| 1–0 | 72.3 | 73.0 | 73.8 | 74.0 | 74.0 | 75.2 | 75.5 | 74.6 | 77.3 | 73.2 |
| 1–6 | 78.8 | 79.5 | 80.6 | 81.4 | 80.2 | 81.7 | 82.6 | 81.6 | 84.0 | 81.0 |
| 2–0 | 84.6 | 84.0 | 86.5 | 87.4 | 85.5 | 88.8 | 88.7 | 88.2 | 89.5 | 87.6 |
| 2–6 | 89.1 | 87.2 | 91.0 | 91.6 | 89.9 | 93.2 | 92.9 | 92.6 | 93.9 | 92.0 |
| 3–0 | 93.2 | 90.4 | 94.5 | 95.8 | 93.8 | 97.1 | 96.5 | 96.5 | 98.5 | 96.2 |
| 3–6 | 96.7 | 93.5 | 98.3 | 99.6 | 97.8 | 101.4 | 100.3 | 102.0 | 102.4 | 103.0 |
| 4–0 | 100.1 | 96.8 | 102.4 | 103.5 | 103.9 | 104.9 | 104.0 | 103.8 | 105.8 | 104.3 |
| 4–6 | 103.5 | 100.2 | 106.0 | 106.7 | 105.8 | 108.6 | 107.5 | 107.4 | 109.4 | 108.0 |
| 5–0 | 106.8 | 103.5 | 108.9 | 109.9 | 109.1 | 111.6 | 110.9 | 111.0 | 112.6 | 111.7 |
| 5–6 | 110.0 | 107.0 | 112.2 | 113.2 | 112.0 | 114.8 | 114.4 | 114.2 | 115.8 | 115.4 |
| 6–0 | 113.2 | 110.2 | 115.0 | 116.2 | 115.0 | 118.2 | 117.8 | 117.3 | 119.1 | 118.8 |
| 6–6 | 116.1 | 113.4 | 117.8 | 119.4 | 117.6 | 121.6 | 121.2 | 120.8 | 122.6 | 122.3 |
| 7–0 | 118.8 | 116.5 | 120.6 | 122.4 | 120.2 | 124.4 | 124.4 | 124.0 | 125.0 | 125.5 |
| 7–6 | 121.7 | 119.4 | 123.5 | 125.7 | 122.9 | 127.6 | 127.6 | 127.3 | 127.8 | 128.7 |
| 8–0 | 124.6 | 122.4 | 126.3 | 128.8 | 125.8 | 130.7 | 130.8 | 130.2 | 130.8 | 132.0 |
| 8–6 | 127.3 | 125.5 | 129.4 | 131.8 | 128.5 | 133.8 | 133.8 | 133.4 | 133.9 | 135.0 |
| 9–0 | 130.1 | 128.6 | 132.2 | 134.7 | 131.4 | 137.1 | 136.7 | 136.6 | 137.0 | 138.2 |
| 9–6 | 132.7 | 131.6 | 135.6 | 137.5 | 134.2 | 140.2 | 139.8 | 139.8 | 139.9 | 140.9 |
| 10–0 | 136.0 | 135.1 | 139.0 | 140.3 | 136.9 | 143.8 | 142.9 | 143.1 | 143.8 | 143.6 |
| 10–6 | 139.1 | 138.5 | 142.3 | 143.2 | 140.0 | 147.4 | 146.0 | 146.6 | 147.4 | 146.4 |
| 11–0 | 141.9 | 141.6 | 145.9 | 146.0 | 143.4 | 150.3 | 149.0 | 149.6 | 151.3 | 149.4 |
| 11–6 | 145.0 | 144.8 | 149.4 | 148.9 | 146.6 | 153.2 | 152.1 | 152.8 | 155.3 | 152.2 |
| 12–0 | 148.0 | 147.8 | 152.8 | 151.8 | 150.3 | 156.4 | 155.2 | 155.8 | 159.0 | 154.9 |
| 12–6 | 150.8 | 151.1 | 155.8 | 154.4 | 154.0 | 159.0 | 158.2 | 158.8 | 161.1 | 158.0 |
| 13–0 | 152.9 | 154.2 | 158.8 | 157.0 | 157.0 | 161.0 | 161.1 | 161.7 | 162.3 | 160.5 |
| 13–6 | 154.5 | 157.2 | 161.0 | 159.1 | 159.0 | 163.0 | 163.3 | 164.0 | 163.0 | 162.5 |
| 14–0 | 155.4 | 158.8 | 161.7 | 160.9 | 160.4 | 163.7 | 165.0 | 165.9 | 163.9 | 164.1 |
| 14–6 | 155.7 | 159.4 | 162.2 | 162.5 | 161.5 | 164.0 | 166.2 | 167.4 | 164.5 | 165.5 |
| 15–0 | 155.9 | 159.8 | 162.6 | 163.7 | 162.2 | 164.0 | 167.1 | 168.4 | 165.0 | 166.5 |
| 15–6 | 156.1 | 160.1 | 162.7 | 164.7 | 162.9 | 164.0 | 167.5 | 169.2 | 165.3 | 167.8 |
| 16–0 | 156.0 | 160.5 | 162.8 | 165.5 | 163.4 | 164.1 | 167.8 | 169.7 | 165.5 | 168.7 |
| 16–6 | 156.1 | 160.7 | 162.9 | 166.1 | 163.8 | 164.2 | 167.8 | 170.3 | 165.6 | 169.4 |
| 17–0 | 156.2 | 160.8 | 163.0 | 166.5 | 164.0 | 164.3 | 167.9 | 170.9 | 165.7 | 170.0 |
| 17–6 | 156.2 | 160.9 | 163.0 | 166.9 | 164.2 | 164.4 | 167.9 | 171.4 | 165.7 | 170.4 |
| 18–0 | 156.2 | 161.0 | 165.0 | 167.2 | 164.3 | 164.4 | 167.9 | 171.8 | 165.7 | 170.8 |

Reproduced by permission from Garn SM, Rohmann CG: Interaction of nutrition and genetics in the timing of growth and development. *Pediatr Clin North Am* **13**:357, 1966.

# Table A-11. Height Prediction Tables for Average Boys: Percentages and Estimated Mature Heights for Boys with Skeletal Ages within One Year of Their Chronological Ages

Skeletal Ages 7 Through 12 Years

| Ht. (inches) / Skeletal Age | 7-0 | 7-3 | 7-6 | 7-9 | 8-0 | 8-3 | 8-6 | 8-9 | 9-0 | 9-3 | 9-6 | 9-9 | 10-0 | 10-3 | 10-6 | 10-9 | 11-0 | 11-3 | 11-6 | 11-9 | 12-0 | 12-3 | 12-6 | 12-9 |
|---|---|---|---|---|---|---|---|---|---|---|---|---|---|---|---|---|---|---|---|---|---|---|---|---|
| % of Mature Height | 69.5 | 70.2 | 70.9 | 71.6 | 72.3 | 73.1 | 73.9 | 74.6 | 75.2 | 76.1 | 76.9 | 77.7 | 78.4 | 79.1 | 79.5 | 80.0 | 80.4 | 81.2 | 81.8 | 82.7 | 83.4 | 84.3 | 85.3 | 86.3 |
| 42 | 60.4 | | | | | | | | | | | | | | | | | | | | | | | |
| 43 | 61.9 | 61.3 | 60.6 | 60.1 | | | | | | | | | | | | | | | | | | | | |
| 44 | 63.3 | 62.7 | 62.1 | 61.5 | 60.9 | 60.2 | | | | | | | | | | | | | | | | | | |
| 45 | 64.7 | 64.1 | 63.5 | 62.8 | 62.2 | 61.6 | 60.9 | 60.3 | | | | | | | | | | | | | | | | |
| 46 | 66.2 | 65.5 | 64.9 | 64.2 | 63.6 | 62.9 | 62.2 | 61.7 | 61.2 | 60.4 | | | | | | | | | | | | | | |
| 47 | 67.6 | 67.0 | 66.3 | 65.6 | 65.0 | 64.3 | 63.6 | 63.0 | 62.5 | 61.8 | 61.1 | 60.5 | | | | | | | | | | | | |
| 48 | 69.1 | 68.4 | 67.7 | 67.0 | 66.4 | 65.7 | 65.0 | 64.3 | 63.8 | 63.1 | 62.4 | 61.8 | 61.2 | 60.7 | 60.4 | 60.0 | | | | | | | | |
| 49 | 70.5 | 69.8 | 69.1 | 68.4 | 67.8 | 67.0 | 66.3 | 65.7 | 65.2 | 64.4 | 63.7 | 63.1 | 62.5 | 61.9 | 61.6 | 61.3 | 61.0 | 60.3 | | | | | | |
| 50 | 71.9 | 71.2 | 70.5 | 69.8 | 69.2 | 68.4 | 67.7 | 67.0 | 66.5 | 65.7 | 65.0 | 64.4 | 63.8 | 63.2 | 62.9 | 62.5 | 62.2 | 61.6 | 61.1 | 60.5 | | | | |
| 51 | 73.4 | 72.6 | 71.9 | 71.2 | 70.5 | 69.8 | 69.0 | 68.4 | 67.8 | 67.0 | 66.3 | 65.6 | 65.1 | 64.5 | 64.2 | 63.8 | 63.4 | 62.8 | 62.3 | 61.7 | 61.2 | 60.5 | 59.8 | |
| 52 | 74.8 | 74.1 | 73.3 | 72.6 | 71.9 | 71.1 | 70.4 | 69.7 | 69.1 | 68.3 | 67.6 | 66.9 | 66.3 | 65.7 | 65.4 | 65.0 | 64.7 | 64.0 | 63.6 | 62.9 | 62.3 | 61.7 | 61.0 | 60.3 |
| 53 | 76.3 | 75.5 | 74.8 | 74.0 | 73.3 | 72.5 | 71.7 | 71.0 | 70.5 | 69.6 | 68.9 | 68.2 | 67.6 | 67.0 | 66.7 | 66.3 | 65.9 | 65.3 | 64.8 | 64.1 | 63.5 | 62.9 | 62.1 | 61.4 |
| 54 | 77.7 | 76.9 | 76.2 | 75.4 | 74.7 | 73.9 | 73.1 | 72.4 | 71.8 | 71.0 | 70.2 | 69.5 | 68.9 | 68.3 | 67.9 | 67.5 | 67.2 | 66.5 | 66.0 | 65.3 | 64.7 | 64.1 | 63.3 | 62.6 |
| 55 | 79.1 | 78.3 | 77.6 | 76.8 | 76.1 | 75.2 | 74.4 | 73.7 | 73.1 | 72.3 | 71.5 | 70.8 | 70.2 | 69.5 | 69.2 | 68.8 | 68.4 | 67.7 | 67.2 | 66.5 | 65.9 | 65.2 | 64.5 | 63.7 |
| 56 | 80.6 | 79.8 | 79.0 | 78.2 | 77.5 | 76.6 | 75.8 | 75.1 | 74.5 | 73.6 | 72.8 | 72.1 | 71.4 | 70.8 | 70.4 | 70.0 | 69.7 | 69.0 | 68.5 | 67.7 | 67.1 | 66.4 | 65.7 | 64.9 |
| 57 | | | 80.4 | 79.6 | 78.8 | 78.0 | 77.1 | 76.4 | 75.8 | 74.9 | 74.1 | 73.4 | 72.7 | 72.1 | 71.7 | 71.3 | 70.9 | 70.2 | 69.7 | 68.9 | 68.3 | 67.6 | 66.8 | 66.0 |
| 58 | | | | | 80.2 | 79.3 | 78.5 | 77.7 | 77.1 | 76.2 | 75.4 | 74.6 | 74.0 | 73.3 | 73.0 | 72.5 | 72.1 | 71.4 | 70.9 | 70.1 | 69.5 | 68.8 | 68.0 | 67.2 |
| 59 | | | | | | 80.7 | 79.8 | 79.1 | 78.5 | 77.5 | 76.7 | 75.9 | 75.3 | 74.6 | 74.2 | 73.8 | 73.4 | 72.7 | 72.1 | 71.3 | 70.7 | 70.0 | 69.2 | 68.4 |
| 60 | | | | | | | | 80.4 | 79.8 | 78.8 | 78.0 | 77.2 | 76.5 | 75.9 | 75.5 | 75.0 | 74.6 | 73.9 | 73.3 | 72.6 | 71.9 | 71.2 | 70.3 | 69.5 |
| 61 | | | | | | | | | | 80.2 | 79.3 | 78.5 | 77.8 | 77.1 | 76.7 | 76.3 | 75.9 | 75.1 | 74.6 | 73.8 | 73.1 | 72.4 | 71.5 | 70.7 |
| 62 | | | | | | | | | | | 80.6 | 79.8 | 79.1 | 78.4 | 78.0 | 77.5 | 77.1 | 76.4 | 75.8 | 75.0 | 74.3 | 73.5 | 72.7 | 71.8 |
| 63 | | | | | | | | | | | | | 80.4 | 79.6 | 79.2 | 78.8 | 78.4 | 77.6 | 77.0 | 76.2 | 75.5 | 74.7 | 73.9 | 73.0 |
| 64 | | | | | | | | | | | | | | 80.9 | 80.5 | 80.0 | 79.6 | 78.8 | 78.2 | 77.4 | 76.7 | 75.9 | 75.0 | 74.2 |
| 65 | | | | | | | | | | | | | | | | | 80.8 | 80.0 | 79.5 | 78.6 | 77.9 | 77.1 | 76.2 | 75.3 |
| 66 | | | | | | | | | | | | | | | | | | | 80.7 | 79.8 | 79.1 | 78.3 | 77.4 | 76.5 |
| 67 | | | | | | | | | | | | | | | | | | | | | 80.3 | 79.5 | 78.5 | 77.6 |
| 68 | | | | | | | | | | | | | | | | | | | | | | 80.7 | 79.7 | 78.8 |
| 69 | | | | | | | | | | | | | | | | | | | | | | | 80.9 | 80.0 |

## Table A-11. (Continued)

Skeletal Ages 13 Years to Maturity

| Skeletal Age | 13-0 | 13-3 | 13-6 | 13-9 | 14-0 | 14-3 | 14-6 | 14-9 | 15-0 | 15-3 | 15-6 | 15-9 | 16-0 | 16-3 | 16-6 | 16-9 | 17-0 | 17-3 | 17-6 | 17-9 | 18-0 | 18-3 | 18-6 |
|---|---|---|---|---|---|---|---|---|---|---|---|---|---|---|---|---|---|---|---|---|---|---|---|
| % of Mature Height | 87.6 | 89.0 | 90.2 | 91.4 | 92.7 | 93.8 | 94.8 | 95.8 | 96.8 | 97.3 | 97.6 | 98.0 | 98.2 | 98.5 | 98.7 | 98.9 | 99.1 | 99.3 | 99.4 | 99.5 | 99.6 | 99.8 | 100.0 |
| **Ht. (inches)** | | | | | | | | | | | | | | | | | | | | | | | |
| 53 | 60.5 | | | | | | | | | | | | | | | | | | | | | | |
| 54 | 61.6 | 60.7 | | | | | | | | | | | | | | | | | | | | | |
| 55 | 62.8 | 61.8 | 61.0 | 60.2 | | | | | | | | | | | | | | | | | | | |
| 56 | 63.9 | 62.9 | 62.1 | 61.3 | 60.4 | | | | | | | | | | | | | | | | | | |
| 57 | 65.1 | 64.0 | 63.2 | 62.4 | 61.5 | 60.8 | 60.1 | | | | | | | | | | | | | | | | |
| 58 | 66.2 | 65.2 | 64.3 | 63.5 | 62.6 | 61.8 | 61.2 | 60.5 | | | | | | | | | | | | | | | |
| 59 | 67.4 | 66.3 | 65.4 | 64.6 | 63.6 | 62.9 | 62.2 | 61.6 | 61.0 | 60.6 | 60.5 | 60.2 | 60.1 | | | | | | | | | | |
| 60 | 68.5 | 67.4 | 66.5 | 65.6 | 64.7 | 64.0 | 63.3 | 62.6 | 62.0 | 61.7 | 61.5 | 61.2 | 61.1 | 60.9 | 60.8 | 60.7 | 60.5 | 60.4 | 60.4 | 60.3 | 60.2 | 60.1 | 60.0 |
| 61 | 69.6 | 68.5 | 67.6 | 66.7 | 65.8 | 65.0 | 64.3 | 63.7 | 63.0 | 62.7 | 62.5 | 62.2 | 62.1 | 61.9 | 61.8 | 61.7 | 61.6 | 61.4 | 61.4 | 61.3 | 61.2 | 61.1 | 61.0 |
| 62 | 70.8 | 69.7 | 68.7 | 67.8 | 66.9 | 66.1 | 65.4 | 64.7 | 64.0 | 63.7 | 63.5 | 63.3 | 63.1 | 62.9 | 62.8 | 62.7 | 62.6 | 62.4 | 62.4 | 62.3 | 62.2 | 62.1 | 62.0 |
| 63 | 71.9 | 70.8 | 69.8 | 68.9 | 68.0 | 67.2 | 66.5 | 65.8 | 65.1 | 64.7 | 64.5 | 64.3 | 64.2 | 64.0 | 63.8 | 63.7 | 63.6 | 63.4 | 63.4 | 63.3 | 63.3 | 63.1 | 63.0 |
| 64 | 73.1 | 71.9 | 71.0 | 70.0 | 69.0 | 68.2 | 67.5 | 66.8 | 66.1 | 65.8 | 65.6 | 65.3 | 65.2 | 65.0 | 64.8 | 64.7 | 64.6 | 64.5 | 64.4 | 64.3 | 64.3 | 64.1 | 64.0 |
| 65 | 74.2 | 73.0 | 72.1 | 71.1 | 70.1 | 69.3 | 68.6 | 67.8 | 67.2 | 66.8 | 66.6 | 66.3 | 66.2 | 66.0 | 65.9 | 65.7 | 65.6 | 65.5 | 65.4 | 65.3 | 65.3 | 65.1 | 65.0 |
| 66 | 75.3 | 74.2 | 73.2 | 72.2 | 71.2 | 70.4 | 69.6 | 68.9 | 68.2 | 67.8 | 67.6 | 67.3 | 67.2 | 67.0 | 66.9 | 66.7 | 66.6 | 66.5 | 66.4 | 66.3 | 66.3 | 66.1 | 66.0 |
| 67 | 76.5 | 75.3 | 74.3 | 73.3 | 72.3 | 71.4 | 70.7 | 69.9 | 69.2 | 68.9 | 68.6 | 68.4 | 68.2 | 68.0 | 67.9 | 67.7 | 67.6 | 67.5 | 67.4 | 67.3 | 67.3 | 67.1 | 67.0 |
| 68 | 77.6 | 76.4 | 75.4 | 74.4 | 73.4 | 72.5 | 71.7 | 71.0 | 70.2 | 69.9 | 69.7 | 69.4 | 69.2 | 69.0 | 68.9 | 68.8 | 68.6 | 68.5 | 68.4 | 68.3 | 68.3 | 68.1 | 68.0 |
| 69 | 78.8 | 77.5 | 76.5 | 75.5 | 74.4 | 73.6 | 72.8 | 72.0 | 71.3 | 70.9 | 70.7 | 70.4 | 70.3 | 70.1 | 69.9 | 69.8 | 69.6 | 69.5 | 69.4 | 69.3 | 69.3 | 69.1 | 69.0 |
| 70 | 79.9 | 78.7 | 77.6 | 76.6 | 75.5 | 74.6 | 73.8 | 73.1 | 72.3 | 71.9 | 71.7 | 71.4 | 71.3 | 71.1 | 70.9 | 70.8 | 70.6 | 70.5 | 70.4 | 70.4 | 70.3 | 70.1 | 70.0 |
| 71 | | 79.8 | 78.7 | 77.7 | 76.6 | 75.7 | 74.9 | 74.1 | 73.3 | 73.0 | 72.7 | 72.4 | 72.3 | 72.1 | 71.9 | 71.8 | 71.6 | 71.5 | 71.4 | 71.4 | 71.3 | 71.1 | 71.0 |
| 72 | | 80.9 | 79.8 | 78.8 | 77.7 | 76.8 | 75.9 | 75.2 | 74.4 | 74.0 | 73.8 | 73.5 | 73.3 | 73.1 | 73.0 | 72.8 | 72.7 | 72.5 | 72.4 | 72.4 | 72.3 | 72.1 | 72.0 |
| 73 | | | 80.9 | 79.9 | 78.7 | 77.8 | 77.0 | 76.2 | 75.4 | 75.0 | 74.8 | 74.5 | 74.3 | 74.1 | 74.0 | 73.8 | 73.7 | 73.5 | 73.4 | 73.4 | 73.3 | 73.1 | 73.0 |
| 74 | | | | | 79.8 | 78.9 | 78.1 | 77.2 | 76.4 | 76.1 | 75.8 | 75.5 | 75.4 | 75.1 | 75.0 | 74.8 | 74.7 | 74.5 | 74.4 | 74.4 | 74.3 | 74.1 | 74.0 |
| 75 | | | | | 80.9 | 80.0 | 79.1 | 78.3 | 77.5 | 77.1 | 76.8 | 76.5 | 76.4 | 76.1 | 76.0 | 75.8 | 75.7 | 75.5 | 75.5 | 75.4 | 75.3 | 75.2 | 75.0 |
| 76 | | | | | | | 80.2 | 79.3 | 78.5 | 78.1 | 77.9 | 77.6 | 77.4 | 77.2 | 77.0 | 76.8 | 76.7 | 76.5 | 76.5 | 76.4 | 76.3 | 76.2 | 76.0 |
| 77 | | | | | | | | 80.4 | 79.5 | 79.1 | 78.9 | 78.6 | 78.4 | 78.2 | 78.0 | 77.9 | 77.7 | 77.5 | 77.5 | 77.4 | 77.3 | 77.2 | 77.0 |
| 78 | | | | | | | | | 80.6 | 80.2 | 79.9 | 79.6 | 79.4 | 79.2 | 79.0 | 78.9 | 78.7 | 78.5 | 78.5 | 78.4 | 78.3 | 78.2 | 78.0 |

**Table A-12. Height Prediction Tables for Average Girls: Percentages and Estimated Mature Heights for Girls with Skeletal Ages within One Year of Their Chronological Ages**

Skeletal Ages 6 Through 11 Years

| Skeletal Age<br>% of Mature Height<br>Ht. (inches) | 6-0<br>72.0 | 6-3<br>72.9 | 6-6<br>73.8 | 6-10<br>75.1 | 7-0<br>75.7 | 7-3<br>76.5 | 7-6<br>77.2 | 7-10<br>78.2 | 8-0<br>79.0 | 8-3<br>80.1 | 8-6<br>81.0 | 8-10<br>82.1 | 9-0<br>82.7 | 9-3<br>83.6 | 9-6<br>84.4 | 9-9<br>85.3 | 10-0<br>86.2 | 10-3<br>87.4 | 10-6<br>88.4 | 10-9<br>89.6 | 11-0<br>90.6 | 11-3<br>91.0 | 11-6<br>91.4 | 11-9<br>91.8 |
|---|---|---|---|---|---|---|---|---|---|---|---|---|---|---|---|---|---|---|---|---|---|---|---|---|
| 37 | 51.4 | | | | | | | | | | | | | | | | | | | | | | | |
| 38 | 52.8 | 52.1 | 51.5 | | | | | | | | | | | | | | | | | | | | | |
| 39 | 54.2 | 53.5 | 52.8 | 51.9 | 51.5 | 51.0 | | | | | | | | | | | | | | | | | | |
| 40 | 55.6 | 54.9 | 54.2 | 53.3 | 52.8 | 52.3 | 51.8 | 51.2 | | | | | | | | | | | | | | | | |
| 41 | 56.9 | 56.2 | 55.6 | 54.6 | 54.2 | 53.6 | 53.1 | 52.4 | 51.9 | 51.2 | | | | | | | | | | | | | | |
| 42 | 58.3 | 57.6 | 56.9 | 55.9 | 55.5 | 54.9 | 54.4 | 53.7 | 53.2 | 52.4 | 51.9 | 51.2 | | | | | | | | | | | | |
| 43 | 59.7 | 59.0 | 58.3 | 57.3 | 56.8 | 56.2 | 55.7 | 55.0 | 54.4 | 53.7 | 53.1 | 52.4 | 52.0 | 51.4 | | | | | | | | | | |
| 44 | 61.1 | 60.4 | 59.6 | 58.6 | 58.1 | 57.5 | 57.0 | 56.3 | 55.7 | 54.9 | 54.3 | 53.6 | 53.2 | 52.6 | 52.1 | 51.6 | 51.0 | | | | | | | |
| 45 | 62.5 | 61.7 | 61.0 | 59.9 | 59.4 | 58.8 | 58.3 | 57.5 | 57.0 | 56.2 | 55.6 | 54.8 | 54.4 | 53.8 | 53.3 | 52.8 | 52.2 | 51.5 | | | | | | |
| 46 | 63.9 | 63.1 | 62.3 | 61.3 | 60.8 | 60.1 | 59.6 | 58.8 | 58.2 | 57.4 | 56.8 | 56.0 | 55.6 | 55.0 | 54.5 | 53.9 | 53.4 | 52.6 | 52.0 | 51.3 | | | | |
| 47 | 65.3 | 64.5 | 63.7 | 62.6 | 62.1 | 61.4 | 60.9 | 60.1 | 59.5 | 58.7 | 58.0 | 57.2 | 56.8 | 56.2 | 55.7 | 55.1 | 54.5 | 53.8 | 53.2 | 52.5 | 51.9 | 51.6 | 51.4 | 51.2 |
| 48 | 66.7 | 65.8 | 65.0 | 63.9 | 63.4 | 62.7 | 62.2 | 61.4 | 60.8 | 59.9 | 59.3 | 58.5 | 58.0 | 57.4 | 56.9 | 56.3 | 55.7 | 54.9 | 54.3 | 53.6 | 53.0 | 52.7 | 52.5 | 52.3 |
| 49 | 68.1 | 67.2 | 66.4 | 65.2 | 64.7 | 64.1 | 63.5 | 62.7 | 62.0 | 61.2 | 60.5 | 59.7 | 59.3 | 58.6 | 58.1 | 57.4 | 56.8 | 56.1 | 55.4 | 54.7 | 54.1 | 53.8 | 53.6 | 53.4 |
| 50 | 69.4 | 68.6 | 67.8 | 66.6 | 66.1 | 65.4 | 64.8 | 63.9 | 63.3 | 62.4 | 61.7 | 60.9 | 60.5 | 59.8 | 59.2 | 58.6 | 58.0 | 57.2 | 56.6 | 55.8 | 55.2 | 54.9 | 54.7 | 54.5 |
| 51 | 70.8 | 70.0 | 69.1 | 67.9 | 67.4 | 66.7 | 66.1 | 65.2 | 64.6 | 63.7 | 63.0 | 62.1 | 61.7 | 61.0 | 60.4 | 59.8 | 59.2 | 58.4 | 57.7 | 56.9 | 56.3 | 56.0 | 55.8 | 55.6 |
| 52 | 72.2 | 71.3 | 70.5 | 69.2 | 68.7 | 68.0 | 67.4 | 66.5 | 65.8 | 64.9 | 64.2 | 63.3 | 62.9 | 62.2 | 61.6 | 61.0 | 60.3 | 59.5 | 58.8 | 58.0 | 57.4 | 57.1 | 56.9 | 56.6 |
| 53 | 73.6 | 72.7 | 71.8 | 70.6 | 70.0 | 69.3 | 68.7 | 67.8 | 67.1 | 66.2 | 65.4 | 64.6 | 64.1 | 63.4 | 62.8 | 62.1 | 61.5 | 60.6 | 60.0 | 59.2 | 58.5 | 58.2 | 58.0 | 57.7 |
| 54 | | 74.1 | 73.2 | 71.9 | 71.3 | 70.6 | 69.9 | 69.1 | 68.4 | 67.4 | 66.7 | 65.8 | 65.3 | 64.6 | 64.0 | 63.3 | 62.6 | 61.8 | 61.1 | 60.3 | 59.6 | 59.3 | 59.1 | 58.8 |
| 55 | | | 74.5 | 73.2 | 72.7 | 71.9 | 71.2 | 70.3 | 69.6 | 68.7 | 67.9 | 67.0 | 66.5 | 65.8 | 65.2 | 64.5 | 63.8 | 62.9 | 62.2 | 61.4 | 60.7 | 60.4 | 60.2 | 59.9 |
| 56 | | | | 74.6 | 74.0 | 73.2 | 72.5 | 71.6 | 70.9 | 69.9 | 69.1 | 68.2 | 67.7 | 67.0 | 66.4 | 65.7 | 65.0 | 64.1 | 63.3 | 62.5 | 61.8 | 61.5 | 61.3 | 61.0 |
| 57 | | | | | | 74.5 | 73.8 | 72.9 | 72.2 | 71.2 | 70.4 | 69.4 | 68.9 | 68.2 | 67.5 | 66.8 | 66.1 | 65.2 | 64.5 | 63.6 | 62.9 | 62.6 | 62.4 | 62.1 |
| 58 | | | | | | | | 74.2 | 73.4 | 72.4 | 71.6 | 70.6 | 70.1 | 69.4 | 68.7 | 68.0 | 67.3 | 66.4 | 65.6 | 64.7 | 64.0 | 63.7 | 63.5 | 63.2 |
| 59 | | | | | | | | | 74.7 | 73.7 | 72.8 | 71.9 | 71.3 | 70.6 | 69.9 | 69.2 | 68.4 | 67.5 | 66.7 | 65.8 | 65.1 | 64.8 | 64.6 | 64.3 |
| 60 | | | | | | | | | | 74.9 | 74.1 | 73.1 | 72.6 | 71.8 | 71.1 | 70.3 | 69.6 | 68.7 | 67.9 | 67.0 | 66.2 | 65.9 | 65.6 | 65.4 |
| 61 | | | | | | | | | | | | 74.3 | 73.8 | 73.0 | 72.3 | 71.5 | 70.8 | 69.8 | 69.0 | 68.1 | 67.3 | 67.0 | 66.7 | 66.4 |
| 62 | | | | | | | | | | | | | | 74.2 | 73.5 | 72.7 | 71.9 | 70.9 | 70.1 | 69.2 | 68.4 | 68.1 | 67.8 | 67.5 |
| 63 | | | | | | | | | | | | | | | 74.6 | 73.9 | 73.1 | 72.1 | 71.3 | 70.3 | 69.5 | 69.2 | 68.9 | 68.6 |
| 64 | | | | | | | | | | | | | | | | | 74.2 | 73.2 | 72.4 | 71.4 | 70.6 | 70.3 | 70.0 | 69.7 |
| 65 | | | | | | | | | | | | | | | | | | 74.4 | 73.5 | 72.5 | 71.7 | 71.4 | 71.1 | 70.8 |
| 66 | | | | | | | | | | | | | | | | | | | 74.7 | 73.7 | 72.8 | 72.5 | 72.2 | 71.9 |
| 67 | | | | | | | | | | | | | | | | | | | | 74.8 | 74.0 | 73.6 | 73.3 | 73.0 |
| 68 | | | | | | | | | | | | | | | | | | | | | | 74.7 | 74.4 | 74.1 |

## Table A-12. (Continued)

Skeletal Ages 12 Through 18 Years

| Skeletal Age → Ht. (inches) ↓ / % of Mature Height | 12-0 92.2 | 12-3 93.2 | 12-6 94.1 | 12-9 95.0 | 13-0 95.8 | 13-3 96.7 | 13-6 97.4 | 13-9 97.8 | 14-0 98.0 | 14-3 98.3 | 14-6 98.6 | 14-9 98.8 | 15-0 99.0 | 15-3 99.1 | 15-6 99.3 | 15-9 99.4 | 16-0 99.6 | 16-3 99.7 | 16-6 99.8 | 16-9 99.9 | 17-0 99.9 | 17-6 99.95 | 18-0 100.0 |
|---|---|---|---|---|---|---|---|---|---|---|---|---|---|---|---|---|---|---|---|---|---|---|---|
| 47 | 51.0 | | | | | | | | | | | | | | | | | | | | | | |
| 48 | 52.1 | 51.5 | 51.0 | | | | | | | | | | | | | | | | | | | | |
| 49 | 53.1 | 52.6 | 52.1 | 51.6 | 51.1 | | | | | | | | | | | | | | | | | | |
| 50 | 54.2 | 53.6 | 53.1 | 52.6 | 52.2 | 51.7 | 51.3 | 51.1 | 51.0 | | | | | | | | | | | | | | |
| 51 | 55.3 | 54.7 | 54.2 | 53.7 | 53.2 | 52.7 | 52.4 | 52.1 | 52.0 | 51.9 | 51.7 | 51.6 | 51.5 | 51.5 | 51.4 | 51.3 | 51.2 | 51.2 | 51.1 | 51.1 | 51.1 | 51.0 | 51.0 |
| 52 | 56.4 | 55.8 | 55.3 | 54.7 | 54.3 | 53.8 | 53.4 | 53.2 | 53.1 | 52.9 | 52.7 | 52.6 | 52.5 | 52.5 | 52.4 | 52.3 | 52.2 | 52.2 | 52.1 | 52.1 | 52.1 | 52.0 | 52.0 |
| 53 | 57.5 | 56.9 | 56.3 | 55.8 | 55.3 | 54.8 | 54.4 | 54.2 | 54.1 | 53.9 | 53.8 | 53.6 | 53.5 | 53.5 | 53.4 | 53.3 | 53.2 | 53.2 | 53.1 | 53.1 | 53.1 | 53.0 | 53.0 |
| 54 | 58.6 | 57.9 | 57.4 | 56.8 | 56.4 | 55.8 | 55.4 | 55.2 | 55.1 | 54.9 | 54.8 | 54.7 | 54.5 | 54.5 | 54.4 | 54.3 | 54.2 | 54.2 | 54.1 | 54.1 | 54.1 | 54.0 | 54.0 |
| 55 | 59.7 | 59.0 | 58.4 | 57.9 | 57.4 | 56.9 | 56.5 | 56.2 | 56.1 | 56.0 | 55.8 | 55.7 | 55.6 | 55.5 | 55.4 | 55.3 | 55.2 | 55.2 | 55.1 | 55.1 | 55.1 | 55.0 | 55.0 |
| 56 | 60.7 | 60.1 | 59.5 | 58.9 | 58.5 | 57.9 | 57.5 | 57.3 | 57.1 | 57.0 | 56.8 | 56.7 | 56.6 | 56.5 | 56.4 | 56.3 | 56.2 | 56.2 | 56.1 | 56.1 | 56.1 | 56.0 | 56.0 |
| 57 | 61.8 | 61.2 | 60.6 | 60.0 | 59.5 | 58.9 | 58.5 | 58.3 | 58.2 | 58.0 | 57.8 | 57.7 | 57.6 | 57.5 | 57.4 | 57.3 | 57.2 | 57.2 | 57.1 | 57.1 | 57.1 | 57.0 | 57.0 |
| 58 | 62.9 | 62.2 | 61.6 | 61.1 | 60.5 | 60.0 | 59.6 | 59.3 | 59.2 | 59.0 | 58.8 | 58.7 | 58.6 | 58.5 | 58.4 | 58.4 | 58.2 | 58.2 | 58.1 | 58.1 | 58.1 | 58.0 | 58.0 |
| 59 | 64.0 | 63.3 | 62.7 | 62.1 | 61.6 | 61.0 | 60.6 | 60.3 | 60.2 | 60.0 | 59.8 | 59.7 | 59.6 | 59.5 | 59.4 | 59.4 | 59.2 | 59.2 | 59.1 | 59.1 | 59.1 | 59.0 | 59.0 |
| 60 | 65.1 | 64.4 | 63.8 | 63.2 | 62.6 | 62.1 | 61.6 | 61.3 | 61.2 | 61.0 | 60.9 | 60.7 | 60.6 | 60.5 | 60.4 | 60.4 | 60.2 | 60.2 | 60.1 | 60.1 | 60.1 | 60.0 | 60.0 |
| 61 | 66.2 | 65.5 | 64.8 | 64.2 | 63.7 | 63.1 | 62.6 | 62.4 | 62.2 | 62.1 | 61.9 | 61.7 | 61.6 | 61.6 | 61.4 | 61.4 | 61.2 | 61.2 | 61.1 | 61.1 | 61.1 | 61.0 | 61.0 |
| 62 | 67.2 | 66.5 | 65.9 | 65.3 | 64.7 | 64.1 | 63.7 | 63.4 | 63.3 | 63.1 | 62.9 | 62.8 | 62.6 | 62.6 | 62.4 | 62.4 | 62.2 | 62.2 | 62.1 | 62.1 | 62.1 | 62.0 | 62.0 |
| 63 | 68.3 | 67.6 | 67.0 | 66.3 | 65.8 | 65.1 | 64.7 | 64.4 | 64.3 | 64.1 | 63.9 | 63.8 | 63.6 | 63.6 | 63.4 | 63.4 | 63.3 | 63.2 | 63.1 | 63.1 | 63.1 | 63.0 | 63.0 |
| 64 | 69.4 | 68.7 | 68.0 | 67.4 | 66.8 | 66.2 | 65.7 | 65.4 | 65.3 | 65.1 | 64.9 | 64.8 | 64.6 | 64.6 | 64.4 | 64.4 | 64.3 | 64.2 | 64.1 | 64.1 | 64.1 | 64.0 | 64.0 |
| 65 | 70.5 | 69.7 | 69.1 | 68.4 | 67.8 | 67.2 | 66.7 | 66.5 | 66.3 | 66.1 | 65.9 | 65.8 | 65.7 | 65.6 | 65.5 | 65.4 | 65.3 | 65.2 | 65.1 | 65.1 | 65.1 | 65.0 | 65.0 |
| 66 | 71.6 | 70.8 | 70.1 | 69.5 | 68.9 | 68.3 | 67.8 | 67.5 | 67.3 | 67.1 | 66.9 | 66.8 | 66.7 | 66.6 | 66.5 | 66.4 | 66.3 | 66.2 | 66.1 | 66.1 | 66.1 | 66.0 | 66.0 |
| 67 | 72.7 | 71.9 | 71.2 | 70.5 | 69.9 | 69.3 | 68.8 | 68.5 | 68.4 | 68.2 | 68.0 | 67.8 | 67.7 | 67.6 | 67.5 | 67.4 | 67.3 | 67.2 | 67.1 | 67.1 | 67.1 | 67.0 | 67.0 |
| 68 | 73.8 | 73.0 | 72.3 | 71.6 | 71.0 | 70.3 | 69.8 | 69.5 | 69.4 | 69.2 | 69.0 | 68.8 | 68.7 | 68.6 | 68.5 | 68.4 | 68.3 | 68.2 | 68.1 | 68.1 | 68.1 | 68.0 | 68.0 |
| 69 | 74.8 | 74.0 | 73.3 | 72.6 | 72.0 | 71.4 | 70.8 | 70.6 | 70.4 | 70.2 | 70.0 | 69.8 | 69.7 | 69.6 | 69.5 | 69.4 | 69.3 | 69.2 | 69.1 | 69.1 | 69.1 | 69.0 | 69.0 |
| 70 | | | 74.4 | 73.7 | 73.1 | 72.4 | 71.9 | 71.6 | 71.4 | 71.2 | 71.0 | 70.9 | 70.7 | 70.6 | 70.5 | 70.4 | 70.3 | 70.2 | 70.1 | 70.1 | 70.1 | 70.0 | 70.0 |
| 71 | | | | 74.7 | 74.1 | 73.4 | 72.9 | 72.6 | 72.4 | 72.2 | 72.0 | 71.9 | 71.7 | 71.6 | 71.5 | 71.4 | 71.3 | 71.2 | 71.1 | 71.1 | 71.1 | 71.0 | 71.0 |
| 72 | | | | | | 74.5 | 73.9 | 73.6 | 73.5 | 73.2 | 73.0 | 72.9 | 72.7 | 72.7 | 72.5 | 72.4 | 72.3 | 72.2 | 72.1 | 72.1 | 72.1 | 72.0 | 72.0 |
| 73 | | | | | | | 74.9 | 74.6 | 74.5 | 74.3 | 74.0 | 73.9 | 73.7 | 73.7 | 73.5 | 73.4 | 73.3 | 73.2 | 73.1 | 73.1 | 73.1 | 73.0 | 73.0 |
| 74 | | | | | | | | | | | | 74.9 | 74.7 | 74.7 | 74.5 | 74.4 | 74.3 | 74.2 | 74.1 | 74.1 | 74.1 | 74.0 | 74.0 |

Reprinted from Bayer LM, Bayley N: *Growth Diagnosis*, Appendix 2, pp. 226 and 229, by permission of the University of Chicago Press, copyright 1959 by the University of Chicago, published 1959, composed and printed by the University of Chicago Press, Chicago, Illinois, USA.

## Neuromuscular Maturity

| | 0 | 1 | 2 | 3 | 4 | 5 |
|---|---|---|---|---|---|---|
| Posture | | | | | | |
| Square Window (wrist) | 90° | 60° | 45° | 30° | 0° | |
| Arm Recoil | 180° | | 100°-180° | 90°-100° | <90° | |
| Popliteal Angle | 180° | 160° | 130° | 110° | 90° | <90° |
| Scarf Sign | | | | | | |
| Heel to Ear | | | | | | |

## Physical Maturity

| | | | | | | |
|---|---|---|---|---|---|---|
| Skin | gelatinous red, transparent | smooth pink, visible veins | superficial peeling, &/or rash few veins | cracking pale area rare veins | parchment deep cracking no vessels | leathery cracked wrinkled |
| Lanugo | none | abundant | thinning | bald areas | mostly bald | |
| Plantar Creases | no crease | faint red marks | anterior transverse crease only | creases ant. 2/3 | creases cover entire sole | |
| Breast | barely percept. | flat areola no bud | stippled areola 1-2mm bud | raised areola 3-4mm bud | full areola 5-10mm bud | |
| Ear | pinna flat, stays folded | sl. curved pinna; soft c̄ slow recoil | well-curv. pinna; soft but ready recoil | formed & firm c̄ instant recoil | thick cartilage ear stiff | |
| Genitals ♂ | scrotum empty no rugae | | testes descending few rugae | testes down good rugae | testes pendulous deep rugae | |
| Genitals ♀ | prominent clitoris & labia minora | | majora & minora equally prominent | majora large minora small | clitoris & minora completely covered | |

## MATURITY RATING

| Score | Wks. |
|---|---|
| 5 | 26 |
| 10 | 28 |
| 15 | 30 |
| 20 | 32 |
| 25 | 34 |
| 30 | 36 |
| 35 | 38 |
| 40 | 40 |
| 45 | 42 |
| 50 | 44 |

**Figure A-1.** Newborn Maturity Rating: Estimation of gestational age by maturity rating. (Reproduced by permission from Ballard JL, Kazmaier K, Driver M: A simplified score for assessment of fetal maturation of newly born infants. *J Pediatr* **95:**769, 1979.)

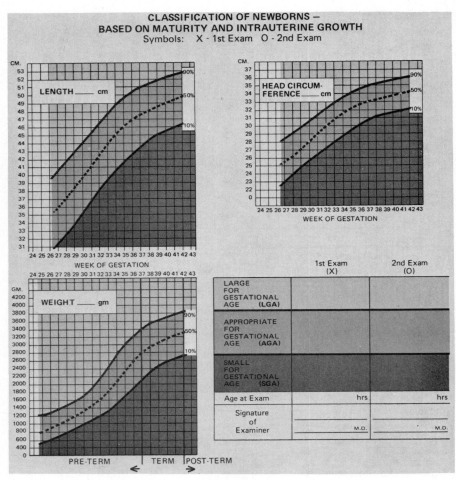

**Figure A-2.** Classification of newborns based on maturity and intrauterine growth. (Adapted by permission from Lubchenco LC, Hansman C, Boyd E: Intrauterine growth in length and head circumference as estimated from live births at gestational ages from 26–42 weeks. *Pediatrics* **37**:403, 1966, copyright American Academy of Pediatrics 1966, and Battaglia FC, Lubchenco LO: A practical classification of newborn infants by weight and gestational age. *J Pediatr* **71**:159, 1967.)

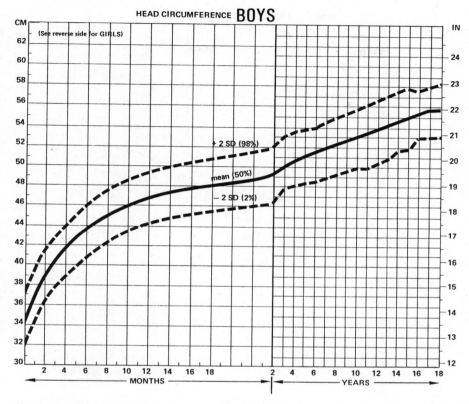

**Figure A-3.** Head circumference boys: birth to 18 years. (Reproduced by permission from Nellhaus G: Composite international and interracial graphs. *Pediatrics* **41:**106, 1968, copyright American Academy of Pediatrics 1968.)

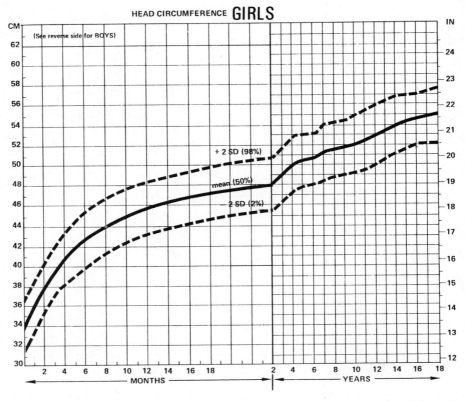

**Figure A-4.** Head circumference girls: birth to 18 years. (Reproduced by permission from Nellhaus G: Composite international and interracial graphs. *Pediatrics* **41:**106, 1968, copyright American Academy of Pediatrics 1968.)

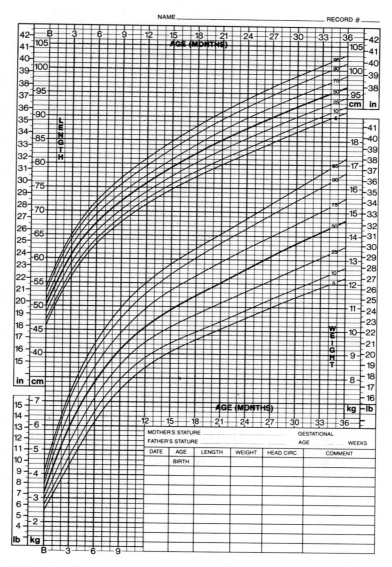

**Figure A-5.** Growth chart for boys birth to 36 months. Physical growth percentiles for length and weight. (Adapted by permission from Hamill PVV, Drizd TA, Johnson CL, et al: Physical growth: National Center for Health Statistics percentiles. *Am J Clin Nutr* **32:**607, 1979. Data from the Fels Research Institute, Wright State University School of Medicine, Yellow Springs, Ohio, courtesy of Ross Laboratories, copyright 1982.)

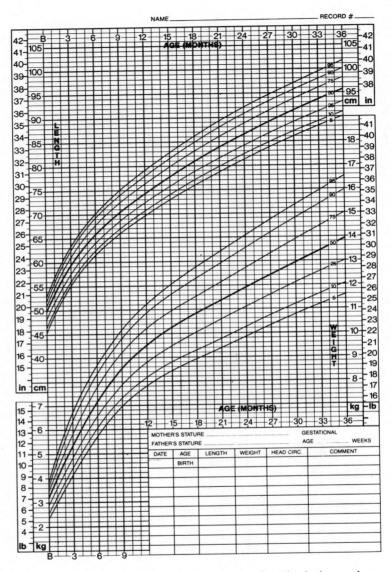

**Figure A-6.** Growth chart for girls birth to 36 months. Physical growth percentiles for length and weight. (Adapted by permission from Hamill PVV, Drizd TA, Johnson CL, et al: Physical growth: National Center for Health Statistics percentiles. *Am J Clin Nutr* **32:**607, 1979. Data from the Fels Research Institute, Wright State University School of Medicine, Yellow Springs, Ohio, courtesy of Ross Laboratories, copyright 1982.)

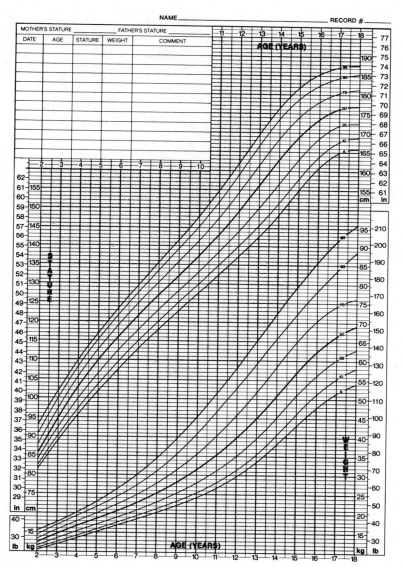

**Figure A-7.** Growth chart for boys ages 2–18 years. Physical growth percentiles for height and weight. (Adapted by permission from Hamill PVV, Drizd TA, Johnson CL, et al: Physical growth: National Center for Health Statistics percentiles. *Am J Clin Nutr* **32**:607, 1979. Data from the Fels Research Institute, Wright State University School of Medicine, Yellow Springs, Ohio, courtesy of Ross Laboratories, copyright 1982.)

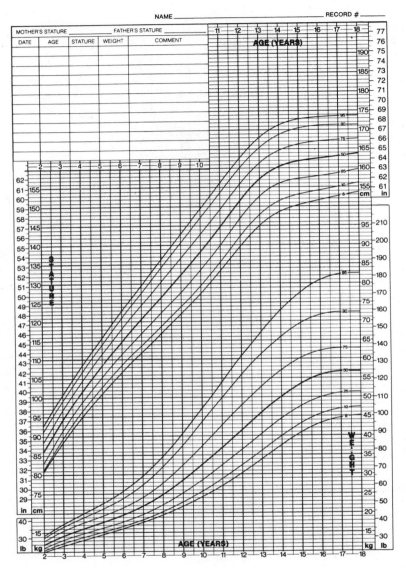

**Figure A-8.** Growth chart for girls ages 2–18 years. Physical growth percentiles for height and weight. (Adapted by permission from Hamill PVV, Drizd TA, Johnson CL, et al: Physical growth: National Center for Health Statistics percentiles. *Am J Clin Nutr* **32:**607, 1979. Data from the Fels Research Institute, Wright State University School of Medicine, Yellow Springs, Ohio, courtesy of Ross Laboratories, copyright 1982.)

462

# Index

## DATE DUE

| | | | |
|---|---|---|---|
| NOV 9 1987 | | | |
| NOV 21 1988 | | | |
| MAY 28 1989 | | | |
| DEC 19 1989 | | | |
| NOV 13 1990 | | | |
| DEC 12 1991 | | | |
| NOV NOV 2 9 2002 18 2010 | | | |
| | | | |
| | | | |
| | | | |

DEMCO 38-297